Nutrition:
The Cancer Answer II

by
Maureen Kennedy Salaman

STAFFORD PUBLISHING

THIS BOOK MAY SAVE YOUR LIFE...

Every new idea goes through three phases:

Phase 1: It is ignored...

Phase 2: It is ridiculed...

Phase 3: The establishment claims it as their own discovery.

Forty years ago holistic medical practitioners warned that smoking leads to cancer. Orthodox medical and government establishments had the same facts and information, yet for twenty-five years they not only withheld this information but financed studies to prove smoking is safe.

Only since 1960 have the American Cancer Society (ACS) and the primary influences in government, industry and medicine grudgingly admitted - **as if they had discovered it** - that smoking is bad for your health.

Nutritionally-knowledgeable health professionals have long known something else. All the while being rejected and ridiculed by orthodox medicine, they have held to their well-researched belief that cancer can be prevented and treated through diet and good nutrition.

Finally in 1982, the prestigious National Academy of Science (NAS) published a report recognizing the vital connection between diet and cancer.

However, the NAS stated that it will take twenty years or more to formulate their findings into practical application! What they mean is it will take twenty years or more before the Food and Drug Administration (FDA) and others recognize nutrition as a valid factor in cancer prevention and treatment.

In the meantime, effective, low-cost and time-tested treatment methods are being rejected and denied by health insurance companies and conventional medicine, limiting our options and guaranteeing our premature deaths.

This book presents, in understandable detail, the discoveries and cancer prevention information contained in the National Academy of Science report, together with a practical plan to put this undeniably correct nutritional information to work for you NOW, not twenty years from now.

Meditrends 1991-1992, a report published by the American Hospital Association, predicts that more than 1.6 million people will be diagnosed with cancer each year throughout the '90s and will account for 20 percent of the nation's total health care costs. If something isn't done NOW, by the year 2000, cancer will surpass heart disease as the leading cause of death.

Most of the estimated 526,000 Americans (according to the ACS) who will die of cancer this year could have lived with the information contained in this book.

Nutrition: The Cancer Answer II is the result of 16 years of vigorous research by a well-known author in the field of health and cancer prevention.

Nutrition: The Cancer Answer II will:

1. Give you research-based proof cancer can be prevented and controlled.
2. Rid you of the fear of ever contracting cancer in your lifetime.
3. Present carefully researched studies of various societies which enjoy cancer-free lives.
4. Show you how you can enjoy exuberant good health untouched by the cancer epidemic. Included is a "gourmet guide" to cancer prevention filled with easy and delicious recipes for vibrant good health.

Nutrition: The Cancer Answer II
By Maureen Kennedy Salaman

This Edition 2002
By Maureen Kennedy Salaman
Original Edition 1995
By Maureen Kennedy Salaman

© Copyright 1995
by Maureen Kennedy Salaman

Library of Congress No. 94-073919

ISBN:0-913087-19-X

Original Edition, 1995

Published by:
MKS, Inc./Statford Publishing
1259 El Camino Real, Suite 1500
Menlo Park, California 94025
www.mksalaman.com
(650) 854-3922 phone
(650) 854-5779 facsimile

Distributed by:
Maximum Living, Inc.
20071 Soulsbyville Road
Soulsbyville, California 95372-9748
www.maximizeyourlife.com
(209) 536-9300 phone
(800) 445-4325 phone
(209) 536-9375 facsimile

Printed in the United States of America

IMPORTANT NOTICE
This book is neither a medical guide nor a manual for self-treatment. It is instead
intended as a reference work only. The information in this book is meant to help you
make informed choices about your health, but is not intended as a substitute for any
treatment that may be prescribed or recommended by your doctor or health care
practitioner. If you should suspect that you suffer from a medical condition or problem,
you should seek competent medical care without delay.

DEDICATION

To those pioneers of Christian Television
whose inspiration feeds the souls
of millions including my own.

To Russ Bixler whose scalpel like editing
of this book strengthened the words
that remain.

ACKNOWLEDGMENTS

My acknowledgments start with the late Dr. Ross Gordon, whose healing brilliance was so rare and real that without him I would not have walked away from a serious injury. He helped me to be more myself, more the person God intended me to be, and it is possible that without him I would never have recognized myself, or grown to be what it is in me to be.

To my son Sean who started me on my search for truth.

My special thanks to Hope Daly for every one of life's little drudgeries that you bear cheerfully for me and for your insistence on excellence in all you do.

To my inimitable friend and researcher Julia Bauer--the sagacity of your work lights my path and brightens the lives of so many.

My thanks also go out to Shirley Osward for your years of help, support and devotion.

I point with pride to the commitment, loyalty and assiduousness of my staff. For them, selfishness and personal glory are subordinate to team effort and team glory. The success I have achieved as an individual has been because I am part of this dedicated team.

To the officers, board members, staff and membership of the National Health Federation: I have served them with passion and dedication for over two decades and for the last 17 years as their President. May God continue to make them brave and keep them true.

To my brother Lt. Col. Thomas Gillespie, United States Marine Corp, a man of integrity, honor and brilliance and his family Jackie, Alexandria and Christopher.

Many think of fulfillment as something to be found in money, wealth, success and applause; and don't learn until it's too late that the greatest gift God gives is loving friends. In this I am the wealthiest of people. My friends, who bless my life so richly, are: Julia "Cori" Haskett-Abbruszzese & Stefan Abbruszzese, Joseph & Michele Allioto, Elaine Becker & Charles Zaloumis, Iran & Howard Billman, Heide Van Doren Betz, Norma Bixler, Susan Blais, Freda & Claud Bowers & Family, Helen Gurley Brown, Ellie & Theodore Brown, Linda Cannon, Dr. Richard Casdorph, Toni Casey, Carolyn Chandler, Samantha Duval-Chandler, Angela Coppola, Tony & Bobby Cortesese, Michael Culbert, Katherine Wells-Debs, Betsy Dohrman, David & Linda Swan-Detert, Donna Douglas, Oleen Eagle, Delia Ehrlich, Courtney Eversole, Pastor Kenny & Shirley Foreman, Alisa & Kenny Foreman, Jr, Dawn & Kurt Foreman, Bella Farrow, Charlie Fox, Kathryn Grayson, Dr. Michael & Inga Gerber, Gail & Dr. Harvey Glasser, Joel Goodrich, Fred Haeberlein, Nancy Hamon, Connie & Ron Haus and Family, Fred Hirth, William Holloway, Ana Luz Holloway, Nancy & Jack Horton, Wendy & Frank Jordon, Sally Jordan, Evelyn Kean, Betty Kimball, Dr. Alan Konce, Dr. Hans Kugler, Dr. Richard Kunin & Mathilda, Nick Lampros and Family, Margaret Lawrence, George Mateljan, Howard & Gretchen Leach, Dr. Ralph Miranda & Billie, Dave McAllister, Ruth & Merl McAnich, Michael & Hershey McKenna, Scotty Morris, Caral Ann & Martin Newman, Becky Niven, David Pace, Bob Pritikin, Mary & Dr. Henry Ritter, Jerry Roberts & Family, Dr. Rodrigo Rodriguez & Associates, Janet & Michael Savage, Cynthia Schreuder, Barbara Brookins-Schneider, Patricia Sinclair, Sue & Jimmy Thompson, Krista Tepe, Karen & Scott Tips, Dr. William & Jo Toy, Princess Paul of Romania (Lia Triff), Dr. John Trowbridge, Alan & Barbara Virchow and Tatiana von Witte.

TABLE OF CONTENTS

How Food is Assimilated
The Importance of Fiber
"Civilized" Carcinogens

Introduction

Etched in the memories of generation after generation, Dickens' "It was the best of times; it was the worst of times" stamps "A Tale of Two Cities" as an eternal marker of a major historical shift. Similarly, the Federalist Papers and the Declaration of Independence are the literary symbols of the rise of a new social order out of the destruction of its predecessor.

Now, author Maureen Kennedy Salaman, employing the scientific research of many eminent scientists, has produced this outstanding literary standard, destined to mark the end of the dark age of medical oppression and the beginning of the new era of health freedom.

Her historical critique of the moral bankruptcy of the high priests of modern medicine guarantees this work a secure position alongside the classical documentations of medical deceit, beginning with Koestler's "Case of the Midwife Toad" and extending through a fifty-year period to Joseph Hixon's, "The Patchwork Mouse."

Indeed, the clarity of the Salaman dissertation embarrasses anyone – and certainly me – who ever bought into modern medicine's outrageous belief system.

Maureen Kennedy Salaman offers hope based on rational thought and optimism founded on fundamental principles of human history.

Modern medicine's death-oriented tyranny results from a disastrous rejection of belief in nutrition – in favor of prostitution to the "better living through chemistry" approach, a pathway which directly led to the modern iatrogenic epidemics of cancer, heart disease and stroke.

In contrast, this landmark work offers us the recipe – and the recipes – for health, for life, and for human survival. I emphasize the words "human survival" because modern medicine poses an overwhelming threat, not only to individual lives, but to life itself.

Nutrition: The Cancer Answer II appears just in time to rescue us, personally and nationally, from the iatrogenicide perpetuated by the idolatrous priesthood of the Religion of Modern Medicine. Maureen Kennedy Salaman merits our deepest gratitude.

Robert S. Mendelsohn, M.D.

Although my dear friend Dr. Robert Mendelsohn no longer lives, his words and deeds in the cause of health freedom are alive as ever and a never-ending inspiration for me to carry on the fight for the same cause in his tradition. – Maureen Kennedy Salaman

PART 1:
Foreword

Cancer Prevention And Alleviation In Our Lifetime

I started writing the first edition of this book in 1973 by saying, "There are three phases of any new idea, in the first phase the establishment ignores it; in the second it ridicules it; and in the third it claims the idea as its own." We are now truly in that third stage as far as nutrition being the true cancer answer. Sadly, however, the cancer establishment is just paying lip service to the link between nutrition and cancer; they profess to claim the idea, but they have not acted on it effectively. Progress for them remains at a snail's pace, which means another eleven million Americans have died from cancer since 1973.

Eleven million! If you are impressed by statistics, you will be shocked by this figure. Since the birth of this book, eleven million lives have been laid victim to mankind's most vicious degenerative disease. It's an anguishing number – and one that is especially ironic for me, knowing as I do that the medical philosophy on which this book is based could have saved so many of those lives and prevented most of the victims from ever contracting cancer in the first place.

Friends and critics alike have described the first edition of this book as being 20 years ahead of its time. Make no mistake about it, *Nutri-*

tion: The Cancer Answer II is still 20 years ahead of its time. I wouldn't be surprised if it takes 30 years before conventional medicine recognizes many of the life-saving truths presented in this second edition. The cutting edge information contained within these pages is akin to Bell's telephone before the public saw it in use. Those who didn't understand the telephone condemned it – until everyone else had one.

The fact that the number of cancer deaths are increasing in America, despite the billions of dollars that have gone into cancer research, is nothing less than a disgrace. With just a few exceptions, the medical establishment continues to ignore the real truth of the importance of nutrition in the fight against cancer and still places its faith upon its dismal record of surgery and radiation treatment.

In the first edition of this book, published in the early 1980s, I stressed the hope that the medical philosophy that forms the basis of this book – preventive medicine – could save the lives of my readers. Judging from the letters I have received over the years, it is clear that my book has succeeded beyond my most fervent expectations.

It is interesting to note that when the first edition was published there was absolutely no research, no computer databases to draw from. I had to go out and find the empirical evidence and instigate the research necessary to come up with valid and effective protocols. Dr. Manner's research, when he was head of the biology department at Loyola University, was spearheaded by me, funded by the National Health Federation (NHF). In fact, I personally did hands-on research, working side by side with Dr. Manner. The incredible and daunting backlash of conventional medicine against my efforts would fill this book, so I will save it for another time. Suffice it to say the efforts required serious dedication and heroic determination on the part of the NHF, Dr. Manner and others. I'm happy to report it was all worth it. This early research was heralded by doctors and scientists serious about finding a cure for cancer. Researchers saw the potential, picked up the ball and ran with it. This enabled me to bring you even more effective treatments and preventive protocols in this new edition.

Ten years ago the health food "movement" was considered a fad. Now we know it wasn't just a trend. It was a lot of people seeking a better life. Those who embraced the lifestyle have demonstrated, through good health, youthfulness and longevity, it's more than just healthy food. It is also preventive medicine; officially termed metabolic or holistic medicine. (Perhaps whole-istic, to avoid the religious insinuation and identify it more properly with the whole-being concept of wellness and natural healing espoused by its practitioners and proponents.)

By whatever name, the preventive approach to combating cancer is what this book is all about. And nothing states its basic premise more succinctly than the wise old adage, "An ounce of prevention is worth a pound of cure." This is not to say that cancer is controllable only by preventing it. Even for those who contract it, cancer can be reversed – and in this book I will offer proof of that assertion. More important, however, is that you, as a potential statistic, learn now how to deny cancer a foothold or future in your life. My book will show you how to slam the door on it and send it packing.

Cancer is usually accompanied by a secondary, undiagnosed metabolic dysfunction. Only a physician skilled in whole-istic medicine is capable of programming and supervising a complete regimen to overcome or reverse the cancer, as well as restore the body to its proper state of health. The information within these pages is not meant, therefore, to be a primer for self-treatment of an already entrenched degenerative disease; rather it is an informative guide to your options and choices in cancer treatment.

What this book does include is a doctor's protocol for treatment. It is intended to serve principally as both an outline and an explanation, to the prospective patient, of the metabolic physician's general procedure. This does not preclude the implementation, by those of us who are well, of a proven prevention program as detailed in the chapters to follow. When adhered to, in conjunction with the normal health care advice of a holistic physician and/or nutritionist, it may likely help to keep you or a loved one from becoming a victim of cancer. At the heart of this program are two simple but all-important essentials: natural foods and nutritional supplements in the form of vitamins and minerals.

The program you will learn about in this book is specifically addressed to cancer prevention. I will introduce you to my Bio-X Diet, the effectiveness of which is based on the addition or restoration to the diet of a daily intake of those foods and nutrients that have heretofore been neglected in otherwise good nutritional programs. As you will learn later, the Bio-X Diet's applicability is not contraindicated by any but the most unusual metabolic diseases. Best of all, it is a diet that can be added to or integrated with all otherwise nutritionally-adequate regimens.

For all its pronouncement of breakthrough discoveries, conventional medicine is still in the embryonic stages of investigating the relationship between nutrition and cancer. While this beginning is certainly welcome and long overdue, it will be many deadly years before the medical establishment in general will finally be forced to accept the realities that have been known to the health movement for so long, and which are described in the pages of this book. The American Cancer Society (*Cancer Facts & Figures 1993*) has estimated "526,000 Americans will die in 1994 of cancer." This estimation is based on their treatment recommendations, not mine. For you, this book offers hope, and a chance to turn around these figures. Just say NO! to statistics and use the nutritional regimens and logic contained here to fight for your lives. We can no longer afford to be guinea pigs in conventional medicine's laboratory. Instead, we must apply what is already known about nutrition and cancer to our daily lives.

Some years ago, the Committee on Diet, Nutrition and Cancer of the prestigious National Research Council (the principal operating agency of the National Academy of Sciences) released a preliminary report of its findings about the relationship between cancer and nutrition. This research was commissioned in June, 1980, by the National Cancer Institute (NCI), a federal government organization. Actually, NCI had commissioned two reports on the subject. The first was merely to determine whether there was any evidence to link cancer with nutrition and diet. The second was to suggest directions for future research along these lines.

The National Research Council (NRC) assigned the task to the executive office of its Assembly of Life Sciences (ALS), which created a 13-member committee with experts from the fields of biochemistry, microbiology, embryology, epidemiology, experimental oncology, internal medicine, microbial genetics, molecular biology, molecular genetics, nutrition, nutrition education, public health and toxicology. This blue-ribbon panel of conventional "experts" did not study or evaluate nutrition in relation to cancer therapy but only addressed itself to diet and nutrition in relation to the cause and prevention of cancer. After two years of labor, this is what the experts found and published:

"It has become absolutely clear that cigarettes are the cause of approximately one quarter of all the fatal cancers in the United States. If the population had been persuaded to stop smoking when the association with lung cancer was first reported, these cancer deaths would not now be occurring. Twenty years ago the 'stop smoking' message required some rather cautious wording. Today, the facts are clear, and the choice of words is not so important... The public is now asking about the causes of cancers that are not associated with smoking... We are in an interim stage of knowledge similar to that for cigarettes 20 years ago. Therefore, in the judgement of the committee, it is now the time to offer some interim guidelines on diet and cancer."

In other words, to read between the lines, it may be another 20 years before orthodox medicine is as willing to recognize the relationship between diet and cancer as they now recognize the relationship between smoking cigarettes and cancer. It's interesting to look at history and see how far we've come in our attitudes toward smoking.

A report issued by Drs. Eon McDonald and Henry Garland on behalf of the California Medical Association, as late as 1953, assured the public that smoking a pack of cigarettes a day was "a harmless pastime." Doctors who say this today would be laughed out of practice. Those of us who are not at an advanced stage of senility remember when magazines carried full page color pictures of doctors leaning over operating tables poised with cigarettes between their fingers. The slogan of the campaign I'm thinking of proclaimed "More doctors smoke Camels than any other cigarette." Then there was the familiar "T" zone the handsome doctor told us would be soothed with cigarettes. But can we wait another 20 years to apply the rules of sound nutrition in the battle against cancer while hundreds of thousands of people die for lack of knowledge? The only humane answer is a resounding **"absolutely not!"**

In its first report, the NRC committee said it would be another year before they could make recommendations for future research. They could not even speculate on how many years it would take before funding was obtained for the research. The research itself has already been done, and the conclusions, if any, were published. And after publication of the results of the research on diet and cancer, how many further years are to elapse as the old school of thought about cancer treatment battles stubbornly with the new?

Some highlights of the NRC report:

"The Committee concluded that the differences in the rates at which various cancers occur in different human populations are often correlated with differences in diet. The likelihood that some of these correlations reflect causality is strengthened by laboratory evidence that similar dietary patterns and components of food also affect the incidence of certain cancers in animals. In general, the evidence suggests that some types of diets and some dietary components tend to increase the risk of cancer, whereas others tend to decrease it."

The Committee made some tentative conclusions as to the dietary elements associated with cancer development and those associated with cancer prevention. These conclusions are consistent with what you will learn in the following pages.

Every once in a while logic and reason win out. The National Cancer Institute has recently accepted the role of fiber in colon cancer, according to *The University of San Diego Nutrition Book* (Little,

Brown and Company, 1993). The NCI now recommends Americans double their intake of fiber from the current average of 10 grams, to 20 grams a day, since "populations that consume approximately 20-35 grams of dietary fiber have a lower rate of cancers of the colon and rectum."

Further evidence of the growing awareness of the relationship between nutrition and cancer is a chapter entitled "Nutrition and Cancer" in the *Mount Sinai School of Medicine Complete Book of Nutrition* (St. Martin's Press, NY, 1990, p. 469).

It starts out with a disclaimer meant to forewarn the reader, "Over the past few years, many groups of scientists have formulated guidelines for a diet that they believe is consistent with good nutritional practice and, at the same time, likely to reduce the risk of cancer. Most of these guidelines are still the subject of fierce debate."

This manual of orthodox medicine discusses numerous studies showing a relationship between diet and cancer:

"At least five studies in humans have shown that the incidence of gastric (stomach) cancer falls as people consume more fresh vegetables and fruits, especially citrus fruits.

"In animals, high doses of vitamin A decrease the numbers of tumors induced by some carcinogens, slow the growth of those tumors that do appear, and lead to tumor regression.

"Some studies in humans with malignant or premalignant changes in the skin have shown that topical applications of vitamin A may reverse these lesions."

The book, used in many different universities, not just for Mt. Sinai medical students, is careful, however, to discourage free-thinkers from considering nutritional therapies.

"...The debate rages on between megavitamin enthusiasts and more responsible physicians."

The unenthusiastic response from the Mount Sinai doctors is not surprising. Modern medicine and orthodox science have always been slow to accept new ideas. It took them decades to finally admit the correlation between smoking and lung cancer. Millions of lives were lost while they ignored the obvious. We cannot afford to wait again for the medical establishment to finally recognize the miraculous way nutrition prevents cancer and, in some cases, reverses the entrenched disease. Each year of delay in the application of what we already know about the relationship between cancer and nutrition results in more than 500,000 dead Americans. It is imperative that the message of good nutrition be spread NOW. While the doctors, scientists and medical journals vacillate, we in the nutrition field must educate the public with what we know about cancer and diet.

For my part, I fervently believe *Nutrition: The Cancer Answer II* can play a major role in the battle with cancer. To achieve that worthy goal, this book is written.

CHAPTER 1:

The Catastrophe of Cancer

"A clean glove often aides a dirty hand"

-English proverb

During one month of each year (April) nearly every family in the U.S. will be called on by an American Cancer Society (ACS) volunteer. They will be asked to contribute money to "fight cancer with a check-up and a check." Reinforced by a sophisticated multi-media campaign and a proclamation by the President declaring April "Cancer Control Month," this unprecedented mobilization stands to gross the ACS $150 million.

When it was founded in 1913, ACS described itself as a "temporary" organization; it would cease to exist once cancer had been eradicated. Seven decades later, ACS is the richest private charity in the world. And cancer is more of a problem than ever before. In the past 10 years alone, while the organization collected more than $1 billion from a cancer-fearing American public, the cancer death rate climbed 12 percent.

According to one disgruntled volunteer, the ACS has become "a self-perpetuating vested interest" and "a very profitable one" for many of those involved. Not many years ago, the National Information Bureau (NIB), a respected independent charity-watchdog

1

organization, listed ACS among the groups which do not meet its standards. Nonetheless, ACS has consistently been the loudest voice of the cancer establishment, and today it remains entrenched in the front lines of the government's war on cancer.

Like other large bureaucracies of the health care delivery system, ACS is not representative of the public at large. Many of its directors and members of its scientific committees have direct financial links to chemical industries and drug companies. Its medical advisors, meanwhile, are drawn exclusively from the fields of orthodox cancer treatment (i.e., surgery, radiation and chemotherapy). Not surprisingly, the society emphasizes treating cancer rather than preventing it.

In addition to its anti-prevention and pro-industry stance, ACS, according to its critics, spends its lavish budget improperly, blacklisting promising research that is not confined to conventional avenues.

During my 25 years of lobbying in every state of the union for freedom of choice to employ natural cancer remedies, I paid my own way while FDA/ACS spokespeople spent as much as $80,000 per hearing to oppose me.

ACS executives loudly proclaim it is a "people-benefit kind of organization with by far the major proportion of its resources spent for caring and rehabilitating the cancer patient."

Analysis of the ACS annual budget reveals an average of five to six percent goes to "assistance to individual patients." Salaries and benefits paid to the ACS staff of more than 3,000 people (large for a "volunteer organization" that conducts no research) exceeds ACS's expenditures for research and patient care put together. Between 50 and 60 percent of ACS's annual budget goes toward its own administrative and office expenses, fund-raising, office supplies and postage. Incredibly, an excess of $10,000 a day is spent in telephone calls alone!

The ACS also lobbies vigorously to suppress new ideas within the medical community, where it wields tremendous power. Science journalist Robert Houston explained how the process works. "Independent, unconventional research," he said, "tends to be clocked by the actions of the ACS, by their whole system of blacklisting and vilification of new therapies. ACS maintains an official blacklist: "Unproven Methods of Cancer Management," 'unproven' being their code word for 'quack.' Once you are on this list, it is very difficult, if not impossible, to get off. And some of the most promising cancer research has landed on that list."

Among the many reputable researchers and clinicians summarily blacklisted by ACS are the late Max Gerson, M.D. (of whom Dr. Albert Schweitzer wrote, "I see in him one of the most eminent geniuses in the history of medicine"); Andrew Ivy, M.D., Ph.D. (former vice president of the University of Illinois); and Ernst Krebs, Jr., Ph.D., (the co-discoverer of Laetrile and vitamin B15). In *The Cancer Syndrome* (Grove), Ralph Moss, Ph.D., documents how blacklisted researchers lose official funding sources. Not surprisingly, the unconventional approaches are rarely tested. Robert Houston emphasized, "It should be noted that 'unproven' is not synonymous with 'disproven'."

It seems incredible that an organization such as ACS, established to champion new cancer research, should in fact spend much of its budget actively suppressing new ideas.

Cancer: A Modern Medicine Phenomenon

Cancer was recorded by the early Greeks and from time to time throughout European history. In 1765, Johann Philip published a treatise at Frankfurt am Main, attributing cancer to an excess of acidic substances in food and drink. The earliest statistical evidence (as opposed to scattered reporting) was probably collected by the Registrar General of England and Wales for the period between 1838 and 1859. The death rate of approximately 20 per 100,000 noted at that time was not significant and certainly no greater than from many other diseases.

During the late 19th century it became evident to many medical observers that cancer was on the rise throughout the world, especially in the industrialized parts of Europe and North America. This increase exploded in the 20th Century. Not, however, as the result of improved medical diagnosis, or more accurate collection and inter-pretation of statistical evidence. The increase was real.

In 1900 only 41,000 Americans died of cancer. Since then every decade has seen a gigantic 23 to 60 percent increase in the death rate.

They admit it: "There has been a steady rise in the cancer mortali-ty rate in the U.S. in the last half-century. The age-adjusted rate in 1930 was 143 per 100,000 population. It rose to 152 by 1940, to 163 in 1970 and was 171 in 1989. About one in three, according to pre-sent rates, or about 85 million Americans now living will eventually have cancer" (*"Cancer Facts & Figures – 1993,"* American Cancer Society, Inc.).

When ACS talks about the cancer "cure" rate, keep this in mind: for most forms of cancer, five years without symptoms following treat-ment is what they consider "cured."

Keep in mind, also, that cure rates may be skewed in order to jus-tify the $1 billion-a-year national cancer program. This is exactly what the Government Accounting Office (GAO) determined regard-ing a 1986 NCI cancer survival rate report.

The GAO, a Congressional investigative agency, produced a 131-page special report in 1988, stating federal health officials lied and misled the public about the progress made in treating cancer in the U.S. For the majority of the twelve most common forms of cancer, the report concluded, there was "little or no improvement from 1950 to 1982 in the rate by which patients survived their disease."

More people now die of cancer each year in the United States than the combined fatalities of the Korean and Vietnamese Wars. Worse, still, the death rates from cancer are still increasing, and more people are dying of cancer at an early age than at any time in the history of the world.

The multi-billion dollar "war on cancer" instituted by President Richard Nixon in the early 1970s focused only on the use of orthodox treatments by the medical establishment: surgery, radiation and chemotherapy – the cut, burn and poison approach. In other words, kill the body to kill the cancer. If the cancer doesn't get you, the cure will. The result of this political and medical inertia has been the dis-astrous increase in cancer deaths.

In addition, there has been little change in the five-year survival rate for cancer since 1955. A slight statistical improvement from the 1930s to 1955 can be attributed to improvements in operating room procedures rather than to cancer research. The introduction of antibiotics and blood transfusions have enabled more patients to survive surgery in general. Since 1955 the cancer survival rate has flattened out as the benefits from improved procedures were absorbed.

Orthodox Treatment of Cancer

Cancer statistics in the U.S. yield one irrefutable conclusion: the incidence of cancer is increasing. At the same time, cancer research expenditures are also increasing and have been throughout this century.

The American Cancer Society's overall annual research expenditure has grown steadily from $1 million in 1946 to approximately $89 million in fiscal year 1992. This incredible sum represents only slightly over 25 percent of their total expenditures. To date, ACS has invested more than $1.5 billion in cancer research (*Cancer Facts & Figures – 1993*).

These two sets of statistics force us to come to a basic conclusion: medical research has failed utterly to come to grips with the problem of cancer. Surgery, radiation and chemotherapy may, in certain individual cases, appear to arrest cancer, but since modern medicine cannot pinpoint the cause(s) of cancer, it's no closer to the cure. Nor can it seemingly prevent the increase in cancer deaths.

If we believe the media, the United States is the healthiest country in the world. We have the finest trained doctors (no foreign doctor is allowed to practice here without additional training); our nurses have masters degrees and some are even Ph.D.s; we have superb medical, diagnostic and health care equipment; and our hospitals are the last word in architectural design and efficient treatment of the sick.

These glowing contentions do not tell the whole story. The United States is fast becoming one of the sickest countries in the world and in some diseases, such as cancer, the United States already ranks among the sickest.

It is true that some virus-caused diseases, so-called pathogenic diseases, have been eliminated or controlled by medical technology. However, when it comes to diseases of the whole body, the metabolic diseases, which, as we shall show, include cancer, billions of dollars worth of research and specialized equipment have not begun to identify the causes, much less establish cures.

A basic premise held by most orthodox medical practitioners is that cancer is not caused by a breakdown or flaw in the body, but rather is like a localized burn in that a carcinogen (a cancer-causing irritant) causes the cancer cells to form locally. If the cancer "burn," in the form of a bump or lump, is removed before cancer cells invade adjacent tissues, the cancer can be cured. Research that attempts to improve on this limited concept ignores the reason the cells formed in the first place.

While early surgeons were content to remove the tumorous mass, it later became common to remove not only the tumorous mass, but also a great amount of normal tissue in the adjacent area. In breast surgery, for example, a mastectomy (removal of the breast) removes not only the tumor itself, but also muscle, connective tissue and lymph glands in the auxiliary area. More recently, surgeons have become more ambitious; to stop one slow-growing tumor, a full quarter of a man was removed. In one extreme case, a man was actually cut in two, losing both legs, the hips, and all of the external reproductive organs.

A second type of localized treatment is to radiate the tumor site with powerful rays known to kill cancer cells. The first objective of radiation is to kill the tumor, and the second is to kill a portion of the adjacent normal tissue into which cancer cells may have infiltrated. The major problem with radiation is that the rays are in no way selective. Burn damage, therefore, will occur in normal as well as cancerous tissues. Hair loss also frequently accompanies radiation due to a disruption of protein metabolism.

A third type of treatment, chemotherapy, is designed to selectively kill cancer cells by taking advantage of their high rate of reproductive activity. Doctors literally inject poisons into the body in order to destroy cancer cells. These poisons are so toxic that masks, gowns and gloves are worn by the medical technicians.

Chemotherapeutic agents are non-selective; they also affect other organ systems of the body with naturally-high cell reproduction. The list of undesirable side effects is long. These side effects differ depending upon the individual and the specific agent used, but include loss of hair, sterility, and reduced ability to assimilate food, resulting in malnutrition. Quality of life is all but destroyed and, in many cases, death results from the agent instead of from the disease.

Conventional cancer treatments are unnatural to the human body, working against it instead of with it. They work to mutilate, burn and poison the host in order to destroy the cancer parasite. The success rate of these treatments has been anything but spectacular. They are lengthy and painful. Often the patient has to choose between a slow death through treatments or a quick one by allowing the cancer to take its course. The logical alternative to this option is contained within these pages.

Crisis Medicine vs. Preventative Medicine

Most American doctors are dedicated men and women who, along with their loved ones, are vulnerable to the ravages of cancer. It would be unrealistic to imply they are not as individually concerned as all of us in curing this dread disease. No doubt the surgeon wielding his talented scalpel during a mastectomy, the highly trained radiologist burning his target with beams of cobalt, or the well-trained chemotherapist mixing his poisons believe they are providing the best care medical science has to offer.

To the extent of the training and knowledge these practitioners have received, this is true. Unfortunately, as you will discover, the knowledge at their command is supplied by a powerful medical-industrial-governmental axis whose multiple-vested interests make cancer prevention unprofitable and total cure financially ruinous.

America has the best equipped and most heavily financed institutions of medical learning in the world. Our medical students are brainwashed into believing that the subsidized education they receive is based upon exacting science. Instead of encouraging free thinking and exploratory medicine, medical schools place emphasis on convention. Nutritional solutions are not investigated or explored; they are discouraged and rejected. There is a dubious reason for this.

Major institutions of medical learning in the U.S. are, without exception, subsidized by the foundations and grants of a multi-billion-dollar drug industry. This industry is repaid for its largesse with countless prescriptions written by its student protéges. This drug-financed educational program has a post-graduate extension where a myriad of drug company salesmen continue to educate the practicing doctors in the latest drugs and machines available, through them, to their patients.

Thus, we see that it is sound business practice, not philanthropy, that ordains the funneling of drug company profits into education and even directs financial support of the AMA itself, through AMA journal advertising. The result is a medical community that thrives on sickness. The entire financial circle depends upon the continuing flow of high-priced drugs, modalities and procedures to be prescribed when the patient becomes sick.

CHAPTER 2:

Prevention vs. Treatment — The Undercover War

"With superior knowledge the physician cures before the illness is manifested...with inferior knowledge the physician can but attempt to care for the illness he was unable to prevent."

Ancient Chinese proverb

Fortunately, there is a growing body of physicians who believe that the Creator, the greatest healer of all, has designed the human body for wellness, not sickness. If we just look we will find, within our own bodies and the biological environment surrounding us, preventives against metabolic disease, as opposed to the crisis medicine of orthodoxy – where treatment commences only when symptoms appear. In cancer, the symptom is a lesion, a lump, or a bump. In this book we will emphasize preventive medicine and how to help avoid and reverse the symptoms that make us candidates for crisis medicine.

The normal state of the human body is one of health: an efficiently-functioning organic system. It is a steady state, a state of no disease, known to doctors as homeostasis.

When this normal state is disturbed by environmental pollutants, junk food, smoking, alcohol, or other drugs and poor eating habits,

9

normal cellular function is altered. Due to our body's innate ability to heal, one cigarette or one cola drink only temporarily effects this body balance.   However, chronic, long-term exposure is a continuing assault on the body's natural balance that breaks down the system and ultimately leads to metabolic disease. One of these diseases is cancer.

Since it is normal for the body to be healthy, it will continually try to maintain that state. If that normality is thrown off balance or out of rhythm in any way, the body's own homeostatic mechanisms will bring it back. When we get a cold or flu, we know that, given enough time, our body will restore itself to health. We may take aspirin for body aches or drink liquids to help cleanse the body of toxins, but we know that basically we can wait for our body to cure itself. Orthodox medicine knows this, but it bends to the challenge to alleviate symptoms. They spend millions of dollars making drugs to alleviate symptoms, instead of concentrating on ways to boost the body's natural ability to heal itself. The homeostatic mechanism of the body not only works for colds, it works for all afflictions of the body, including cancer.

The body can stand a certain amount of junk food. You can eat marshmallow-filled goodies for breakfast, TV dinners at night, be subjected to all kinds of stress and environmental pollutants, and the body will make adjustments to stay healthy. Unfortunately, the homeostatic mechanisms in the human body are not inexhaustible – they wear out.

Junk food, stress and a toxic environment can be tolerated only so long. Eventually our protective mechanisms will stop, and the result is disease. Maintaining homeostasis is very important. It seeks balance. Stress from any source depletes strategic vitamins and minerals (B1, B3, B6, B12 and chromium) from the body in an attempt to make up for what cannot be obtained from incomplete foods.

As a young World War II army lieutenant, Paul Wedel, M.D., himself a recovered cancer patient, was put in charge of rescuing and rehabilitating the victims of one of the largest Nazi concentration camps. His first order to his troops upon reaching the camp was not to give the former prisoners any food. He realized that their bodies were in a severe state of imbalance and had to be carefully attended to. The prisoners had been living only on water used in cooking cabbage, and some carrots. Many were barely alive. Some of the U.S. soldiers disobeyed Wedel's order and slipped candy bars to the inmates, thinking they were being merciful. As a direct result of this misplaced kindness, approximately 300 inmates died. The last of the vitamins and minerals in their systems were depleted in their bodies' attempt to compensate for the ingestion of this tempting non-food.

In most instances we are better off eating nothing than eating a sugary snack which will actually leach out vital vitamins and minerals during the digestive process. Consider some of the manufactured non-foods we dignify with the name "food."

Powdered non-dairy creamer, for example. We know what it is not: milk. But what is it? The ingredients listed are: sugar, partially hydrogenated vegetable oil, corn syrup solids, sodium caseinate (a milk derivative – that's cheating), dipotassium phosphate, mono- and diglycerides, salt, natural and artificial flavor. What they are really doing is turning the coffee from a dark color to a lighter color with chemicals made palatable with sugar.

Next time you go to the supermarket take along a piece of paper – you will need a long one – and write down the names of the chemicals in the prepared foods you customarily purchase.

Take fig cookies, for example. Read the label. Regardless of who manufacturers them, there is artificial flavor added. Why add artificial fig flavor to something that tastes as good as figs? Because they either pick the figs when they are unripe and have little nutrition or no flavor – or they pick them ripe and the processing is so drastic it destroys the naturalness of everything. So, flavor is added.

How about white and "wheat" bread? White bread is refined white flour, but if you look at some so-called wheat breads, they are refined white flour with caramel color added. If you assembled on a plate all the things you had eaten in a week, plus all the chemicals in them, you would not feed it to an animal.

Non-food or junk food is causing an unprecedented increase in the breakdown of the homeostatic mechanism. When the mechanism breaks down, the body becomes diseased. Metabolic degenerative diseases used to be diseases of the aged. Not any more. We now have people under 30 with arthritis, arteriosclerosis, heart disease, osteoporosis and cancer – all diseases of the elderly. This adds credence to the fact that it is not time that ages us; it is disease. Old age is not a number, it is a feeling, and those with poor health feel it much sooner.

As long as the American people continue to consume junk non-foods and chemicals, and the medical establishment insists on treating symptoms not problems, we come to an inevitable conclusion: there is no health care in the United States today. What we have is disease care, or crisis medicine.

"Currently, the emphasis in medicine is more on the treatment of disease than on the maintenance of health," Andrew McNaughton, head of the McNaughton Foundation and pioneer researcher.

The Failure of Establishment Research

That modern medical research, with all its sophisticated techniques and vast investment of money and skills, has failed to resolve the disease of cancer is undeniable. Moreover, the failure was recognized many years ago – almost 60, in fact. A book by M. Beddow Bayle entitled *Cancer: The Failure of Modern Research* was published in 1936. As we noted in the preceding chapter, cancer mortality rates have risen considerably since the 1930s. By 1925 a medical journal reported, "Of all the people alive on this globe today, more that 100 million are doomed to die from cancer" (*Surgery, Gynecology and Obstetrics*, 1925). A year later, in 1926, a British surgeon wrote, "To show how little use medical research has been in this direction, one need only call attention to the fact that, within the last three years, an important research body, confirmed by eminent opinion, stated that food has nothing to do with cancer" (*Sunday Express*).

In the 1920s, eminent medical opinion dismissed any possibility nutrition might be related to cancer. While ignorance may be understandable in the 1920s, it is remarkable that it continues into the '90s.

One articulate enemy of the metabolic and nutritional approach to cancer research is Victor Herbert, M.D., Professor of Medicine at State University, New York, and a speaker at conferences sponsored by the food industry. Dr. Herbert argues, "Inspect any medical school's textbook of medicine or ask your doctor. They will tell you that most diseases have nothing to do with diet" (Herbert). This is prima facie evidence to "scientific" minds like Dr. Herbert's.

On the other hand, as early as 1915 a book by Frederick L. Hoffman, *The Mortality from Cancer Throughout the World*, discussed the links between nutrition and cancer: "Based upon more general considerations, the opinion has frequently been advanced by ancient and modern writers that there is a direct relationship between diet and cancer frequency, and particularly in the case of excessive consumption of salt and meat. The per capita rise in the meat consumption of the principal civilized countries has often been referred to as a causative factor in the corresponding rise in the cancer death rate."

Another early writer, W.R. Williams, in *The Natural History of Cancer*, also reported a link between cancer and diet: "It may be well to recall the fact that although cancer is remarkably rare in vegetarian communities, complete exemption cannot be claimed for such; and the same is true of herbivorous (plant-eating) communities as compared with carnivorous (meat-eating) groups." Williams is, however, convinced by overwhelming evidence "that the incidence of cancer is largely conditioned by nutrition" (Williams).

Famed scientist Albert Schweitzer made a related comment, although its significance has been lost on the medical world: "On my arrival in Gabson, in 1913, I was astonished to encounter no cases of cancer. I saw none among the natives two-hundred miles from the coast.

"I cannot, of course, say positively that there was no cancer at all, but, like other frontier doctors, I can only say that if any cases existed they must have been quite rare. This absence of cancer seemed to be due to the difference in nutrition of the natives, as compared to the Europeans" (Bergulas).

In recent times, it has become widely known that people with specific types of diets are remarkably cancer-free. For example, Utah has a lower cancer death rate than any other state in America. According to the American Cancer Society, the total number of deaths in 1993 is estimated at 52,000 for California and 2,000 for Utah. If you think this is because California is so much bigger, Massachusetts' death rate is 13,700. Cancer *cases* in 1993 were estimated at 4,500 for Utah, 120,000 for California and 88,000 for New York.

The Evidence in Favor of Diet

Why this differential? A plausible explanation may be the concentration of Mormons in Utah and their mandated diet. The Mormon Church's doctrine includes a law of health (the 'Word of Wisdom') that counsels against the use of tobacco, alcoholic beverages, tea and coffee, and emphasizes the use of grains, wholesome herbs and fruits "for the benefit and health of man."

Another possible factor is revealed by the unique research of Gerhard Schrauzer, Ph.D., University of California at San Diego, on the presence or absence of selenium in the soil. It is Schrauzer's conviction, based on depth of research, that if our soils, and, consequently, the food grown in our soils, contained adequate selenium, cancer would be reduced by an astounding 75 percent. Much of Utah's soil has a higher than average selenium content.

We can find observations extending back over a century from numerous sources suggesting some relationship between cancer and diet – certainly enough to compel medical research to explore the relationship. The failure of modern cancer research is essentially its failure to break out of the tunnel-vision search for viral causes of cancer and explore the possibility of a nutritional cause.

Only now, after fires have been built under them for decades, is the American Cancer Society beginning to invest in research on diet and nutrition as a contributory cause of cancer.

The inability or unwillingness of orthodox medicine to consider nutrition in their search for cancer answers is just the tip of the iceberg. Even when established medicine has bowed to pressure and conducted research, any positive results have been suppressed.

"It is an open secret that there exists in the U.S.A. for incomprehensible reasons – or rather, very comprehensible ones – considerable opposition against prevention of malignancies with nitriloside therapy." – Dr. Hans A. Nieper in Krebsgeschehen, 1972/4.

The Amygdalin Answer

A classic example is the work of Kanematsu Sugiura, M.D., at Memorial Sloan-Kettering Cancer Institute. Some years ago, Dr. Sugiura was intrigued by the apparent usefulness of amygdalin, a nitriloside. This natural substance, also called Vitamin B17, is included in the controversial alternative cancer treatment, Laetrile. It is contained in many edible seeds (Laetrile is made from apricot seeds) and plants that have mostly been eliminated from modern man's diet.

Following is a summary conclusion from one of Dr. Sugiura's early experiences which notes "inhibition of growth," "regression" of tumors, and "better health and appearance" in mice under amygdalin treatment.

"Amygdalin in i.p. doses of 1000-2000 mg/kg/day causes significant inhibition of spontaneous mammary tumors in a highly inbred mouse. There is significant inhibition of the formation of lung metastases. It possibly prevents, to an uncertain degree, the formation of new tumors, regardless of the age of the mouse. Greater inhibition of tumor growth was seen in smaller spontaneous tumors of this strain.

"In Swiss Webster albino females with both large and small spontaneous mammary tumors, amygdalin caused regression in 80 percent of animals studied and complete regression in 40 percent. The complete regressions occurred only in small tumors on non-inbred mice.

"All treated animals maintained better health and appearance than the controls."

What was the fate of this promising work? Sloan-Kettering announced that the results were not significant and suppressed the report. Fortunately, individuals within Sloan-Kettering had a more sensible concept of scientific freedom and "leaked" the report to the outside world.

Profitability of Cancer Drugs

Why would established medicine suppress and ignore a promising research path? The simplest answer is there is no profit in nutrition for drug companies, which are locked into an association with orthodox medical research and practice. A more abstract answer would be pride, prejudice and vested interest.

The production and sale of drugs for cancer treatment is a gigantic and profitable business in contrast to the low profits generated by natural foods and substances. Antineoplastic agents, the narrowest possible definition of cancer drugs, including anesthetics, hormonal preparations affecting neoplasms and other cancer-related drugs, puts the cancer drug industry in the $1 billion-a-year category.

Cancer treatment drugs are produced by a dozen or so major pharmaceutical firms whose annual financial statements confirm this is a highly profitable business. Syntex, manufacturer of the chemotherapy Cytovene, had 1993 fiscal sales of $2.1 billion. Bristol-Myers Squibb, manufacturer of at least six chemotherapeutic agents, had 1993 worldwide sales of $11.4 billion. Fifty-seven percent of Bristol's sales are from pharmaceuticals.

When we look in detail at the anti-cancer drugs produced and sold by these and other drug companies, it is extraordinary that their products received FDA approval as being safe for human use. The toxic effects of anti-cancer drugs brings to mind a statement once made by Dr. Ernst Krebs, Jr.:

"Chemotherapy and radiation will make the ancient method of drilling holes in a patient's head to permit escape of demons to cure madness look relatively advanced...toxic chemotherapy is a hoax. It is premeditated murder. Use of cobalt and other methods of cancer treatment popular today closes the door on cure."

The cost to the patient of orthodox cancer "treatment" is horrendous. Anybody who has spent even a day or two in the hospital knows this. Costs continue to skyrocket. There's no point in quoting figures, inasmuch as they're old as soon as they're new.

Anti-Cancer Drugs: Toxic and Useless

Proponents of orthodox chemotherapeutic treatment for cancer continually allude to purported toxic reactions caused by the natural foods we will recommend in this book. Included in their unsupported list of dangerous items are amygdalin, vitamin A and lentil bean enzymes, all of which are nontoxic when taken in appropriate amounts.

Chart 1 lists some of the well-known and widely prescribed anti-cancer drugs used by orthodox medical practitioners. Manufacturers, brand names, efficacy and toxicity are as recorded in orthodoxy's own *Physician's Desk Reference* (p. 671).

Two observations can be made about the anti-cancer drugs listed in Chart 1:

1. These "anti-cancer" drugs are less than efficacious and, in many cases, not curative at all.

2. These drugs are highly toxic, sometimes fatal, yet they receive FDA approval as "safe" drugs.

The following detailed excerpts of a few selected drugs from the Physician's Desk Reference exemplify their extremely limited value and highly-dangerous side effects.

Leukeran

The alklyating agent Leukeran (chlorambucil) is a derivative of nitrogen mustard, under U.S. Patent No. 2,994,079, manufactured by Burroughs Wellcome Co. It is described as a "potent" drug used in the treatment of leukemia. It is not curative but produces "striking remissions" and is used with warnings: "Excessive or prolonged dosage will produce severe bone marrow depression. Severe neutropenia (abnormally small numbers of neutrophils in circulating blood) is related to dosage in a significant number of cases and there

Chart 1
DRUGS USED FOR CANCER
(according to the National Cancer Institute)

GENERIC NAME	BRAND NAME	MANUFACTURER	EFFICACY, according to Physicians Desk Reference	TOXICITY
BUSULFAN (sulfonic ester, alkylating agent)	"MYLERAN"	Burroughs, Wellcome	"Of value, not curative"	"Toxic effects"
CHLORAMBUCIL (alkylating agent)	"LEUKERAN"	Burroughs, Wellcome	"not curative but produces remissions"	"a potent drug… patients must be followed carefully to avoid irreversible damage to the bone marrow"
CYTOXAN (Cyclophosphamide)	"CYTOXAN"	Mead, Johnson	"interferes with growth of cancer (and normal cells). Has oncogenic (cancer creating) possibilities"	"Numerous adverse reactions including "severe, even fatal" reactions"
PIPOBROMAN	"VERCYTE"	Abbott	Mechanism not known, "useful"	"Adverse reactions reported: Nausea, vomiting, cramping, diarrhea, skin rash"
TRIETHYLENETHIO-PHOSPHORAMIDE	"THIOTEPA"	Lederle	Widely used with "varying results"	"Complications can cause death unless checked promptly"
CYTARABINE	"CYTOSAR"	Upjohn	"Few with solid tumors have benefited from the drug"	"Highly toxic and numerous reactions"
5-FLUOROURACIL	"5-FU"	Hoffman-LaRoche	"Effective in palliative management of some cancers… not for patients in poor nutritional state."	"Possibility of "severe toxic reactions""
MERCAPTOPURINE	"PURINETHOL"	Burroughs, Wellcome	"Believed to interfere with nucleic acid biosynthesis"	"Severe toxic reactions with no known acid biosynthesis antagonist."
METHOTREXATE		Lederle	"Inhibits growth of cell tissue"	"Highly toxic, deaths have been reported"
THIOGUANINE		Burroughs, Wellcome	"Not effective against solid tumors"	"Toxic, no known antagonist."
VINGLASTINE SULFATE	"VELBAN"	Eli Lilly	"Relieves pain, has produced temporary reduction in tumors"	"Some adverse reactions"
VINCRISTINE SULFATE	"ONCOVIN"	Eli Lilly	"Indicated in acute leukemia"	"Adverse reactions are reversible but overdose can have fatal outcome."

is a real risk of causing irreversible bone marrow damage."

Leukeran has FDA approval as a safe drug.

Cytoxan

Cytoxan (cyclophosphamide) is a synthetic drug related to the nitrogen mustards, classified as an alkylating agent (defined as "one which destroys tumor cells by altering their chemical composition"), manufactured by Bristol-Meyers. It interferes with the growth of cancer "and, to some extent, certain normal tissues." Among warnings for its use is "Cytoxan has been reported to have oncogenic activity in rats and mice" (it can cause cancer). It is recommended that "the possibility it may have oncogenic potential in humans should be considered." The adverse reactions for Cytoxan are numerous. Leukopenia is an "expected effect." Nausea and vomiting are common. Sterile hemorrhagic cystitis can result from Cytoxan: "This can be severe, even fatal, and is probably due to metabolites in the urine. Other complications can occur."

Cytoxan has FDA approval as a safe drug.

Vercyte

Vercyte (pipobroman) is another alkylating agent, manufactured by Abbott Laboratories. According to the Physician's Desk Reference, "The mechanism of action is unknown and the metabolic fate and route of excretion are unknown." However it is known that Vercyte frequently causes "bone marrow depression." It is not recommended for use in children under age 15 "because no significant clinical effect has been shown with patients in this age group."

Vercyte has FDA approval as a safe drug.

Thiotepa

Thiotepa is an alkylating agent used in conventional treatment of cancer, manufactured by Lederle Laboratories. It is used "with varying results" in a wide variety of neoplasms. It is "highly toxic," can create serious complications which "unless checked promptly...may lead to death." There is no known antidote for an overdose of Thiopeta and the numerous adverse reactions include local pain, nausea, dizziness, headache.

Thiotepa has FDA approval as a safe drug.

Cytosar

Cytosar was synthesized simultaneously by University of California Laboratories and the Upjohn Company. The results in the first 389 cases used are summarized in Chart 2. Almost 60 percent indicated no beneficial response and only 6.7 percent of cases had "complete remission." On the other hand, there are major known toxic effects and an extremely high percentage of patients report adverse reactions. Experimental studies indicated that some transplanted mouse tumors were inhibited, but there is no activity against rat tumors. Further studies show that Cytosar is immunosuppressive: it suppresses the body's natural immunological responses and is a potent bone marrow depressant. Other effects reported were:

Leukopenia 65.9 percent

Bone Marrow Suppression 19.4 percent

Nausea 15.6 percent

Vomiting 14.2 percent

"Given large doses, patients are frequently nauseated and may vomit for several hours post injection."

Cytosar has FDA approval as a safe drug.

5-Fluorouracil

The antimetabolite 5-FU is manufactured by Hoffman-La Roche Laboratories, and used as a palliative in some cancers that cannot be treated surgically. 5-FU is very toxic and has to be used with extreme caution, treatment being discontinued if any one of several adverse effects appear. It is described as a "highly toxic drug with a narrow

Chart 2
Results of Tests with Cytosar (First 389 Cases)

Total Number Patients Treated	Complete Remission	Partial Remission	Improved	No Beneficial Response	Inadequate Trial
235 adults (acute leukemia)	19	30	22	137	27
154 children (Leukemia)	7	40	9	89	9
TOTALS					
389	26	70	31	226	36
100 percent	6.7%	18.0%	8.0%	58.1%	9.2%

margin of safety." Fatalities may be encountered even in patients in relatively good condition. It is so dangerous it is recommended that therapy be discontinued at the end of the 12th day even if no toxicity has become apparent.

Its efficacy is rather questionable: the effect may be to "create a thiamine deficiency which provokes unbalanced growth and death of the cell."

5-Fluorouracil has FDA approval as a safe drug.

Mercaptopurine

Manufactured by Burroughs, Wellcome Co. under the brand name Purinethol, Mercaptopurine is a potent drug used in treatment of acute leukemia. The drug is toxic and effects may be delayed even with highly lethal doses. Numerous adverse reactions have been recorded and there is no known drug which will counter Mercaptopurine.

Mercaptopurine has FDA approval as a safe drug.

Methotrexate

Methotrexate, manufactured by Lederle Laboratories, is a highly-toxic antimetabolite. Side effects include the possibility of fatal toxic reactions and, sure enough, deaths have been reported. The drug is supposed to prevent the growth of malignant tissues without irreversible damage to normal tissue, and it has been used as a palliative in leukemia.

Methotrexate has FDA approval as a safe drug.

Readers are reminded that the foregoing statements of toxicity on FDA-approved drugs are not our opinion, but are taken directly from the Physician's Desk Reference, a volume used to guide the practicing physician in his choice of treatment.

Throughout this book, we will advocate the cancer-preventive properties of natural vitamins, including B17 and amygdalin.

Many of the advocates and users of the previously listed dangerous chemicals have the temerity to tell their patients vitamins and amygdalin are toxic and should, therefore, be avoided. They choose to ignore even the FDA's admission amygdalin is "harmless to both man and beast when used as an essential part of the metabolic approach to cancer" (Moertal).

Although Laetrile (vitamin B17 or amygdalin) is not listed in the *Physician's Desk Reference*, the following reactions have been reported by physicians using the pure, natural form of amygdalin, based on clinical human use: "temporary lowering of blood pressure, pain reduction, complete pain elimination, increased appetite, weight gain, increased mental acuity, increased energy, subjective remission, objective remission, total remission." Laetrile can be legally obtained.

CHAPTER 3:

The Cancer Conglomerates

"There is a growing awareness among the American people that orthodox medicine is not working because the solutions lie outside accepted patterns of thought."

—Marilyn Ferguson

In recent years, a new and unorthodox school of thought has emerged which views cancer as a metabolic disease that can be prevented. Millions of private individuals and public professionals have proven to their own satisfaction that cancer is a nutritional deficiency. Alternative medical practitioners as well as an indignant and dissatisfied public are in strident daily battle with mainstream medicine in a war that rages in the news, courts and doctors' offices. Through my books and the efforts of the National Health Federation, the largest and oldest health freedom organization in America, and fueled by mainstream medicine's failures, the notion that diet can affect disease has become a populist movement.

Opponents of the preventive, nutritional approach include the American Medical Association, the Food and Drug Administration, the American Cancer Society, the Memorial Sloan-Kettering Institute and the National Cancer Institute. However, public and political pressure, started by these early pioneers, are forcing them to reluctantly modify their stands.

The war reflects an underlying basic difference in the interpretation of the nature of cancer. Established medicine acknowledges it does not know the nature of the disease and, therefore, can expect only limited success in treatment. At the same time its approach reflects an underlying assumption that each type of cancer is a biologically distinctive phenomenon – that all cancers are different. They contend there are many types of cancer cells and, therefore, many varying explanations and treatments of the phenomenon. Mainstream medicine continues to spend billions of dollars seeking out a biological enemy that causes cancer, instead of examining the reasons cells mutate to cancer, and working within this biological framework.

Researchers are now discovering what I've been saying all along: cancer cells are an aberration of a naturally-occurring cell, one that exists in the body as a natural part of the life cycle, but which has malfunctioned and is not influenced by normal body defenses. Because cancer is an internal aberration rooted in DNA, genes, enzymes and proteins, as epidemiologists, oncologists and geneticists are now finding out, as long as those aberrations exist, cancer can occur anywhere in the body. This latter position is referred to as the unitarian thesis of cancer.

The orthodox interpretation and the challenging unitarian thesis are irreconcilable. Either cancer is unitary or it is non-unitarian. In the words of unitarian pioneers, "The malignant component in all cancer is the same. This component is not spontaneously created, but is the most primitive cell in the life cycle, the trophoblast cell gone awry." (Dr. Ernst Krebs, discoverer of B17, Laetrile).

The Diet, Nutrition and Cancer Program (DNCP) of the National Cancer Institute is only lightly funded, and has but a few faltering projects underway. While a river of gold provided by your taxes is pumped into the mammoth cancer establishment, and fails to produce results, metabolic medicine researchers proceed without government money. The results of their investigations are so overwhelmingly positive that the second half of this book is dedicated to offering you a cookbook for a healthy life – a dietary guide to healthy living in which cancer cannot exist.

Research Beneficiaries

Cancer research and treatment is riddled with conflicts of interest, giving rise to a situation in which there is no incentive to explore new avenues of research, and the financial advantage is to maintain a status quo – an inertial languor that kills 500,000 Americans annually.

The board directors of pharmaceutical companies manufacturing chemotherapeutic cancer drugs are sprinkled with academics and researchers supposedly involved in the unbiased search for a cancer cure.

Merck & Co., Inc., the world's largest pharmaceutical company, makes two of the commonly-prescribed chemotherapies: Mustargen (a relative of mustard gas) and Cosmegen. It also produces the highly-promoted Proscar, a treatment for prostate enlargement. According to the company's 1993 Annual Report, Proscar has annual sales exceeding $100 million.

Included among Merck's board of directors are Richard S. Ross, M.D., Dean Emeritus of the Medical Faculty, Johns Hopkins University School of Medicine; William N. Kelley, M.D., Chief Executive Officer, University of Pennsylvania Medical Center and Health System; and Lloyd C. Elam, M.D., Professor of Psychiatry Mebarry Medical College. With that kind of representation, no wonder Proscar does so well.

Syntex Corporation, manufacturer of Ganclovir (cytovene), boasts two esteemed educators on its board of directors: Julius R. Krevans, M.D., Chancellor Emeritus, University of California, San Francisco and Kenneth Melmon, M.D., Department of Medicine, Stanford University. Dr. Melmon serves on the corporation's Committee on "Science" (Syntex Corporation 1993 Annual Report).

The Abbott Laboratories' board of directors include: K. Frank Austen, M.D., Professor of Medicine, Harvard Medical School; and Boone Powell Jr., President and CEO, Baylor Health Care System and Baylor University Medical Center, and Vice President Baylor University (Abbott Laboratories 1993 Annual Report). Abbott makes Pipobroman, used in treatment of leukemia.

In brief, supposedly unbiased cancer researchers have an unhealthy link to and pecuniary interest in cancer drug-producing companies. If only subconsciously, they cannot dismiss the devastating financial effect a nutritional solution to cancer will have on the drug industry.

The Rockefeller Family Interest in Cancer

The link between the production and sale of toxic, useless drugs for cancer treatment and the medical establishment is nowhere more clear than in the case of the Rockefeller family. The family has pecuniary interests in drug production and at the same time trusteeship in cancer research and hospital facilities.

In 1949, the late Nelson Rockefeller became a member of the board of the Memorial Sloan-Kettering Institute for Cancer Research, and later was named Chairman of the Board.

Rockefeller also claimed to have tried to increase federal participation in the fight against cancer, and served six years on the National Cancer Advisory Board.

This powerful, aristocratic family has a significant influence on cancer research. In 1976 the Rockefeller Brothers Fund contributed $2.5 million toward the building program at Memorial Sloan-Kettering Cancer Center, the key U.S. cancer research complex. Lawrence Rockefeller is chairman of Sloan-Kettering. During U.S. Senate hearings on the nomination of Vice President Nelson Rockefeller, it was revealed that the Rockefeller Brothers Fund was heavily invested in Merck & Co. (manufacturers of the cancer drug Mithracin), Pfizer, Inc. (manufacturers of antibiotics used in cancer treatments) and Squibb Corporation (manufacturer of the cancer drug Hydrea).

More importantly, the Rockefeller family interests have close associations with drug companies. These relationships were summarized in the Congressional report on the nomination of Nelson Rockefeller for Vice President, as follows:

– Ralston Purina, manufacturers of lab chow to feed testing mice: two associations with the Rockefeller family.

– Colgate Palmolive (subsidiary in Kendall). Eighteen percent of its earnings come from surgical products: four associations with the Rockefeller family.

– Bristol Myers: two associations with the Rockefeller family through Bristol Labs and Mead Johnson, manufacturers of BCNU, Vepefid, Mutamycin, Paraplatin and Carboplatin.

– Warner Lambert: two associations with the Rockefeller family (through Parke Davis and Warner Chilcott Labs).

– Eli Lilly: two associations with the Rockefeller family; manufactures Velban, Drolban and Oncovin.

Cancer Research More Profitable Than Cancer Cure

Let us suppose the metabolic-nutritional approach to cancer prevention were to become widespread and were not restricted to those estimated 50,000 Americans willing to risk harassment by bureaucrats and medical associates. What would be the results?

Certainly the size and commercial influence of the lucrative cancer research industry would be drastically reduced. The American Cancer Society, the numerous academics who serve on cancer research boards, the fund raisers and the public relations people would be looking for other work. Manufacturers of radiation equipment, X-ray machines and cobalt machines would suffer drastic cuts in production and revenue. Most alarming (for the drug firms), a whole range of dangerous toxic drugs would no longer be required. A multi-billion-dollar industry would be devastated.

To compound the prejudicial problems of these already heavily-vested interests, according to one study by the Office of Technology Assessment, the cost of developing a new drug is estimated to be $359 million. Other studies show the development process can take up to 12 years from the time a new compound is first identified.

Amygdalin and other natural substances are in the public domain and cannot be patented. No one is going to invest that kind of money on a substance that cannot be patented and made profitable.

Thus, the FDA acts as little more than a protection racket benefiting drug companies that can well afford these huge sums. Only because 54 percent of the American people (these figures are escalating daily) have opted for alternatives are there cracks in the well-heeled cancer establishment dike. They can't afford to lose face completely by revealing their hidden agenda.

In conclusion, there is more profit, and therefore incentive, in *looking* for a cancer cure than in *finding* it.

CHAPTER 4:

Nutrition:
The Right Direction

*"If a patient dies of cancer without being informed that there are
alternative treatment methods to those of established medical opinion,
I believe it would be appropriate for his survivors to sue the doctors
who failed to inform him."*
—*Robert C. Atkins, M.D., Nutrition Breakthrough.*

Backed by an educated, indignant and dissatisfied public, a small
but vocal group of enlightened physicians has concluded, empirically and logically, that cancer is a dietary deficiency disease.
Research has shown it involves specific cellular-level deficiencies of
pancreatic enzymes, amygdalin (vitamin B17), and other vitamin and
minerals including A, E and C. The logic of this position is supported by the fact that, without exception, the cure for chronic metabolic
diseases, when finally discovered, has been made by supplying a
missing food factor in the same molecular form as available in nature.
There is no logical reason to believe cancer is an exception.

Scurvy: Cured by Vitamin C

Several centuries ago, scurvy, a disease characterized by weakness
and hemorrhaging of tissues and pain-racked joints, was a common,
often fatal disease among sailors, explorers, and the inhabitants of

communities lacking fresh food. So many artificially-fed infants develop scurvy that the dread disease once known as the "sailor's calamity" became known as the "baby's calamity."

Today scurvy is relatively rare, but before 1700, thousands of people suffered through catastrophic widespread epidemics. People of all walks of life in many nations were wracked by the painful, raging throes of terminal scurvy. In 1498, Vasco de Gama sailed around the Cape of Good Hope in South Africa. Out of his crew of 160, fully one-quarter succumbed to it.

About the end of the 16th Century it was randomly observed that fresh fruit and vegetables had immediate curative effects on scurvy. In 1593, during his voyages in the South Seas, Sir Richard Hawkins noted and later published his observation that natives of the area ate sour oranges and lemons as a cure for scurvy, with the same result noted among his crew. Yet, for nearly two centuries European doctors refused to consider this simple treatment, used so effectively on island natives and Hawkins' crew. Instead, they continued to search the dark, dank hulls of ships for some strange undiscovered source of the disease.

Finally, in 1754, Dr. James Lind, surgeon at the Royal Naval Hospital, Haslar, England, wrote *Treatise on the Scurvy*, in which he described experiments on sailors using oranges and lemons to prevent and cure scurvy. It still took 50 more years for British physicians to accept the nutritional solution and recommend lime juice be included in sea rations.

Lind's perceptive observations can be applied to present day cancer treatment considerations. We find it impossible to believe that something as simple as diet could be responsible for something as painful and deadly as cancer. Like cancer today, scurvy killed millions of people in its day. Doctors then could not be brought to believe the answer was as simple as citrus fruit.

The practical effects of fresh fruit on scurvy were known before there was an understanding of the reason for the cure. For two centuries ships carried oranges, lemons and vegetables as a preventive against scurvy without understanding the principle of vitamins. In

1804, regulations were introduced into the British Navy requiring use of lime juice in the absence of fresh fruits. This measure was eventually enacted into law by the British Board of Trade in 1865, leading to almost entirely eliminating scurvy.

While the empirical cure for scurvy was known, it was not realized until the early 20th Century that vitamin C was the specific anti-scurvy element at work. In summary, it took two centuries to translate empirical observation into action and more than another century before the curative element for scurvy was identified as vitamin C.

Beriberi: Cured by Vitamin B1 (Thiamine)

For thousands of years, beriberi was a major disease in the Far East and other areas with high consumption of polished rice. No exception to this dietary rule was the food given to Japanese sailors. On one naval voyage there were 169 cases of beriberi out of a total crew of 376, of which no fewer than 25 died. In 1882, a Japanese Navy doctor, Takaki, empirically determined beriberi to be a dietary deficiency. On the next training ship voyage, Takaki substituted a high-protein diet, accidentally containing sufficient vitamin B1 to eliminate beriberi. In 1878, 1,485 cases of beriberi were reported in the Japanese Navy. By 1888, it was completely eliminated. Similar results were reported from the Dutch East Indies, the Philippines and even inside the United States. It was found by Eijkman in 1897 that beriberi could be induced by feeding polished rice to chickens, and by Funk in 1911 that pigeons could be cured of beriberi by feeding them rice polishings (the part removed in rice processing).

In 1927, vitamin B was isolated by two Dutch researchers, Jansen and Dunath, and in 1936, vitamin B1 was synthesized. As in the case of vitamin C, we find that the cure for beriberi was determined empirically and then the substance was isolated and synthesized in the laboratory, but not until many years had passed.

	Chart 3		
Vitamin Deficiency Diseases and Their Cures			
Disease	Empirical observation of "cures" for the disease	Testing and hypothesizing	Generally accepted as a vitamin deficiency disease
Scurvy	During 16th and 17th centuries	British navy in late 18th century, Holst & Frolich (1907-1912)	Early to mid-19th century
Beriberi	Takaki in 1877	Tested in Japanese Navy 1886; Suzuki, Funk, Jansen & Dunath (1912-1926)	Early 20th century
Rickets	Guenn (1838) to Dibbelt (1909) (concentrating on calcium in diet)	Testing of cod liver oil at London Zoo. Later experiments with rats in U.S.	Early 1922 with separation of Vitamin A into A and D
Pellagra	Goldberger in U.S. noted relationship of pellagra to diet	Voegtlin (1920) Goldberger (1927)	Early 1930's Vitamin B$_3$ accepted anti-pellagra component.

Pellagra: Cured by Vitamin B3 (Niacin)

As recently as 50 years ago, pellagra was a common disease in the Southern United States. In 1917, for example, there were more than 170,000 cases in the South, and in South Carolina pellagra ranked second as a cause of death. In 1920, it was found that a diet rich in vitamin B-complex would cure pellagra. In 1927, Dr. J. Goldberger identified the differences between pellagra and beriberi, and determined that vitamin B-complex was pellagra's cure. This eminent medical scholar was ignored by the medical establishment, which was concentrating its own research on finding a viral cause of the disease. Dr. Goldberger's clinical studies proved conclusively that the disease was concentrated in the Southern United States, where the diet of blacks and poor whites was heavy in maize meal, molasses and meat, which contained insufficient vitamin B3 to prevent pellagra.

Is Cancer a Dietary Deficiency?

Most research programs start with random empirical observations. These seemingly casual observations link a postulated cause to an observed effect and form a preliminary pattern in the mind of the investigator. It is this preliminary pattern which gives rise to the process of hypothesizing, or outlining possible explanations.

In the assault on scurvy, beriberi and pellagra, this cycle of empirical observation, development of explanatory patterns, derivation of and testing of hypotheses, is seen clearly.

In cancer today, establishment science admittedly knows of no general cause for the lumps or bumps it calls cancer. The establishment "cure" for cancer is to remove the lump or bump by surgery, radiation, or chemical means. Orthodox medicine cannot guarantee cancer will not recur, nor can it control the cancer once it has grown beyond a certain point.

On the other hand, for the past century there have been numerous random observations linking cancer to nutrition; paralleling the observations made between the 16th and 18th centuries linking nutrition to scurvy, beriberi and, later, rickets to sunshine and vitamin D deficiency. These preliminary patterns of cause-and-effect developed into the science of hypothesizing and, ultimately, resolution.

How extensive then are the empirical observations linking cancer to nutrition? Why has modern research ignored nutrition as a cancer factor? More than 60 years ago, medical journals reported significant results from controlled experiments on the relationship between diet and cancer. Several researchers confirmed this important relationship that cried out for further investigation. The research was continued by individuals such as biochemist Ernst Krebs, but Krebs' work has been arbitrarily rejected by modern medicine.

In 1911, Peyton Rous reported in the *Proceedings of the Society for Experimental Biology and Medicine*: "Experimental work shows that the development of tumor grafts can in many cases be prevented or retarded by underfeeding the host or by putting it on a special diet." Further work along these lines was reported by Rous in the *Journal of Experimental Medicine*.

In 1913, three researchers reported similar findings in the *Journal of Biological Chemistry,* citing the unfavorable influence of poor nutrition on tumor growth.   In the article, authors Sweet, Corson-White and Saxon refer to other researchers who noted in their studies the effects of feeding rats combinations of pure vegetable protein, and a number of diets that completely retarded the normal growth of the animals.   These findings concluded that susceptibility to transplantable tumors can be influenced positively or negatively by diet.

This early experimental evidence, discovered under controlled conditions, was ignored by establishment medicine and government reporters.

Observational evidence cannot be ignored, however, and today conventional medicine is admitting that diet has a role in the development of cancer.   Organizations interested in seeing the public at large reduce its cancer risk are recommending preventive dietary guidelines.

In 1992, the National Cancer Institute estimated that following its dietary guidelines for cancer prevention could result in a 50 percent reduction in colon cancer and a 25 percent reduction in breast cancer.

Even the American Cancer Society is admitting to the important role nutrition plays in preventing cancer, advocating a high fiber, low saturated fat diet. I don't know about you, but when someone tells me what to do, I like to know why. Here's one reason why these organizations make these recommendations.

For one thing, a high meat and animal (saturated) fat diet tends to be deficient in whole grains and other high-fiber foods. Fiber moves waste through quickly, with less time for the body to absorb chemicals contained in the food.   In fact, when protein putrefies in a lazy colon, 3-methylcholanthrene, a powerful carcinogen, is formed. Another explanatory factor is recent research that points to the excess free radical formation that develops when quantities of unsaturated oil-containing foods are consumed.   Free radicals in the body are believed to contribute to cancer cell formation and the effects of aging. Antioxidants (vitamins A, E and C) are believed to counter this effect.

Keep in mind that water is another important element in bowel transit time. Drink lots of clean, fresh, pure spring water to cleanse the body of cancer-causing toxins.

In the meantime, millions of people are contracting cancer and conventional medicine does nothing to help. Doctors prescribe cancer-causing chemicals to treat it, then can't be sure whether it was the original cancer or a new one caused by the chemicals that brought it back for the fatal blow. Based on history, another generation will be dying of cancer before conventional medicine considers nutrition for treating it.

If diet can prevent cancer, how farfetched is it that it can also treat it? The closest they've come is this new interleukin immuno-therapy that boosts the body's immunity against cancer cells. But they still won't abandon profitable "burn and poison" therapies that tragically lower the body's immune-boosting ability in the first place.

With the exception of the suppressed Sloan-Kettering experiment, modern research is notable for its lack of interest in the nutritional approach. Yet, established medicine is well aware of scientific criteria and quote them at length when it's to its own benefit.

Only by overcoming the prejudicial quackery of consensus medicine have pernicious metabolic diseases been conquered. In every case the cause has been nutritional deficiency and the cure has been in the reversal of that deficiency. The final resolution of cancer will likewise be found in nutrition.

The Geography of Cancer

The monumental failure by established medicine to come to grips with cancer suggests that over the past century medical research has taken a wrong turn. The response in Washington has been to throw money at the problem. This approach may make good politics but it makes bad cancer research. If the basic approach is in error, then the investment of more funds will compound, rather than solve, the cancer problem. (Good money thrown after bad!)

The common-sense approach, for both scientists and laymen, is to step back and take a fresh look at cancer. If cancer deaths have been increasing over the past century, and at an accelerated rate during the past two decades (all this acceleration occurring while waging a massive research attack), then we have to logically assume:

(1) present treatments are, in effect, no cure; and

(2) some pervasive causative factor is at work, is increasing, and establishment research has no awareness of cancer's true nature or its workings.

The medical establishment maintains a monopoly on medical research. It refuses to allow, or even test, what it calls "unproven methods." There is a monopoly of thinking in medical research which inhibits new directions. The attacks on "unproven methods," and, in the U.S., the use of police power to forcibly prevent and imprison any doctor or researcher who attempts to probe "unproven methods," is a sign of uncertainty – the establishment's inability to find a solution within its own framework of analysis and past knowledge.

The very vehemence of the attacks by orthodox medicine on therapies not originated by the establishment is not only a rejection of free choice but a sign of self-admitted failure.

This bias in favor of well-worn research paths was explained to a congressional committee by a Washington representative of the National Health Foundation in 1971:

"Bias can occur in very honest and sincere people. I have never met an unbiased person in my life and I hope I never do. It is a myth that scientists are less biased than politicians or people with strong religious convictions.

"We have assumed, and have actually been taught, that there is something in science that removes bias, and this simply is not so." (That today's medical science is still biased against vitamin and nutritional research, there can be no doubt.) "The American cancer establishment has looked only at highly toxic chemotherapeutic agents.

"The minute an agent gets to the gentleness of a natural food or vitamin, the research stops. What is more important, laws stop it from being tried on others."

Decades have gone by without a solution. It's time to take a new direction. One does not have to be a medical researcher to identify the logical direction needed or to identify bias. We cannot undertake the research ourselves, but we can make initial observations and draw initial conclusions.

Our observations have to go further than a general recommendation to eat more fiber. The point is that certain kinds of fiber foods, and the nutrients contained within them, are not only cancer-preventatives but cancer antagonists. They work to reverse cancer, not just prevent it. Scientists need to go one step further in examining foods by looking at the effect they have on the body and cancer specifically.

It has long been recognized that Mormons in Utah have a lower cancer rate than the general population. This is a widely-dispersed group. Every member of it breathes the same air, uses the same soaps, is subjected to the same environmental hazards as we all are. There is one outstanding exception: their nutritional preferences, member-for-member, substantially include whole grains and food made therefrom.

Many native tribesmen in Nigeria are cancer-free. Their staple diet is cassava, rich in nitrilosides. Amygdalin is a nitriloside. Nigerian people eat very little or no processed food. The work of Dr. Oake, of the University of Ile-Ifa in Nigeria, confirms this observation.

"Western progress in agriculture has caused the abandonment of natural vitamins. We have abandoned millet, which is rich in nitrilosides and went on to wheat. We quit eating the seeds of the common fruits as our affluence grew. The reduction in the incidence of cancer appears proportional to the amount of nitrilosides (amygdalin) included in the diet of certain geographical populations" (Dr. Ernst Krebs, Jr.).

Conventional medicine tells us if we eat a variety of foods, and enough vegetables and fruits, we will be getting enough of all the nutrients to stay healthy. What they don't explain, and perhaps don't know, is that our soils are so depleted, we aren't getting adequate nutrition from our food.

The fact is, today's agricultural techniques are robbing our soils of nutrients. Instead of natural fertilizers, they use man-made chemicals which alter the plant's chemistry and often result in infertility. So, more chemicals are added and the problem goes on.

Charles Walters Jr. and C.J. Fenzau, in their book *An Acres USA Primer* examine the state of today's agriculture techniques and what farmers can do to improve the nutrition and yield of their crops without chemicals and poisons. They also emphasize the importance of soil and soil health in human health.

"Man, the Bible tells us, was a mere handful of clay into which the Creator has blown his warm breath. Even in such early thinking some consideration was given to the possibility that the soil has something to do with the construction of the human body" (William A. Albrecht, Ph.D., p. 78).

"We are exhausting the quality of our soils. As we do so the quality of our plants goes down. And we are accepting this" (p. 148).

We eat plants, we eat animals, yet we feed them not to make them nutritious, but to make them fat. The bottom line? We are probably nutritionally deficient because our food is. The geographical differences in cancer rates probably has a lot to do with local soil fertility and the nutrients available and missing from the crops grown on it.

The appropriate study of human nutrition includes soil science, agriculture and animal health, for we are inextricably intertwined.

CHAF

Digestive System: First Line of Defense

"Wastebasket diagnosis abounds in medicine. The excuse often given by the medical profession is that a 'label' on the patients' illness saves the patients' (or their families) money in that they do not go shopping around among doctors for a cure that does not exist! However, the search for more effective treatment should never be relaxed by patient, parent or doctor."

–Carl C. Pfeiffer, Ph.D., M.D.

Why this chapter? What does our digestive system have to do with cancer? Just everything. All body systems are intertwined, but the digestive and the immune systems even more. Our body can be our best friend or our worst enemy. If it is healthy, it cures itself. If it is sick, it gets sicker. It is your digestive system that allows your body to be nourished. Without nourishment the immune system breaks down and we get sick and die. It's as simple as that.

Take flatulence, for example. Harmless gas, right? Wrong. If it smells, it could mean bacteria in your colon are turning your waste into life-threatening carcinogens. Painful gas or bad breath can mean your body isn't breaking down and assimilating your food. You could be malnourished and not even know it. When symptoms are chronic, consider the cause.

Low Stomach Acid Common

"Quick fix" antacids are made for people who have too much stomach acid. But most people with pain in the gut have too little stomach acid, according to world-famous alternative physician Jonathan Wright, M.D., of Kent, Washington.

A lack of hydrochloric or stomach acid is called hypo-acidity or hypochlorhydria. Without adequate gastric acid in the stomach, proteins are not digested, and essential amino acids, nutrients and minerals such as iron and B12 are not absorbed. Without diagnosis and treatment, malnutrition and death can result.

This lack of acid is more common than we think and can cause all of the symptoms that appear when the stomach contains too much gastric acid. Doctors warn that people should not take antacids too readily as heartburn, gas, bloating after eating and even constipation can all be symptoms of hypoacidity. The burning sensation common to too much acid is also present when the stomach is too alkaline, and can be made worse by antacids. Other physical signs of low secretion of hydrochloric acid include split, peeling nails, hair falling out, and dilated capillaries on cheeks and nose when not drinking heavily. Dr. Jonathan Wright estimates every third adult he sees in his Tahoma, Washington clinic secretes too little hydrochloric acid.

Researchers at the Mayo Clinic and Johns Hopkins University pumped the stomachs of over 3,000 individuals and analyzed their contents. It was determined that by the age of 60 years, 60 percent had a significant decline in hydrochloric acid.

Antibiotics are designed to kill bacteria – the good and the bad. Certain bacteria are essential to the breakdown and assimilation of food. Always when taking antibiotics, supplement with a lactobacillus acidophilus "chaser." It won't interfere with the antibiotics and will keep your internal body chemistry at peak performance. Acidophilus can be purchased in pill, powder or liquid form in health food stores or in yogurt with active cultures.

An interesting albeit ethically-questionable study was performed in 1935 by psychiatrists at St. Elizabeth's Hospital, a hospital for the criminally insane in Washington, D.C. Doctors there rounded up patients with chronic schizophrenia and low amounts of hydrochloric acid and gave them all prefrontal lobotomies – surgery that removes the possibility of stress (and free-thinking). Rather extreme measures, obviously, but the patients' normal gastric acidity did return.

Other causes of low secretion of hydrochloric acid are hypothyroidism, thyroid toxicosis, autoimmune disorders such as Addison's disease, diabetes, and, among others, heart attacks. Dr. Jonathan Wright estimates 85 to 95 percent of rheumatoid arthritis to be associated with hypoacidity.

Inasmuch as a lack of hydrochloric acid in the stomach prevents absorption of minerals, even super-supplementation with minerals will not help. Instead, Doctor Wright and his associate, Dr. Alan R. Gaby, recommend intramuscular injections of vitamin B12, small then larger doses of pepsin, Betaine Hydrochloride with or without pepsin, acquired at health food stores, or Glutamic Acid HCl with or without pepsin.

Eating Right

Dr. Wright says there are many causes for digestive disorders: eating too fast and inadequate chewing, food allergies and milk sensitivity; inability to produce enough stomach acid and, one of the most common reasons, a high fat, low fiber, high sugar junk food diet. Eating the right foods is important, but no less important is eating right.

The mouth is where it all begins. Biochemist Bruce Pacette, Ph.D., recommends we chew each mouthful of food at least 20 times and meat at least 30 times, almost liquefying it before swallowing.

The idea is to chew food to a near liquid state, which is the form in which it is best absorbed in the stomach. As soon as food touches the taste buds and releases its appealing odors, our network of nerves transmits the message for the release of saliva in the mouth and digestive juices in the stomach. Saliva lubricates the food for easy swallowing and contains enzymes, including those that start the digestive process.

One way to slow down your eating and step up your digestion is to play soft, slow music as you eat. There's an added bonus: you'll lose weight. Mona Simonson, Ph.D., director of the Health, Weight and Stress Clinic at Johns Hopkins University, carried out an experiment showing that musical munching actually works. Not only does slow, soothing music slacken your eating pace, but it makes you less likely to desire seconds. Simonson found that when a calming flute instrument played while eating, the study volunteers slowed their chewing to 3.2 bites per minute – much smaller bites too – and lingered over the meal for almost an hour. Not one of the diners requested seconds.

As the salivary glands secrete the digestive enzyme ptyalin and food in the mouth starts breaking down, the system prepares for complete digestion. All the parts: the stomach, pancreas, liver, gall bladder, small and large intestine, rectum and anus, begin moving and secreting enzymes in anticipation.

Those who do not masticate, nature castigates. If you do not chew your food thoroughly prior to swallowing, part of the digestive process is lost, and can result in painful gas from swallowing air, or constipation, as well as the loss of essential nutrients. The esophagus, using a slow, wavelike motion called peristalsis, moves the partially digested food into the stomach. Digestion begins in the middle of the stomach, where food is mixed with gastric juices containing hydrochloric acid, water, and enzymes that break up protein and other substances. These stomach acids, important to efficient breakdown of food, are extremely caustic. If the mucous barrier that protects the stomach breaks down or too much acid is produced too often, which happens during stress, this lining is eroded and an ulcer can develop.

After one to four hours, depending upon the combination of foods ingested, peristalsis (a push and pull movement) moves the food, now in the liquid form of chyme, out of the stomach and into the small intestine in the following order: carbohydrates, protein, and fat – each according to the time required for digestion. A suggestion: eat your vegetables before your meat because meat takes longer to digest.

The chyme enters the small intestine, breaks down further and eventually is absorbed. First, the pancreas secretes its digestive juices. If fats are present in the food bile, an enzyme produced by the liver and stored in the gallbladder is also secreted. Bile reduces the fat to small droplets so the pancreatic enzymes can break it down. The pancreas also secretes a substance that neutralizes the digestive acids in the food and secretes additional enzymes that continue the breakdown of proteins and carbohydrates. You can see how important the liver, gallbladder and pancreas are in the digestive process. The loss of some or all of their functions can make a significant difference in your health.

The small intestine absorbs nutrients as follows: glucose from carbohydrates, amino acids from protein, and fatty acids and glycerol from fats. These essential nutrients are taken up by minute fingerlike projections in the small intestine called villi. These contain tiny blood vessels, or capillaries, and are the principal channels for absorption. When flattened or damaged, as may happen with food allergies or illness, the villi are limited in their ability to absorb, and health is jeopardized. This happens more easily and more often than people realize.

Fiber – An Important Food Additive

After all possible nutrients have been absorbed through the walls of the small intestine, a watery mix of undigested fiber should be left. This essential residue of fecal matter is propelled toward the large intestine, or colon. The large intestine absorbs excess water from the fiber and stores the feces, eventually evacuating it through the last portion of the colon, the rectum, and discharging it through a muscular canal called the anus.

If little fiber is present at this stage, the waste matter becomes small and hard to move. Anything in the feces that the small intestine can't absorb into the body is also stored here: man-made chemicals, particulates from polluted air, even objects swallowed by children. Without adequate fiber to move the waste through, this undigested garbage sits, and the large intestine continues to absorb water and any chemicals contained in it. It is here that carcinogens can be created by the body's bacteria. The longer it sits, the better the chance carcinogens will form, not to mention the harder it will be to expel. Anybody troubled with constipation knows how uncomfortable this can be.

Today's Civilized Disorders

Digestion end-products – glucose and amino acids – are necessary for tumor survival and growth. Like normal tissue, tumors use glucose as fuel. The tumor is apparently able to capture and use from five to 10 times more glucose than normal cells. This is how tumors rob cancer victims of body warmth and energy.

Both normal and malignant cells need amino acids to synthesize protein. Tumors steal nitrogen from the patient to multiply cancer cells, at the expense of the health and integrity of normal cells.

Unlike healthy cells, cancer cells do not use and then recycle amino acids. They hoard them to speed up multiplication of cancer cells.

Cutting-edge research on cancer cell metabolism was performed by Otto Warburg, a two-time Nobel Prize winner. In 1931, Warburg discovered oxygen-transferring enzymes of cell respiration and, in 1944, discovered the active groups of the hydrogen-transferring enzymes.

Warburg believed the onset of anaerobic glycolysis – air-deprived glucose formation – is the forerunner to cancer development. If this is true, he hypothesized, the cause of cancer can be determined by discovering the reason for a change in metabolism by a normal cell to anaerobic glycolysis.

In 1966, Warburg found that a 35 percent decrease in oxygen causes embryonic cells to change into cells with malignant characteristics. Based on these findings, he proposed that vitamin E be taken as a possible deterrent for cancer. Inasmuch as vitamin E reduces the cells' need for oxygen, a cell may be able to tolerate lesser amounts of available oxygen without changing its metabolic pattern from normal to cancer-causing. Since Warburg, scientists have discovered that vitamin E is a powerful antioxidant, reducing the damaging effects of environmental poisons including carbon monoxide from cigarettes and ultraviolet radiation, which is believed to contribute to cancer. In one study, vitamin E was found to help protect against bowel cancer (Stahelin, p. 1463). As discussed in the foreword of this book, other research has found vitamin A to be useful in skin cancer and studies with animals found high doses of vitamin A decreased the number of tumors.

The nutritional program presented in this book provides a cancer preventive program based on your digestive system requirements, together with changes in diet and the addition of supplemental vitamins and enzymes, to counteract the assault from chemicals that invite cancer.

Carcinogens

There are many different carcinogens, and their sources vary. Some are in the water we drink, others are in the food we eat and still others in the air we breathe.

In present day society, the number of carcinogens entering or affecting our bodies is increasing. It is foolhardy to believe that, even with the most stringent environmental protection plans, we can decrease environmental carcinogens to a safe level. Research money in large amounts is awarded each year by governmental granting agencies to identify carcinogens. Suspect carcinogens are applied to animals to determine the increase in the number of tumors. This research is valid. We should, as much as possible, eliminate contact with any known carcinogen.

However, carcinogens alone do not cause cancer. Even orthodox medicine finally agrees carcinogens are merely the irritant that determines the location of the lump or bump the medical establishment recognizes as cancer. In reality, lumps and bumps are only the symptom or final manifestation of an underlying metabolic imbalance or weakness in our body's intrinsic defense against disease. Carcinogens change the body's normal trophoblast cells into rapidly-proliferating cancer cells that it either has not protected itself from or cannot (Krebs, E.T., Jr).

The Immune System

If cancer was simply caused by the carcinogens we breathe and eat, we would all get cancer. But we don't. Why some do and some don't is a major clue to the puzzle. The cancer cell is a foreign body and should be cast out by the immune system. One person in an auditorium full of people has a contagious flu virus. After the group leaves, some have contracted it, some have not (assuming all have been sprayed by the person's flu-laden sneezes). How do you spell relief? R-E-S-I-S-T-A-N-C-E. Some are resistant – their bodies' immune systems are working well – and some are not.

Even when subjected to carcinogens, the immune system attempts to keep the body in a steady state. The body's normal condition is one of health. Anything that enters the system – a virus, bacteria, or foreign protein – causes a reaction that will lead to a rejection of the invader. The cancer cells, once formed, should logically be eliminated. In some instances, the body is so weakened that the immune system fails to reject the cancer cell. When not rejected, cancer cells divide rapidly, ultimately forming the lump or bump medical science has come to recognize.

Most of us are born with an efficient immune system. But an alarming percentage of us are slowly destroying our bodies. We get no exercise, we smoke, drink excessively, and eat foods laden with chemicals and fats. We've accepted this fact of nature to such a point we've coined the terms "couch potato" and "junk food," as though this habit of eating were normal. We eat junk food knowing full well it is nutritionally worthless. Excessive stress of everyday life also takes its toll in lengthy work hours with little time for recreation, play or exercise. All these factors lead to a lowered efficiency of the immune system. The end result, all too often, is a metabolic or degenerative disease.

The principal mechanism of the body's defense against foreign substances is its continually circulating reserve of white blood cells. White blood cells have the ability to destroy invading viruses, or even errant deviating cells if they are recognized. The first malignant can-

cer cell should be destroyed in the bloodstream befor
chance to multiply and attach to tissues and organs. Scien.
ognizes the cancer cell wraps itself in a protein coating having the
same electrical charge as the white cells. The two identical charges
repel each other. The cancer cell, in this clever protective disguise,
could remain free to proliferate were it not for another marvelous
mechanism: enzymes. Enzymes circulate in our bloodstreams and are
able to dissolve the protein coat from around the malignant cell. Once
robbed of their protective coating, the cancer cells are recognized and
overwhelmed by white cells. This, then, is the body's intrinsic
method of ridding itself of cancer.

Thankfully, in most of us this enzymatic second line of defense
proves adequate. However, logic recognizes that different bodies will
vary in their ability to function. What of those individuals who have
perhaps inherited a weak immune system or, for reasons we will outline later, have insufficient enzymes available? Our Creator, the
Master Engineer, has designed an extrinsic protective system in the
foods available for us to eat.

It is these foods, and their nutrients, which compose our extrinsic
defense against cancer.

At this point I should say: **you are not what you eat, but rather
what your system is able to digest, absorb or utilize**. This explains
why one person can eat junk food and look and feel comparatively
well while another can eat all the "right foods" and be sick. The well
person's first line of defense (his or her remarkable body) may be better capable of deriving the nutrients needed to stay well than the
well-fed sickly person.

While all the nutrients necessary for good health should be available from proper diet, supplementation may still be required. In some
areas needed foods aren't available at certain times of the year. The
local soil may be deficient, making the food deficient. Lifestyle
choices like birth control pills, cigarette smoking or a high stress job
necessitate specific supplementation. Or illness, heredity, advancing
age or allergy may make nutrient assimilation difficult to achieve.
The holistic or metabolic physician is capable of evaluating the indi-

vidual's state of health and recommending supplementation to put the body back into peak performance.

Something else to keep in mind about supplementation: taking supplements that follow the government's recommended daily allowances (RDA) is probably not enough. RDAs are self-admittedly neither minimal nor optimal levels. They are purposely low to take in account the large variation between people. RDAs are not determined to improve life; merely to sustain it.

CHAPTER 6:

Vitamins, Inner Warriors

*"The American public is being sold a bill of goods about cancer...
today the press releases coming out of the National Cancer Institute
have all the honesty of the Pentagon."*
                              –Dr. James Watson, Nobel Prize winner

Vitamins are organic substances contained in foods in minute
quantities. They are both fundamental and essential for the
well-being and healthy operation of our bodies.

The identification and isolation of vitamins is comparatively recent,
beginning only in this century. Our knowledge is still far from complete, although we do know that human need for certain nutrients has
increased tremendously because of pollution, stress, increased consumption of refined foods, and other factors. While most animals can
create their own vitamin C, man cannot. It is likely we are deficient
in one or more vitamins and just as likely we are unaware of it.
Protection is simple – make our diets as close to that of nature as possible, include unrefined and unprocessed natural foods, and supplement nutrients in which we may be deficient.

Table of Vitamins

Vitamins are designated by letters and subscripts. Chart 4 (page
50) lists known vitamins with a letter designation, name of the specific compound and its function in the human body. Those vitamins

Chart 4
TABLE OF VITAMINS

Table of Properties (stability)	Biological Function
Vitamin A — Carotene fat soluble; stable to heat; unstable to air; destroyed by ultraviolet	Essential for growth of young; increases resistance to urinary and respiratory infection; lactation and reproduction; night vision (visual purple); proper appetite and digestion; skin health
Vitamin D — Calciferol fat soluble; stable to light, heat and air	Absorption and metabolism of calcium and phosphorus; clotting; heat action; and proper gland and nerve function; tooth and bone formation; skin respiration
Vitamin E — Tocopherol stable to visible light, heat, acid & alkali; destroyed by u.v. light; rancid fats reduce its potency	Blood flow to heart; fertility; lung protection; male potency; prevents toxemia of pregnancy; pituitary regulation; reduces blood cholesterol; retards aging
Vitamin K — Menadione fat soluble	Blood clotting (prevents hemorrhage); vital for normal liver function; vitality and longevity factor
Vitamin B_1 — Thiamine water soluble; unstable to ultra-violet; destroyed by boiling in acidic solution, heat	Absorption and digestion; appetite; blood building; carbohydrate metabolism; corrects and prevents beriberi; learning ability; promotes growth, resistance to infection and proper nerve function
Vitamin B_2 — Riboflavin water soluble; stable to air, heat; unstable to visible light, u.v.; destroyed by alkalies	Antibody and red blood cell formation; aids iron assimilation and protein metabolism; healthy skin and digestive tract; prolongs life; promotes growth and general health; vision
Vitamin B_3 — Niacin water soluble; stable to heat; light, air, acid and alkali	Circulation; hormone (sex) production; growth; hydrochloric acid production; maintenance of nervous system; metabolism; reduces cholesterol level; respiration
Vitamin B_5 — Pantothenic Acid water soluble; unstable to heat; destroyed by acid & alkali (vinegar — baking soda)	Antibody formation; carbohydrate metabolism; growth stimulation; healthy skin and nerves; maintains blood sugar level; stimulates adrenals; vitamin utilization
Vitamin B_6 — Pyridoxine water soluble; stable in heat; unstable in light	Antibody formation; controls level of magnesium in blood and tissues; digestion; maintains sodium/potassium balance; cholesterol levels; metabolism of fats
Vitamin B_{12} — Cyarocobalamin water soluble	Appetite; blood cell formation; cell longevity; normal metabolism of nerve tissue; protein; fat and carbohydrate metabolism, glandular and nervous system
Vitamin B_{15} — Pangamic Acid water soluble	Cell oxidation and respiration; stimulates glucose, fat, protein metabolism, glandular and nervous system
Vitamin B_{17} — Amygdalin destroyed by heat and light	Cell protection; protects cells against environmental and internal toxicity; unlocks immune system's ability to destroy malignant cancer cells

most important to the prevention and treatment of cancer are described.

The Antioxidants

One way to combat the breakdown of the body's immune system, scientists think, is to trap damaging agents before they can do the body harm. At the top of researchers' list of biochemical outlaws is a group of dangerous chemicals called "free radicals," discovered by Denham Harmon in 1954.

Some of these extremely reactive compounds hail from environmental sources, such as radiation and smog, but the bulk are generated as by-products in the body's normal course of converting sugar and oxygen to energy, a job performed in every cell by structures called mitochondria. Thousands of these tiny powerhouses wander through cells' interiors, leaking free radicals that burn holes in membranes and leave hot spots of so-called oxidative damage in their wake, says John Carney of the University of Kentucky in Lexington. Free radicals mangle not only vital protein enzymes and molecules carrying the genetic code but also the energy-generating mitochondria themselves, half of which may be dysfunctional in old animals (Schmidt, p.66).

Since 1954, scientists have discovered substances that can reverse the effect of free radical damage. They are called antioxidants, and include vitamin A, beta carotene (a vitamin A precursor), vitamin C and vitamin E.

According to Anthony T. Diplock, Ph.D., of the University of London, England, free radical damage is linked to chronic diseases such as cancer, heart disease, stroke, cataracts and certain neurological disorders.

Epidemiological studies and some clinical trials provide evidence that antioxidants protect against these and other diseases.

I had the pleasure of attending a symposium, "Beyond Deficiency: Vitamin Issues of the '90s," March 27-29, 1992 at Captiva Island, FL. It was there that Harinder S. Garewal, M.D., Ph.D., said recent data suggest antioxidants have a role in inhibiting the development of oral cancers.

Dr. Garewal, who is with the Tucson V.A. Medical Center Hematology and Oncology Research Laboratory in Arizona, has focused on oral leukoplakia, white patches that form on the mucous membranes of the mouth and are thought to precede mouth cancer.

In their pilot study, 70 percent of 25 patients with mouth cancer responded to 30 mg of beta carotene daily. Dr. Garewal reported a trial in Virginia achieved similar results using vitamin E, vitamin C and beta carotene.

Vitamin C Specifics

Gladys Block, Ph.D., of the University of California at Berkeley, another speaker at the conference, said in reviewing more than 90 epidemiological studies, high vitamin C intake was found to significantly reduce the risk of cancer in about three-fourths of the cases.

"Vitamin C acts as an antioxidant in the bloodstream, neutralizing the free radicals that are formed in the body and can damage cells," Dr. Block said. "Cell damage is thought to be one of the first steps in the development of cancer. Vitamin C also works with vitamin E to help restore the latter's ability to function as an antioxidant."

In surveys of more than 6,000 people, cancer mortality was highest in individuals consuming the lowest amounts of vitamin C. Vitamin C has been shown in the laboratory to prevent the formation of nitrosamine, a potent carcinogen formed from nitrates found in food and air.

The most important work was done by Ewan Cameron, M.D., chief surgeon in Vale of Leven Hospital, Loch Lomonside, Scotland. An account of his work, "Supplemental Ascorbate in the Supportive Treatment of Cancer" was published in *Proceedings of the National Academy of Sciences U.S.A.*, October, 1976.

In the clinical trials by Cameron in Vale of Leven Hospital, 100 patients with advanced cancer received 10 grams a day of vitamin C (sodium ascorbate), compared to 100 control patients who were matched for sex, age, type of cancer, and were treated in the same way, except for the ascorbate. The average survival time of the ascorbate-treated patients was over four times that of the controls, and a fraction of these patients have had very long survival times, over 20 times the average for the controls, and no longer showed signs of malignant disease.

Highly significant vitamin C work has been undertaken in recent years at the Linus Pauling Institute in Menlo Park, California. Data show vitamin C in very high doses (100 grams a day) is startlingly effective in reducing the incidence and severity of skin cancer in laboratory mice.

"The incidence of severe lesions in these experiments was caused to vary over a 70-fold range by nutritional measures alone," is the official word from the Institute. "Regardless of the specific nutrition or the specific cancer assay system used, these results support the view that optimum nutrition should be given a high priority in cancer research."

Dr. Robert Cathcart, a California physician, has successfully treated over 15,000 patients with massive doses of vitamin C; curing viral pneumonia, mononucleosis, influenza, colds, hepatitis, shingles, and cold sores with this method. He has developed a guideline for practical application of vitamin C which he refers to as "bowel tolerance."

Dr. Cathcart found that the individual's own body will determine how much vitamin C it requires. The cutoff point is determined by the onset of diarrhea. In an interview in *Public Scrutiny*, Cathcart stated, "The tolerance level in each individual differs. Some days you can tolerate more, some days less, but from general experience I label a cold as a 20-to-30-gram cold, or 60-gram flu, according to how much a person can take before he reaches the bowel tolerance level."

The vitamin C will permeate every cell of the body before it reaches the bowel, according to Dr. Cathcart. He justifies these massive doses by explaining that viruses within the sick cells excrete toxins, rendering them scorbutic (with scurvy).

In short, if you have not reached bowel tolerance (diarrhea), you have not taken enough vitamin C.

These intriguing results obviously demand further research, but the federal government has been consistently unwilling to finance major work into the relationship between nutrition and disease. This prompted the Pauling Institute to run a unique series of advertisements in the *Wall Street Journal*.

The Pauling Institute applied for NCI grants of a paltry $50,000 based on Dr. Ewan Cameron's work. This prestigious institute was refused funds for their research on five different occasions.

Vitamin A and Beta Carotene

Discovered in 1909 and synthesized in 1946, vitamin A is a fat-soluble alcohol known as retinol, and is found in natural form only in animals. Fish liver, for example, is a prime source of vitamin A with up to 300 mg of retinol per hundred grams of liver. Calf liver contains about 15-150 mg per 100 grams. Eggs, milk and butter contain only minute amounts of vitamin A. The U.S. government recommended daily allowance (RDA) is set at 5,000 IU (International Units) per day for a moderately active male. Although the government says anything over 10,000 is highly toxic, experience and statistics do not bear this out. There are, for example, 11,000 IU of vitamin A in a carrot and 43,000 IU in an average size piece of liver.

Vitamin A has been the subject of numerous studies to determine its role in the prevention of cancer. Essential to the growth and differentiation of epithelial tissue, vitamin A has been shown to prevent or inhibit cellular deformation. Diets rich in vitamin A and its analogues, carotenes and retinoids, are associated with a lower incidence of cancer of the bladder, cervix, larynx, lung, and other types that affect soft tissue. Beta carotene, a nontoxic precursor of vitamin A, is being studied as a possible lung cancer preventive. Experiments with animals have demonstrated that vitamin A and its derivatives can protect lung tissue against the carcinogenic effects of cigarette smoke, inhibit dimethylhydrazine-induced colon tumors and prevent the development of cervical cancer. Supplementation with large quantities of the vitamin has been shown to reverse the immunosuppressive effects of chemotherapy, radiation therapy and surgical anesthesia.

The late Harold Manner, Ph.D., conducted a series of tests with vitamin A on mice with tumors. In the initial tests, each experimental
mouse received amygdalin injected intra-muscularly in the rump area,
plus 333,333 IU per kilogram of body weight of emulsified vitamin
A. Enzymes from the pea, lentil, papaya, calf thymus and beef pancreas were used for a preparation injected into and around the tumor
mass every other day.

"The results were dramatic," Dr. Manner reported. "In four to six
weeks the tumors were completely gone in 90 percent of the 84 experimental animals. Tumors on the other 10 percent of the mice were in
regression at the close of the experiment. Animals with completely
regressed tumors were autopsied by the pathologist. No sign of the
tumor remained."

An 8-year, nationwide study involving nearly 90,000 female
nurses conducted by Harvard School of Public Health researchers
found those with the lowest intake of vitamin A had about a 20 percent increased risk of breast cancer, compared to those with higher
consumptions.

The research involved 89,494 women in the ongoing Nurses'
Health Study. From 1980 to 1988, the women – who were aged 34 to
59 and free of cancer when the investigation began – were asked to
fill out questionnaires every two years about their consumption of
food and dietary supplements and the state of their health. The study
found women who ranked in the lowest 5th of participants in vitamin
A intake were about 20 percent more likely to develop breast cancer
than others. Altogether, 1439 women were diagnosed with the disease
during the study period.

As of this writing, 22,000 doctors around the country are popping
daily doses of beta carotene (or a placebo) in a Harvard University
study to see if it will help prevent cancers. Studies have shown that
smokers who remain healthy have more vitamin A in their bloodstream than do those who develop lung cancer.

Vitamin A and beta carotene (which your body converts to vitamin
A) are found in dark-green and dark-orange vegetables like broccoli,
kale, collards, spinach, sweet potatoes, pumpkin, winter squash, car-

rots, bok choy, Swiss chard, Brussel sprouts, cantaloupe and apricots.

Lack of vitamin A has a known effect on animals; in general, loss of appetite, inhibited growth and an increased susceptibility to infection. Substantial deficiencies of A can lead to death. Dry and scaly skin are surface effects of a deficiency. Deficiency can also result in infection of the respiratory or urinary tract.

Vitamin A absorption occurs in the small intestine. In animals, vitamin A is ingested usually in the form of its ester, called retinal palmitate. Not all vitamin A in the oil reaches the liver, its storage organ. (About 90 percent is stored in the liver.)

To avoid the problem of a toxic liver resulting from high amounts of vitamin A (a high amount would be between 300,000 and 3 million IU per day), vitamin A for cancer treatment is used in a water-soluble (emulsified) substance. This allows for rapid and complete absorption into the lymph system, then into the blood.

Vitamin E

Denham Harman, the father of the free radical theory, considers vitamin E his favorite. He calls it "the natural antioxidant," adding, "It's in all our membranes." He cites a study of 5,000 women on the English island of Guernsey. Those with the highest blood levels of vitamin E had the lowest incidence of breast cancer. Harman says it's hard to overdose on E (Teresi, p. 58).

The incredible versatility of vitamin E was amply demonstrated in papers read at a symposium on the vitamin in June, 1990. For example, Joel Schwartz, D.M.D., reported that cancer cells were killed in a test tube with vitamin E and beta carotene, one form of vitamin A. "In studies combining these two nutrients, there is a synergistic anti-tumor effort" (Adams, p. 14).

The B Vitamins

One of the world's foremost authorities on the physiological development and effects of cancer was the late Professor Otto Warburg, two-time Nobel Prize winner and director of the renowned Max Planck Institute for Cell Physiology in Berlin, Germany. Warburg's research led him to the assumption that one primary factor is at work in causing cancer: oxygen starvation. When a cell becomes starved of oxygen it gives up the process of oxidation (burning) of food, and instead tries to gain energy by fermenting sugar, a process that requires no oxygen. It is this fermentation process that encourages the growth of cancer cells.

At the heart of any nutrient that fights cancer is its ability to provide oxygen to the cells. Antioxidants do that, as do certain B vitamins. It was Warburg's contention that three specific B vitamins, riboflavin (B2), niacin (B3) and pantothenic acid (B5), because they are essential to the respiration of the cell, are powerful cancer-preventives (Warburg).

Dr. Loraine Bush and associates found niacin, also known as nicotinamide, to be consistently lacking in cancer cells and always present in normal cells. When the researchers added it to cancer cells, they found it inhibited their growth (Biochemistry).

For many years, pangamic acid (B15), a vitamin discovered by Dr. E.T. Krebs, Jr., has been under scientific investigation, resulting in widespread use in the former Soviet Union. It is probably the vitamin supplement most often deficient, since its chief source, rice bran, is not included in most American diets.

Trained nutritionists, few of whom can be found among medically trained doctors, recognize the tremendous asset this vitamin is to cell metabolism. The contribution of B15 or pangamic acid to physical fitness and body endurance is inestimable. In the specific instance of cancer, the increased blood oxygenation provided by vitamin B15 precludes the low oxygen environment which enables malignancy to flourish.

Developed by Drs. E.T. Krebs, Sr. and Jr., vitamin B17, amygdalin, is the crown jewel in the extrinsic nutritional defense mechanism against cancer.

The word "amygdalin" comes from the Greek "amygdala," or almond. Amygdalin was discovered in bitter almonds, and its taste resembles almonds. Amygdalin was first used by a Chinese herbalist (Pen T'Sao) in the year 2800 B.C. and has been in use since that time, making nonsense of the FDA claim it is a "new drug" and therefore requires FDA approval.

Amygdalin is a cyanogenetic glycoside that occurs naturally in over 1100 edible plants, grasses and seeds. Our most accessible sources are the seeds of the Rosaceae plant family - apricots, peaches, plums, prunes, bitter almonds, cherries, apples and a number of lentils and grasses. Other amygdalin-containing foods are millet, cassava, maize, bean, sweet potato, lima bean, linseed and almond. Amygdalin is one of a family of cyanide-containing substances collectively referred to as nitrilosides. The cassava plant contains these compounds throughout its system, with the richest concentration in the root.

The Pueblo Indians of Taos, New Mexico traditionally eat many foods rich in nitrilosides. Not coincidentally, cancer is rare among this population. Robert G. Houston, who has written several articles on the Pueblo, was given a recipe by them as he researched a book on cancer prevention. In a glass of milk or juice mix a tablespoon of honey with 1/4 ounce or two dozen freshly ground apricot kernels, or one kernel for every ten pounds of body weight. More may be eaten but Houston warns they can upset the stomach if ingested in large quantities. Houston wrote that the drink was so delicious he had it daily. On the third day, he wrote, a funny thing happened. Two little benign skin growths on his arm, which were formerly pink, turned brown. By the seventh day, they were gone (Encyclopedia, p. 351).

Ingested amygdalin is enzymatically broken down in the intestinal tract by way of bacterially-produced beta-glucosidase. The resultant prunasin, mandelonitrile, and other constituents travel via the blood to the liver where they are converted to glucuronide.

Glucuronides have been known to protect against the systemically-toxic side effects of orthodox chemotherapy for many years. Clinical observations by Drs. Mario Soto, Paul Wedel and Donald Cole indicate that when they administer chemotherapeutic therapy combined with amygdalin, the side effects are vastly reduced.

For over 40 years, science has recognized cancer cells contain levels of beta-glucuronidase enzymes many times higher than those of normal cells. Amygdalin has the capability of destroying cancer cells and here's how: the cancer cells' beta-glucuronidase has the unique enzymatic ability to cleave active, deadly cyanide from the cyanogenic glucuronidase molecule released by amygdalin's ingestion process. The cyanide then destroys the cancer cell, leaving normal cells unharmed.

I wish to emphasize that the cyanide contained in naturally-occurring amygdalin is benign and totally nontoxic until it reaches the malignancy, where the cancer cell's singular ability to unlock the poisonous cyanide contributes to its own destruction.

With the exception of suppressed Sloan-Kettering experiments, modern research is notable for its lack of interest in the nutritional approach to cancer control. Yet, established medicine is well aware of scientific criteria and quotes them at length in attacking the use of amygdalin.*

We repeat the scientific axiom fundamental to all scientific research: that a negative proposition cannot be proven. In other words, it is unscientific for orthodox medical practitioners to make the statement, "no diet containing amygdalin prevents cancer." This is a negative statement impossible to support with scientific proof, and ignores empirical evidence available to metabolic physicians.

* For example, California State Board of Public Health, *Quackery: and the Cancer Law.*

What is Laetrile? – Origin and Development

The isolation of amygdalin is a simple extractive procedure. First the kernels or seeds are defatted with ether. Then this fat-free residue is boiled in alcohol, filtered and cooled. Amygdalin is the white crystalline substance separated from other compounds during the cooling and filtering process.

Robiquet and Boutron, in France, first isolated crystalline amygdalin in 1830. Although many cyanogenic glycosides exist, they are, at most, amygdalin-like. There is one, and only one, amygdalin with a chemical specification.

In 1952, Ernst Krebs, Jr., altered the amygdalin molecule synthetically to make an "empirical apricot formula safe for administration to humans." This new compound was patented and called Laetrile. Unlike amygdalin, it contains glucuronic acid in place of glucose. Therefore, Laetrile, with a capital 'L' and a registered patent mark, is not true amygdalin since it does not contain a molecule of glucose. Laetrile is a synthetic derivative of glucuronic acid and, therefore, is a glucuronide. Laetrile was developed at the John Beard Memorial Foundation in San Francisco. It was patented in 1958 by Ernst Krebs, Sr. and Ernst Krebs, Jr. (Brit. Pat. 788,855). Because it is laevorotary (turns polarized light to the left as does amygdalin), Krebs combined the first three letters of the word laevorotary, and the last five letters of the word, nitrile, and coined the trade name Laetrile. As Laetrile became more popular, the word was borrowed to refer to any glycosidic compound containing cyanide and exhibiting the laevorotary power.

Most research and clinical work today uses amygdalin. The glucuronide Laetrile® is scarce and cost-prohibitive. Narrowing the use of such compounds down to basically one substance does minimize the confusion experienced in previous years. However, the importance of knowing the exact structure and purity of any compound tested cannot be stressed enough. Lack of this knowledge in the past has led to an array of results which are extremely contradictory and ultimately useless.

A prime reason for inconsistent results in therapy has been that, until recently – and since the time of the original amygdalin production at the Krebs and Delmar Laboratories – there has been a lack of consistently high extracting and packaging standards among the various amygdalin manufacturers. It is certainly not that the technical definition and specification for Laetrile have not been exacting enough. For over 150 years, these standards were defined in all scientific literature, including the authoritatively-definitive Merck Index. Part of the problem was the extreme instability of amygdalin, once extracted and placed in an aqueous solution. Once in water, unless heavily and unnaturally buffered, amygdalin degrades into subpotency and therapeutically inactive forms. Suffice it to say amygdalin should never, despite various suppliers' claims of stabilization, be purchased or used from a liquid solution of known age. Only pure natural crystalline amygdalin is acceptable.

Vitamin Therapy Lengthens Cancer Survival

Vitamins are like people; they do their best when they work together. Free-thinking doctors, aware of the nutritional advantage, have learned this. Abram Hoffer, M.D., Ph.D., of Victoria, B.C., Canada regularly treats cancer patients with vitamin therapy. He and other Victoria-area doctors have found advanced cancer patients who follow the vitamin program live longer than those who do not.

In 1991, Hoffer asked Nobel laureate Linus Pauling, Ph.D., founder of the aforementioned Pauling Institute and discoverer of the benefits of vitamin C, to statistically compare the survival rates of 101 advanced cancer patients who followed Hoffer's specially-prescribed vitamin regimen with 34 who did not (Challem, p. 20).

Pauling's analysis found patients with cancers of the breast, ovaries, uterus and cervix had a life expectancy 20 times longer when they adhered to Hoffer's regimen. A second study, published in the *Journal of Orthomolecular Medicine* (third quarter 1993, pp. 157-167), confirmed the benefits. A third study followed up the first cancer survivors. Pauling and Hoffer found half of patients with breast, ovarian, uterine and cervical cancer lived at least five years longer and some 15 years longer after being referred to Hoffer. The American Cancer Society considers five years or more of life after cancer as "cured."

The typical Hoffer regimen includes a diet high in fruits and vegetables and the following supplements divided into three doses daily:
Vitamin C – 12 grams (12,000 mg.)
Vitamin B3 – 1.5 to 3 gms
Vitamin B6 – 250 mg.

Folic Acid – 5 to 10 mg.
Other B vitamins – 25 to 50 times the RDA
Vitamin E – 800 IU
Beta carotene – 25,000 to 5,000 IU
Selenium – 0.2 to 0.5 mg.
Zinc – 220 mg.

CHAPTER 7:

Enzymes, Little Known Soldiers For Defense

"If you will tell the utter, absolute truth, it is remarkable how most of your problems are solved. It simplifies life tremendously. If you start telling half the truth or three-quarters of the truth, they will get you."

–Dr. Dean Burke, former head Cytochemistry Department, National Cancer Institute, and one of its original founders

Enzymes are catalysts, specifically proteins. More than two thousand varieties play vital roles in every human physical function. Three enzymes are instrumental in the use of amygdalin (vitamin B17) in cancer therapy: beta-glucosidase, beta-glucuronidase and rhodanase.

Historically, enzyme therapy has been used in cancer treatment many times. Some physicians have been able to obtain beneficial results, while others, due to the enzymes' non-selective proteolytic property, have not. Since early enzyme-therapy experimentation (1900-1915), various enzyme complexes have been synthesized; many of them exhibit a certain specificity for cancerous tissue.

The most important role of this enzyme complex is digestion of the cancer cell's protein coat-camouflage, leaving it open to attack by the body's natural white cell defenses. This is why using vitamin A in conjunction with enzymes has a greater anti-tumor effect.

The pancreas produces digestive enzymes that break down food. These enzymes are secreted in the form of precursors and active enzymes. The precursors are trypsinogen and chymotrypsinogen which convert to their active forms of trypsin and chymotrypsin in the presence of enterokinase, found in the duodenum, and in the presence of trypsin, respectively. These are proteolytic enzymes that break down proteins to polypeptides and amino acids. Two enzymes – pancreatic amylase, which breaks down polysaccharides to disaccharides, and lipase, which converts neutral triglycerides to diglycerides, monoglycerides and free fatty acids – are secreted in their active forms. In this respect they are unlike trypsin and chymotrypsin, which are secreted in their inactive forms.

Backed by Research, Rejected by Orthodoxy

Well over 70 years ago, London and New York doctors noted that injections of trypsin had an anti-cancer effect. This was reported extensively in the medical journals of the time. The studies are worth recording here because their existence casts doubt over the motivation of our modern medical establishment. The considerable anti-tumor effect of enzymes, reported so long ago, is ignored today. Not only are clinical trials not being conducted, but enzyme proponents are scorned and persecuted by the FDA.

Following is a selective listing of these early medical research reports on the anti-tumor effects of enzymes and related treatments and research. The comments on some of the articles are by embryologist John Beard and were published in 1911 (p. 274).

1. Rice, Clarence C., "Treatment of Cancer of the Larynx by Subcutaneous Injections of Pancreatic Extract (Trypsin)," *Medical Record*, New York, November 24, 1906, pp. 812-816.

2. Wiggin, Frederick H., "Case of Multiple Fibro-Sarcoma of the Tongue," *Journal of the American Medical Association*, December 15, 1906, pp. 2003-2006. [Nine months later the patient was examined by two hospital physicians, found free

from malignant disease, and considered cured. A copy of their certificate is in the writer's (Beard) possession.]

3.   Golley, F.B., "Two Cases of Cancer Treated by the Injection of Pancreatic Extract," *Medical Record*, New York, December 8, 1906, pp. 918-919.

4.   Golley, F.B., "Two Cases of Cancer Treated with Trypsin," Supplementary report to the foregoing in *Medical Record*, May 8, 1909, pp. 804-805.

[At the above date the one patient was in "fairly good health," the other – apparently a "scirrhus" cancer of the bowel – died in the summer of 1908...Treatment by injection of trypsin was continued at intervals up to June 1907. There was not much pain up to the last three months. The suffering was nothing like that usually experienced in such cases.]

Other very favorable points are noted in the report – such as an artificial anus never became necessary, and *[the character of the disease changed from an active and rapidly progressive type to a slow and practically stationary one, which not only prolonged life, but shut off the disease from outside irritative influences, making life more bearable and wholesome by the formation of membrane over the raw surfaces. In short, replacing an active loathsome disease by one more durable]*.

In light of our knowledge today, the treatment in this case was carried out with preparations much too weak for their task, and probably far too little amylopsin was employed.

5.   Campbell, James T., "Trypsin treatment of Malignant Disease (Left Tonsil, Base of Tongue, Epiglottis)," *Journal of the American Medical Association*, January 19, 1907, pp. 225-226.

6.   Geoth, Richard A., "Pancreatic Treatment of Cancer with Report of a Cure," *Journal of the American Medical Association,* March 23, 1907, p. 1030.

7. Duprey, H., "Trypsin in Epithelioma of Larynx," *New Orleans Medical and Surgical Journal*, vol. 68, p. 33.

8. Cutfield, A., "Trypsin Treatment in Malignant Disease," *British Medical Journal,* August 31, 1907, p. 525.

9. Dontai, "The Trypsin Treatment of Malignant Disease," (Review of Medicine), *British Medical Journal*, March 2, 1907. (Recurrent sarcoma of testicle.)

10. Marsden, Aspinall, "Carcinoma of Cervix Uteri Successfully Treated with the Pancreatic Ferment," *General Practitioner,* January 11, 1908, p. 22.

11. Meggitt, Henry, "The Pancreatic Treatment of Cancer," *General Practitioner*, March 21, 1908. (Cure in seven months of recurrent cancer of the liver.)

12. Franklin, Byjay & Tirelee, Ritnin, "Correct Approach to Cancer Therapy," *Lotta Workana Research*, March 8, 1908, p. 381. (Reduction of pain in rectal and visceral areas with oral enzyme and ancillary therapies substituted for conventional treatment.)

Note the dates – 1906, 1907, 1908, 1909 – all over eighty-five years ago! Today enzymatic treatment of cancer is rejected by the medical establishment. The American Cancer Society, the American Medical Association and the FDA dismiss such treatments as "quackery." Obviously not because enzymes are unsuccessful. The fear of extensive testing of enzyme treatments suggests that segments of our medical establishment are only too aware cancer can be treated. Failure to recognize this potential treatment therapy exposes certain segments of the orthodox medical establishment as callous charlatans, trading profit for people's lives. So we need to ask the questions: who are the quacks? Who are the charlatans?

Significant Research

In recent years, this early enzyme research has been renewed, expanded and verified by researchers abroad or outside the

AMA-ACS-FDA establishment. In the 1960s and 1970s, several investigators confirmed the anti-tumor effects of vitamin A. In 1971, Dr. Hoefer-Janker in Germany demonstrated that 40 percent of tumors injected with enzyme preparations showed regression. In 1973, Tiscjer, *et al*, treated 119 patients with enzyme preparations and found that cancer cells disappeared in 47 percent of the cases.

In 1978, supported by funds from outside the medical establishment, Dr. Harold Manner, Chairman of the Department of Biology at Loyola University in Chicago, undertook anti-tumor experiments using combined therapy: amygdalin, vitamin A and enzyme complex. In this test 550 breeder mice were divided into 11 groups of 50 animals each. C3H/HeJ retired breeder female mice were used because about 80 percent spontaneously develop malignant mammary tumors between 12 and 17 months of age.

The application of this combined treatment resulted in an 89.3 percent complete remission rate and 100 percent regression rate of various degrees. It was found the enzyme complex attacks the tumor directly and digests the surrounding protein coat, allowing the amygdalin, vitamin A and the body's immune system to fight the cancer cells. Dr. Manner followed this with an experiment to determine the effects of each substance individually. The findings confirmed that for the treatment to be successful all three compounds must be used together, not by themselves. Manner summarized his findings as follows:

"When enzymes and vitamin A are used together we get a retardation of tumor growth, but not regression. When we add Laetrile to it, we get retardation that ends with total regression."

How Do Enzymes Attack Cancer?

Several theories have been proposed to explain the action of the enzyme complex, with its selective destruction of cancer cells. It may well be that a normal functioning pancreas, adequately producing proteolytic enzymes, is the body's best defense against cancer.

This observation has been verified by Drs. Tilscher and Wrba of the Cancer Research Institute of the University of Vienna in Austria, as well as by Dr. Hoefer-Janker in Germany.

G. Stojanows, who tested the toxicity of enzymes, stated "The (protolase) mixture can be regarded as completely atoxic" (without toxicity). He also observed there was no damage to healthy tissues and that animal experiments essentially agree with patient observations made at the clinic.

"The best way to attack cancer is to act before it starts, through the use of raw foods and vitamin supplements. The use of enzymes from these foods or food supplements should not be limited to the treatment of degenerative disease, but also used as protection for those who wish to forestall degenerative diseases."

A combination of beef pancreas, calf thymus, and an extract of the garden pea, lentil bean, and papaya has been found by Dr. Manner to be the most destructive force against cancer cells and/or the protein coat surrounding the cancer cell. Once the protein coat is dissolved, cancer cells are defenseless. The enzymes in these foods are fractionated hydrolysates of the beef pancreas, calf thymus, pisum sativum, lens esculenta and papyotin.

The mode of action of the components most widely used in enzyme therapy are:

Chymotrypsin – reduces inflammation

Trypsin – digests necrotic tissue

Amylase – digests starch

Lipase – digests fat

Papain – de-shields tumor tissue

Bromelain – digests protein

Pancreatin – natural synergistic enzyme mixture

Thymus substance – contains enzymes

Emulsified vitamin A – activates lysosomes and nourishes epithelium

Emulsified vitamin E – antioxidant and cell protectant

In addition to being the primary defense mechanism against malignant cells in the bloodstream, pancreatic enzymes break down and aid digestion of food protein. If heredity has provided a normal pancreas there will be enough enzymes to fulfill both functions. However, a body that requires the use of all pancreatic enzymes for digestion will not have sufficient freely-circulating enzymes to prevent cancer. Unfortunately, a large percentage of people, due to their genetics, are unable to produce enough enzymes for proper digestion. Not only do they have digestive problems, but they have no defense against cancer as well.

Part of the metabolic approach to cancer therapy is to reduce or eliminate the consumption of beef. Beef protein is difficult for pancreatic enzymes to break down and, therefore, requires a large quantity of enzymes, whereas the protein of chicken and fish is far more easily digested. The less demand we make on pancreatic enzymes to digest our food, the more enzymes there will be to function as part of our immune defense.

CHAPTER 8:

Spare the Scalpel

"Internal Medicine was born of witchcraft...surgery is a child of the battlefield."

–Dr. Norman Schumway

A USA Today front page story estimates the '90s decade will see 1.6 million people dead of cancer each year.

In the meantime, a thorough investigation of the medical establishment is long overdue. Unless an aroused electorate put sufficient pressure on Congress, we may well wait a couple of decades before a sluggish government investigates the motives and goals of the American Cancer Society, the American Medical Association, the National Cancer Institute, Memorial Sloan-Kettering Institute and their bureaucratic allies in the Food and Drug Administration. Meanwhile, potential cancer victims must find their own solutions.

Citizens and others concerned about our freedom to choose, as well as about food purity and safety, must remain diligent in opposing those who would restrict our freedoms and jeopardize our health.

Rep. Henry Waxman (D-Calif), from Southern California, is trying to restrict your access to nutrients.

Legislatures in two states, Massachusetts and California, have actually deemed it necessary to pass laws requiring that medical doctors fully inform their breast cancer patients of alternative treatment methods.

People can and are doing for themselves. If we can pressure Congress to put the FDA back in its place and repeal the Harris-Kefauver amendment, the freedoms our forefathers guaranteed us in the Constitution of the United States can include the freedom to choose medical therapies.

Unfortunately, laws cannot be passed that would force the physician to become knowledgeable about all the alternatives. Most doctors are not only unfamiliar with the new and contradictory surgery and radiation techniques within their own field but are hopelessly uninformed, as well, in the preventive/corrective disciplines of immunotherapy and clinical nutrition.

Experimental Systemic Poisons

Toxic chemotherapeutic drugs are, at best, experimental non-specific poisons. Their ill effects often slip past the ravages of the disease and suppress the immune system. The expected results from such lethal poisons has been compared to medical witchcraft. To compare current consensus attitudes against the protocol and treatment advocated by holistic, metabolically-informed physicians, I need to briefly discuss the art (as opposed to science) of surgery in its attack on cancer. I must concede that when the body's natural immune system has been neglected to the point where a tumor threatens an internal organ, surgical trauma to the body cannot be avoided. Mechanical removal of the obstruction then is imperative. But what of the patient whose vital functions are not affected?

An attempt to review the controversies and contradictions throughout the field of oncological surgery is impossible. For the sake of brevity I will restrict myself to breast cancer, the most common malignancy in women, and one I am most often asked to comment upon.

Orthodoxy has traditionally regarded radical surgery as the treatment of choice. This, despite the devastating physical, psychological and often unnecessary side effects of the procedure.

Until the late 1800s, breast cancer was far less common than it is today. No consistent form of therapy was practiced or recognized.

Patients seldom saw their doctors until the malignancy was well advanced.

During the late 1880s, William Halstead, M.D., Johns Hopkins University Hospital, devised the radical mastectomy. In 1902, Dr. Halstead published the results of 133 operations. Although the survival rate was little better than that of untreated patients, the surgical bandwagon was rolling, using as its excuse the fact that tumors seldom recur in the same area once surgically removed. The fact that the area has become surgical offal (waste parts) seems to have escaped consideration – as well as the even-then recognized fact that tumor recurrences are not the usual cause of cancer death. Death occurs when the cancer metastasizes and spreads to other parts of the body.

Halstead's procedure is based on the assumption that cancer is a local disease, one that spreads in a predictable way, first to the lymph vessels and nodes, which for a time act as a defense barrier until they are overwhelmed, then on to adjoining organs and tissues. This principle holds only if cancer cells are indeed an independent entity against which the body has no defense mechanism and, secondly, that it does not spread by way of the blood.

Once these assumptions were made, conventional medicine decided the best way to prevent the spread of the disease (remember, it was assumed to be spread by close contact) was to excise it while it was still localized. The more extensive the operation, including lymph system, pectoral muscles, etc., the greater the chance of intercepting all tumor cells. Sometimes the unfortunate patient, after having limbs or other body parts removed, received the grim news that the cancer had reappeared in another organ. The convenient explanation was that either the operation had not been extensive enough or had been performed too late. We refer to this as the "too bad – I guess we did not get it all" theory of cancer therapy.

Believe it or not, this illogical and already discredited procedure provides the basis for generations of physicians to continue their surgical mayhem, notwithstanding the fact it was statistically proven to have small value from the very beginning.

Until the mid 1950s, the possibility that the blood could serve as the route for metastases received little, if any, consideration. Unquestionably, surgery performed during these years did as much to spread or metastasize the malignancy by way of the blood as to localize it. Fifteen years ago all physicians would have recommended, in diagnosing breast cancer, the entire breast be sacrificed, regardless of the stage or condition of the disease.

Only a few physicians, notably George Crile, Jr., M.D., of Cleveland Clinic and Vera Peters, M.D., of Princess Margaret Hospital in Toronto, Canada, would have dissented, based on their practical experience that many patients survive with far less drastic surgery. Traditional surgical opinion refused to be swayed by their clinical observations.

In 1955, Drs. Edwin R. Fisher and Rupert Trunbull discovered cancer cells in the blood. This was confirmed shortly thereafter by other investigators, spurring Dr. Fisher to continue investigation of tumor metastases. Unfortunately, the surgical grip on the female breast remained so firm that radical mastectomies continued, despite contradictory research questioning their value.

The continuing work of Dr. Fisher and his brother, Dr. Bernard Fisher, has ultimately resulted in orthodoxy's recognition of a fact logic made obvious decades before: the bloodstream, not just the lymph system, is an important route for the cancer cell. Researchers still refuse to recognize or investigate the possibility that when cancer appears in a second organ, it may be a totally separate manifestation, and the result of an immune system breakdown. In any case, the Drs. Fishers' research has proven to all but the most recalcitrant that a surgical attack on the lymph system, no matter how extensive, has scant hope of eradicating or containing cancer.

Much of orthodoxy has had to reluctantly recognize cancer tumors are not autonomous. Malignant cell growth is directly related to the condition of the body, principally the strength of the body's immunosuppressive system. More and more physicians (only a few surgeons among them) are belatedly admitting that cancer, rather than being a local affliction that will spread unless surrounded and eliminated, is a systemic disease. Therefore, any therapeutic approach must be systemic in nature. Despite the preponderance of evidence, the vast majority of orthodoxy prefers to continue in entrenched error.

In 1971, an organized clinical trial to compare radical mastectomy with less extensive surgical treatment was headed by Dr. Fisher. Thirty-four U.S. and Canadian institutions were represented with more than 1,700 patients assigned at random to three separate kinds of mastectomy surgery. These patients were followed for six to nine years. The results have conclusively proven there is no significant difference in longevity between patients on whom radical surgery is perpetrated and those fortunate enough to receive much less severe butchery.

As a result of these tests, in 1979 the NCI brought together a panel of experts to develop surgical protocol. Notice that the trials had already proven dissimilar surgical treatments produce the same dismal results – and evidence continues to pile up that cancer is systemic and not a local disease.

Still, these heads of cancer establishments failed to consider for one moment discontinuing mastectomy surgery altogether. Instead, they noted the "exciting preliminary results" and urged "continued support for such studies." Because of continuing debate between radical and conservative proponents, they still failed to endorse any less drastic surgery than has been performed for the last 90 years.

Not even considered by this group was the eye-opening statistical research of Dr. Hardin Jones of the University of California. His findings indicate women with diagnosed breast cancer who refuse surgery stand an equal, if not better, chance of surviving than patients who have been led to the operating table by their uninformed physicians and establishment-indoctrinated surgeons.

Nor did they consider the results of an autopsy study of women over 70 who died of causes other than cancer. The percentage of those women with microscopically-diagnosable breast cancer was 19 times greater than the actual incidence of overt breast cancer in that age group; evidence that these women had immuno-suppressive systems capable of handling cancer without the surgeon's knife or the radiologist's gun. No doubt had they survived their fatalities, they would have been victims of these procedures had the disease been diagnosed in their lifetimes.

The evidence continues to come in from researchers such as Dr. Veronesi of Italy, Dr. M. Olevski of Helsinki, Finland, and R. Calle, Foundation Curie, Paris. No matter how much or how little surgery is performed, statistically the resulting patient longevity is always the same.

The butchery continues. Surgeons continue to classify their patients into Groups I, II, III, depending upon size of tumor, and debate among themselves which type of operation should be performed: radial mastectomy, modified radical mastectomy, total mastectomy, segmental mastectomy, wide excision, tumor excision, lumpectomy. No matter how you slice it, it's still human vivisection. It offers no statistical evidence of increased survival or cure.

Establishment medicine has failed. It continues to callously persist in methods that generate profits at the cost of hundreds of thousands of lives every year.

The solution, for many, is too late. It may not be too late, however, for you. Prevention is the answer. Nutrition and metabolic therapy is the core of prevention.

The recipes in the second half of this book outline a simple nutritional program that will maintain and build your natural defenses against cancer.

If you already have cancer, nutrition alone may not be enough. The only solution is to seek medical advice from a metabolic-oriented doctor. Under no circumstances should you attempt self-treatment. A preventive diet is common sense but once cancer is suspected, the only course is to see a doctor. There is nothing secret about the course of treatment followed by a doctor oriented to metabolic therapy. There may be some local differences due to harassment by the police power of the state and medical orthodoxy, which finds the profits in surgery and drug dealing too great to allow quick and easy surrender to prevention or nutrition.

The logic and common sense of the protocols of preventive and metabolic medicine in cancer therapy are just as important as technical and theoretical explanations, if not more so. For the sake of easy reading, footnotes and references in this book have been kept to a minimum. All statements contained herein have been thoroughly researched at Chicago's Loyola University and at equally well-equipped and respected research facilities around the world. Therapeutic evaluations and protocols are the results of work by internationally recognized medical and scientific investigators.

CHAPTER 9:

The Alternative Physician's Protocol

"All truth passes through three stages. First, it is ridiculed; second, it is violently opposed; third, it is accepted as being self-evident."
—Schoepenhauer

In revising this chapter, I have included the most recent scientific verification of the principles contained in the first edition of this book. Although those principles were based upon years of successful innovative treatment, the medical establishment chose to dispute them or disregard them. Instead of accepting these new scientific developments, the medical majority have continued with their discredited cut, burn and poison philosophy of cancer treatment, despite its often fatal results.

However, I am happy to report that since this book's first publication, the medical profession is finally awakening to the new world of cancer treatment. An increasing number of physicians are now admitting to the failure of their methods. At last, physicians are recognizing the successes of nutrition and its implementation into the successful therapy and prevention of chronic metabolic disease, which, of course, includes cancer.

In recent years, many practicing physicians have requested information from me that can aid them in treating and advising their patients when a diagnosis of cancer has been made. I hope to provide all the information they need in this chapter. In addition, I hope to answer in the following pages the question most asked of me by readers of my books and viewers of my syndicated TV program, *Accent on Health*.

I regret that some of the products designated herein must, of necessity, be identified by their brand rather than generic names. FDA regulation of these products has been inconsistent and confusing. Quite often, the FDA will arbitrarily ban products from the marketplace. Yet it allows others to be distributed without matching the technical specifications for the item or meeting the standards of good pharmaceutical practice in its preparation. No therapy program can produce consistent clinical results unless the products used are consistent.

The brands mentioned here have been analyzed and used in the laboratory and clinical studies. No doubt other good products are available. However, the purchaser would do well to remember the adage, "If you do not know what you are buying, know whom you are buying it from."

This protocol is solely for the practicing physician. It should in no way be considered a "do-it-yourself" therapy. Professional diagnosis and regular checkups by a holistically-oriented physician are essential to the success of any treatment schedule.

Pre-Treatment

Acknowledging the fact that all chronic metabolic diseases are caused, controlled or corrected by proper nutrition, the treating physician must first become familiar with the patient's dietary history. In addition, primary consideration must be given to a total body examination. Many underlying, as yet undiagnosed, disorders can determine the patient's ability to utilize nutritional treatment. Particular attention should be given to the digestive system and its ability to assimilate nutrients and avoid allergies.

<u>Without exception, cancer patients have an imbalance of minerals to other nutrients</u>. It is probable that selenium levels will be low. Zinc levels must be elevated consistently in the case of prostate cancer.

Molybdenum deficiency seems to be related to cancer of the esophagus. Copper and lead levels are often far above average. The triglycerides and cholesterol in the blood typically must be lowered. Low manganese appears to be linked to high cholesterol levels (Manner).

A hair and blood elemental analysis should be performed to determine the supplementation or eliminations necessary to bring the body as close to normalcy as possible.

Laboratory norms for blood profiles represent an average for the population. As the population becomes sicker, the ranges become greater. The norms usually accompanying the standard blood tests do not represent an ideal condition from metabolic therapy's viewpoint.

We are only now beginning to realize that proper assimilation and balance of minerals in the body is equally if not more important for consistent good health than vitamin assimilation.

The following values are within the acceptable mineral balance:

Calcium 9.7 – 10.1/Potassium "serum" 4.0 – 4.3
Phosphorous 3.1 – 3.5/Chloride "serum" 100 – 104
Glucose 85 – 100/Creatinine "serum" 0.7 – 1.0
Bun 13 – 17/Iron "serum" 95-100
Uric Acid 4.5 – 5.5/Bun/Creatinine ratio 14.5 – 15.5
Cholesterol 185 – 215/Triglycerides 95 – 105
Total Protein 7.2 – 7.5/WBC 5000 – 6000
Albumen 4.0 – 4.4/RBC 4.5 – 5.0 million
Bilirubin 0.5 – 0.7/Hemoglobin 14.5 – 15.0
Alkaline Phosphatase 67.5 – 77.5/Hematocrit 40 – 50
LDH 125/135/Eosinophils 0 – 2
SGOT 18 – 22/Basophils 0 – 2
Total Globulin 2.8 – 3.5/Monocytes 4 – 6
A/G Ratio 2.5 – 3.5/Lymphocytes 34 – 45
Sodium "serum" 140 – 143/Segs 45 – 55

Every effort must be made to remove surplus minerals and toxins. To this end, a physician trained in chelation should be consulted. Chelation is a cleansing procedure performed by an experienced physician. It enables the body to excrete through the urine harmful and excessive amounts of heavy metals and toxic minerals.

To correct mineral deficiencies quickly and regain a homeostatic balance of all body functions, a liquid multi-mineral supplement must be commenced. The specific minerals excluded are as important as those that must be included. The amounts should match the requirement of the normal body equation.

Dissolved minerals in solution are the best delivery system for easy and prompt assimilation. For certain cancers, additional specific mineral supplementation is required. A brand new system for optimum absorption of minerals has been developed, revolutionizing the supplementation market. Look for the method called "Solucell" (which means solution into the cells) in your supplemental formula. Especially important when the body is at less than peak performance, this system of assimilation increases greatly the odds that you get the nutrients your body needs the most.

The diet recommendations of this book will bring the triglycerides and cholesterol to appropriate low levels.

Treatment

Phase 1, First 21 Days:

Commence chelation treatments by a trained specialist in this procedure. Start mineral supplementation as above.

1. FAST. For the first two days, patient intake must be confined strictly to organic, fresh-squeezed fruit and vegetable juices. The more the better. The reasons are threefold.

First, the body must be saturated with a maximum of full-potency, natural vitamins and minerals. Nutritional intake is optimized by eliminating bulk.

Second, the entire gastrointestinal system must quickly be cleansed as thoroughly as possible, eliminating all residue toxins. Physicians recommend adding four or five tablespoons of bran each day to the juices as an additional cleansing agent.

Third, it is essential bowel movements become regular. At least one and preferably two to four movements a day must be achieved. The stool should be soft but well formed.

Body wastes are themselves carcinogenic, so bowel transit time must be reduced to a minimum. Usually the increased intake of juice has a natural laxative effect. After the two-day juice fast, if frequent bowel evacuation has not been achieved, increase the amount of bran taken each day. In addition, two capsules of Lactozyme in a glass of juice taken one hour after meals should be started and continued until normalcy. In extreme cases it may be necessary to use colonic irrigation.

During this initial period, as much of the patient's liquid intake as is possible should be fruit and vegetable juices. When supplemental water is required, it should be pure spring water or distilled water. The chemicals in most tap water are extremely undesirable. Since spring waters vary in mineral content, and because in some cases distilled water will chelate certain minerals from the body, the doctor should give consideration to the type of water recommended.

2. DETOXIFICATION. This crisis nutritional program depends upon a foundation of detoxification as complete as possible, achieved in as short a time as possible. There is absolutely no doubt liver dysfunction is a concomitant phenomenon of cancer. As one of the body's chief organs for the elimination and conversion of toxic substances, the livers of cancer patients are clogged with poisons that should have been eliminated.

Dr. Buckner and Dr. Swaffield reported in *Cancer Research 1973*, "One hundred percent of a group suffering from gastrointestinal cancer suffered liver disorder." Drs. R. Robertson and H. Kahler have reported that laboratory animals in whom they induced liver cirrhosis all developed tumors in sites as varied as lung and bladder. Cancer can be reversed and controlled only if we regenerate the liver.

Fortunately, the liver is the one organ the body is capable of regenerating. A program of regeneration and purification must be immediately begun. This is assisted by the natural diuretic effect of the liquid fruit and vegetable intake. In addition, the purging process will be enhanced and speeded by the daily administration of a coffee-retention enema. In cases of extreme toxemia, which is most common, coffee enemas should be given twice daily.

Prepare the coffee by normal percolation or drip method. Instant coffee is not acceptable. Preferably, the coffee should be as fresh as possible. However, it can be made and stored in the refrigerator for use within a 48-hour period. The enema should consist of a minimum 8-oz cup to a maximum of one quart at body temperature and should be retained for at least 15 to 30 minutes. The body should not be expected to accept the liquid at too fast a rate. So as to avoid cramps, the enema bag should be no higher than six inches above the bowel. Patients will find they are better able to increase both the amount and the time of the retention as they become used to the procedure.

The importance of cleaning out the liver before rebuilding the immune system cannot be over-emphasized. During the period of retention, massage the bowel and maintain a position, if possible, where the trunk of the body is higher than the head. If this is not possible, the patient should lie on the left side. Caffeine stimulates secretion of bile, detoxifying the liver and restoring the alkaline condition of the small intestines. Perhaps it would appear more professional to prescribe a solution of so many grains of caffeine benzoate or caffeine citrate, but coffee has proven to be the simplest and most thorough, and it is most generally available.

In addition to this daily enema, six Tolatihsot capsules should be taken daily to facilitate absorption of nutrients.

It is important that the patient perspire heavily at least 15 minutes each day. The skin is the largest organ of excretion and, as such, acts as a third kidney in eliminating toxins from the body. Exercise is the preferable method to create the sweating condition. When this is not possible, a heated room, heavy sweat clothing or blanketing is acceptable.

3. DIGESTIVE ENZYMES. To decrease the stress placed on the gastric glands and the pancreas, one or two Hydrozyme tablets should be taken with each meal. This compound contains hydrochloric acid, pepsin and enterically-coated pancreatic enzymes. This will ensure proper digestion. The patient should be given a graded litmus paper and instructed to test the first urine in the morning. It should have a pH of about 5.5.

4. ENZYMES. Enzymes are an important part of the complete crisis protocol. A good pancreatic enzyme will vitalize the immune system and expose the cancer cell to attack. We have found Retenzyme E.C. and Intenzyme effective. The recommended amount is three Retenzyme E.C. and one Intenzyme tablet taken together three times daily. These enzymes must be taken when the digestive tract is the most empty. They should be administered midway between breakfast and lunch, lunch and dinner, and dinner and bedtime. The 3:1 ratio must be maintained.

NOTE: If there is a problem with oral administration of the enzyme, or if it is believed additional enzyme therapy is required, a rectal form of the enzyme is available.

5. VITAMIN A. This should be given in an emulsified form to prevent liver involvement. Twenty drops of Bio AE Mulsion Forte are given in morning juice and another 20 drops in evening juice to increase the number of circulating lymphocytes. This will give the patient 500,000 IU daily. Every second day an additional five drops should be added morning and evening. The incidence of headache or dry, scaling skin usually indicates maximum dosage has been exceeded. When these symptoms occur, discontinue vitamin A for one week. Return after one week with a two-week on, one-week off routine employing a 5 a.m. and 5 p.m. dosage of ten drops less than that which caused the toxic reaction. 700,000 IU daily is the usual toxic level.

6. VITAMIN C. Fifteen grams of ascorbic acid (or to bowel tolerance) should be given daily. This amount of ascorbic acid may cause gastric disturbances. For this reason, spread the fifteen grams throughout the day. The dosage may be increased at the discretion of the physician. Some have recommended dosages as high as 50-70 grams daily. A buffered C may be used to minimize any digestive upset that may occur.

Humans are an exception in the animal kingdom in that they do not have the capability of manufacturing vitamin C within their own bodies, as demonstrated by the onset of scurvy (sailors' calamity) when vitamin C is missing from the diet. Our only source is from our food supply, which in many cases is so depleted in this nutrient that many of the colds, skin disorders and infirmities of modern man are nothing more than subclinical scurvy.

It has been laboratory proven that animals under the stress of illness increase the internal synthesis of vitamin C many-fold and supplement with increased intake from external sources.

Similarly, human beings must increase their intake of vitamin C during periods of stress. Normal amounts of the vitamin required during periods of good health must be dramatically increased; the body itself will determine at what level by the bowel tolerance mechanism explained in a previous section on vitamin C.

Vitamin C in a green tea base with green tea extract, polyphenols, lemon and grape bioflavonoids is the best formula for boosting the immune system and help enable it to conquer the cancer.

7. VITAMIN B15. Stimulating cellular oxidation is extremely important. Cancer cells are anaerobic and cannot exist in a normal oxygen environment. Organic B15 (the salts of pangamic acid) should be prescribed; two capsules with each meal — six per day.

8. AMYGDALIN B17. By now the physician has balanced the patient's body chemistry, stimulated and supplemented the immune system with enzymes that will seek out and destroy the protective protein coat surrounding the cancer cell, reduced toxemia, oxygenated the blood and cleansed the liver. Now we supply the amygdalin that helps the body destroy the cancer cell.

The most important supplement in the metabolic program of cancer control is amygdalin, vitamin B17. This naturally occurring nitriloside has either not been sufficiently present in the patient's diet or was inadequately metabolized. Amygdalin tablets will correct this vital deficiency.

In all but extremely severe cases of gastrointestinal cancer, the most successful method for delivering amygdalin to the body is oral administration. At one time I. V. injection was used. However, the observations of experienced physicians over the last decade have determined that tablets or capsules are equally effective and far less stressful to the patient. In addition, there is the advantage that a physician need not always be in attendance during therapy.

Six to nine 500 mg amygdalin tablets should be taken daily, specifically two or three after meals when there is food in the stomach. Some patients may experience light-headedness, but it will quickly pass. Subjective improvement should be noticed within a short period of time. Many doctors regularly prescribe considerably larger amounts of amygdalin, and this may be good. The patients should be closely monitored, however, to determine that no undue stomach distress occurs.

While amygdalin is a dietary supplement, obtained from natural food sources, present FDA regulations have limited its production in the United States. Consequently, many of the tablets obtainable from foreign sources or questionable purveyors contain an unnatural configuration of the amygdalin molecule which is totally ineffective. This is caused by incorrect extraction methods, and these tablets should be avoided as they defeat the entire protocol and offer no protection if taken for prevention.

The amygdalin tablet most often recommended is Laevalin. It is manufactured in the United States and maintains the proper laevo rotation of the amygdalin molecule.

If the patient is unable in ingest the oral tablets, administration may be done rectally by mini enema. Crush six 500 mg Laevaline tablets in 50-100 cc of warm tap water. Agitate until fully dissolved. Using a 100-cc syringe with plastic tube attached, insert into the rectum.

This procedure should be started only after completion of the coffee enema. The liquid should then be retained until the next bowel movement. This compromise method of administration offers the advantages of the IV administration in that the amygdalin is quickly absorbed into the bloodstream via the portal vein directly to the liver. There is no gastrointestinal distress, and usually higher amounts may be taken than with the oral delivery method. The rectal method offers all the advantage of the oral but is accomplished in the bowel.

The disadvantage may be in an extremely high amount of betaglucosidase contained in fecal matter retained in the lower intestines. Such high concentration could precipitate too extensive an enzymatic conversion of the amygdalin, resulting in a toxic reaction. It must be closely monitored, therefore, by the physician. When administration is made after the regular coffee enema, the process should be safe and results have been excellent. This method is often combined with oral administration of Laevalin tablets.

In case of an extreme crisis condition, the physician may recommend intravenous injection: three 3-gram vials injected – IV push. A subjective response should be noted within 48 hours (increased appetite, lower blood pressure, increased feeling of well-being, release from pain). If this response is not noted, increase the injection by three grams each day up to 30 grams or until a definite positive response is achieved. When administered in large amounts, the amygdalin should be placed in a physiological solution and injected within 20 to 30 minutes.

9. It has been stated elsewhere in this book that apricot kernels be ingested on a regular basis for prevention. The betaglucosidase enzyme contained abundantly in the kernel enhances the action of amygdalin, and therefore 10 to 15 kernels a day should be included in the crisis patient's diet to synergistically enhance the action of the Laevalin supplement. They should be taken three or four at a time but separated by a two or three hour interval from the amygdalin tablets.

10. A good therapeutic vitamin preparation should be given morning and evening in addition to the liquid mineral supplement. Quarter-inch organic seed sprouts retain the most concentrated nutrients. Recently a product has been developed that has taken the fluid and fiber from organic vegetables and seed sprouts after harvesting and put them into tablet form. The nutrient power of six beets can be placed on the head of a pin with this unique method of processing. Enzymes are also preserved, allowing greater absorption.

ADDITIONAL SUPPLEMENTS. If there is a past history of radiation or chemotherapy, Dismuzyme should be prescribed, six tablets per day. Vitamin E, as explained in the vitamin chapter, is the best natural antioxidant. RNA and DNA have been found to be extremely beneficial to the cancer patient.

In recent years considerable research has been devoted to sharks' metabolic resistance to cancer. They are one of the few animals that seem totally resistant to this disease. Many doctors have noted a dramatic improvement in patients when seven to ten capsules of refined lyophilized shark cartilage is prescribed per day.

All the vitamins, minerals and enzymes specifically mentioned in this protocol are saliently included in the recommended dietary plan that succeeds the crisis therapy. However, supplementation should continue under the supervision of a nutritionist trained in holistic therapy. Balance is as important in supplementation as in nature.

Vitamins work synergistically, enhancing the effect of each other. So a well balanced continuing vitamin plan should be designed for each patient.

12. DIET. All the foregoing will not result in a control of malignancy unless the proper diet is commenced. This may require a complete change of lifestyle and eating habits. The recipes in the second section will show that this diet, once past the initial phase, need not be unappetizing. Strict adherence must be maintained in the beginning. The slightest deviance may prevent the body from reaching homeostasis and result in failure.

A juice extractor should be purchased, and most of the vegetables in the diet juiced so that all of the naturally-occurring enzymes, minerals and vitamins are present. These fresh juices many be warmed slightly to make a soup, but never heated beyond 107° F, the point at which the enzymes will be destroyed. At least 64 ounces of raw juice each day should be consumed.

It is important to maintain a good fiber content in the system, obtainable in bran as well as in whole, raw vegetables. The amount will be determined by the physician, depending upon the location of the tumor. Other variables will be determined by individual situations and the effects of additional diseases such as diabetes, hypoglycemia, arteriosclerosis, heart problems and allergies.

I once had the sad experience of calling on an acquaintance who had been diagnosed as terminally ill with cancer. Visiting him was one of his personal friends, who happens to be one of the most respected orthodox physicians in our community. This doctor had doubtless been exposed to less than a four-hour course in nutrition during his entire medical education. His wife, through kitchen experience, was probably better qualified to give nutritional information. Yet here was my friend being advised by this ill-informed doctor to build his resistance with increased protein intake of red meat, and to maintain his body weight and energy by drinking milkshakes! Such misguided and presumptuous recommendations are repeated regularly by doctors whose ignorance of cancer's epidemiological link to the foundations of the American diet continues to jeopardize the health of their patients.

The rationale of diet in the prevention of cancer will be more thoroughly explained in the following chapter. Suffice it to say that in crisis situations where cancer symptoms have manifested themselves, we must have a crisis diet.

Fats must be reduced to an absolute minimum in order to reduce bloodstream levels of triglycerides and fatty globules. Both inhibit

Category	Foods Allowed	Foods to Avoid
Beverages	Herb teas; fresh fruit juices; fresh vegetable juice	Alcohol; cocoa; coffee; carbonated and canned drinks; artificial fruit drinks; regular tea
Dairy Products	Raw, skim or non-fat milk on cereal only; non-fat yogurt; non-fat cottage cheese; whole milk and/or cream for sauces only in limited amounts	Butter; margarine; ice cream
Eggs	Egg whites only	No whole eggs in any form
Fish	None (during first three weeks)	All
Fruits	All-fresh, dried, un-sulphured; frozen, whole when possible, including seeds or kernels	Canned; sweetened; avocado
Grains	All whole-grain cereals; millet; buckwheat; oats; rye; wheat; breads made from these without sugar and eggs	Processed grains, such as white rice; refined wheat; crackers, including bran; macaroni; prepared cereals; pita break (if refined flour)
Nuts	All nuts and seeds, preferably raw; dry-roasted, if neces-	Roasted in oil; salted

	sary; sunflower; soy nuts; pumpkin	
Oils	Small amounts of flaxseed oil or walnut oil	Shortening; refined oil, both saturated and unsaturated; margarine; olive oil
Seasonings	Herbs; garlic salt; onion; thyme; cayenne; parsley; marjoram; basil; celery salt; soy sauce; preservative-free salsa; wine flavoring only; seeds; raisins	Salt
Soup	All made from scratch in blender, salt-free; asparagus; bean; tomato; millet	Canned; creamed; bouillon
Sprouts	All, especially millet, soy, lentil, alfalfa, mung	Potato, Tomato
Sweeteners	Frozen fruit concentrates containing no sugar; raisins	Honey; refined sugar, white or brown; syrups
Vegetables	All cooked as little as possible, preferably not over 107°F. (Clean all vegetables thoroughly to eliminate surface contaminants. All beverage and food preparation must be done with only pure bottled water in stainless steel, ceramic or glass utensils. There can be no exceptions.)	All canned, prepared

oxygen transference to the cells. And cholesterol must be totally eliminated in order to ease liver function. (Dr. R. Steiner, in Cancer Research 1942, noted that cholesterol alone was capable of inducing tumors in mice. In humans, impaired cholesterol metabolism is a common cause of cancers, since oleic acid leads to fatty liver generation.) Animal proteins must be completely eliminated from the diet to allow the bowel to establish the proper flora for the generation of beta-glucosidase, which commences the breakdown processes of amygdalin in the nitriloside foods that will be included in the nutritional mix, and also reduce digestive need for pancreatic enzymes. Sugar, caffeine and salt, all of which have been linked to carcinogenic metabolic processes within the body, must be eliminated throughout the first three-week program.

The diet will consist almost exclusively of unrefined carbohydrates. This is a crisis diet for a crisis situation. It must be maintained with no exceptions. Not only is it the foundation for immediate reversal of cancer metabolism, but at the end of the three-week period the patient is going to find that his desire for foods that are toxic, carcinogenic and otherwise metabolically inappropriate has completely disappeared. Moreover, the patient will more easily accept dietary habits that will reinforce and support the immune system for the rest of his life.

Patients on this diet should not lose weight, other than that which is excessive for their height and bone structure. This is extremely desirable. If the weight loss is excessive, the physician should prescribe two to four tablets of free form amino acids taken daily. This will supply amino acids which do not require pancreatic enzymes for body assimilation.

In the past I have been reluctant to recommend predigested proteins due to inconsistencies in their manufacture, and to the high incidence of allergic reaction and loss of bone density during their use. But the recent introduction of free amino acids has been found to overcome these objections and they are recommended where necessary.

For the individual who resists a diet regimen as strict as we outline, let me emphasize again this is a three-week-long crisis diet. We are attempting to overcome the overt symptoms of a killer disease that has been preparing its assault on the body for as long as 15 years. The alternative is an early and probably agonizing demise.

For clarity, this is not strictly a salt-free diet, as celery salt, soya and preservative-free salsas are included. The imaginative cook can make many combinations of tasty herbs, yogurt, and cottage cheese sauces for combined vegetable dishes, and add texture with seeds and sprouts. Fructose sugar is sparingly allowed. Sugar-free fruit concentrate on pita bread or whole-grain muffins is really delicious. Salsa and herb salad dressings can be quite appetizing. Remember, this isn't forever. What is three weeks compared to a lifetime?

Additional Ancillary Therapy

The principal causes of cancer death, although nonexclusive and overlapping are:

1. Mechanical interference with the function of a vital organ.
2. Toxemia.
3. Side effects of chemotherapy and radiation.
4. The depression or destruction of the immune system, allowing an additional chronic or viral disease to invade the body and provide the final coup de grace.
5. Dysfunction of the psyche.
6. Cachexia – the gradual wasting away of the body. The patient becomes mentally listless, physically without energy. The condition is finalized by a rapid loss of weight.

Cancerous tumor cells derive their energy for growth and division from the fermentation of glucose. The malignant cell requires more than 50 times more glucose than a normal cell. This glucose is fermented into lactic acid which returns by way of the bloodstream to the liver and kidneys where it is recycled back to glucose. This process, called gluconeogenesis (gluco-neo-genesis), consumes body energy and is an extremely wasteful metabolism that causes the breakdown of tissue proteins into their amino acids, which are then converted into the glucose the tumor demands for fuel. The tumor grows at the expense of deteriorating muscle and connective tissue throughout the body, which self-destructively degenerates away. This is classic cachexia.

Amygdalin normally increases patient appetite to deter cachexia; the diet is designed to stabilize and reverse this process by increasing blood oxygenation and limiting fermentation.

In cases where the patient comes to the physician in an advanced state of cachexatic deterioration and continues to sink into malaise, immediate therapeutic effects have been achieved by the administration of hydrazine sulfate, which appears to block this devastating metabolism.

Considerable research into the process of gluconeogenesis has been done by Joseph Odlaw, D.Sc., and Joseph Gold, M.D., of Syracuse University, and Dean Burke, Ph.D., formerly with National Cancer Institute. They find this therapy extremely beneficial.

Hydrazine sulfate should be taken on an empty stomach, before dinner, lunch or bedtime. For a person 140 lbs. or over, two 60-mg capsules, one taken in the morning and one at night, is the usual physician-prescribed amount. For a person less than this weight, 30-mg tablets on the same schedule should prove sufficient.

Some doctors recommend dietary inclusion of natural yogurt or acidophilus capsules to seed the intestines with the betaglucosidase necessary for the first enzymatic breakdown of amygdalin. Betaglucosidase is an excretion product of acidophilus bacilli. Where meat is the principle ingested food, these acid bacilli will not be contained in sufficient quantity in the intestine. The prescribed diet of unrefined carbohydrates provides an environment for proper bacterial concentration so additional sources of acidophilus, while welcome, should not be necessary.

Cancer precursors include maladaption to stress, mental as well as physical. Biofeedback, Bible study, anything leading to a relaxed mental attitude, have proven helpful. To the greatest extent possible, the patient's family and friends should be totally supportive and remove as much stress and turmoil from the environment as they can. A patient's good mental attitude is part of the protocol every physician would like to prescribe. Unfortunately, it must originate within the patient.

Metabolic physicians conclude that patients who say, "Doctor, show me how to heal myself," have far better chances for survival than those patients who expect the doctor alone to provide a miracle. The fighters survive. They stick to the diet. They remain faithful to their medication. And their positive attitude provides a climate for self healing. Every possible avenue should be taken to develop in the patient the proper psyche for self healing.

Obviously all carcinogenic substances and environments should be avoided. No smoking. Avoid smog or congested streets and areas whenever possible. Food selected should be as organic as possible, without pesticides and preservatives.

The protocol outlined here for a crisis situation is not designed to fight only an invasive condition, as orthodoxy attempts to do with its radiation, drugs and surgery directed against the lump or bump. Metabolic physicians recognize that these symptoms are just the final result of an underlying metabolic imbalance and weakened immune system. Herein lies the solution.

For the name of a metabolic physician in your area, contact the National Health Federation at 212 West Foothill Blvd., Monrovia, CA 91016. Please be prepared to give a $25 donation for this service since the NHF is a non-profit organization. The donation also includes membership, and I urge every reader of this book to become a member. The NHF is the oldest and largest health freedom organization in America. Your membership dollars will guarantee not only your access to valuable information, courtesy of its publication, *Health Freedom News*, but your dollars help fund the ongoing legislative fight for the right to nutritional and alternative medical choice in America.

CHAPTER 10:

Biological Experience and Cancer Prevention

"Our present system recognizes disease only when it has reached crisis proportions. This is tantamount to saying that a fire is only a fire when it has burst through the roof. When, in actuality, it was a fire when the cigarette butt began to smolder in the rug."
—Carlton Fredericks, author

Cancer, like most diseases, is preceded by a latency period until its symptoms may no longer be ignored. Cancer does not start with a tumor. The tumor is simply the expressed symptom. A chest tumor can be seen by X-ray only after its diameter has reached five to 10 millimeters.

Katakowski and Gerstenberg proved conclusively that some tumors require at least 15 years to grow from the first fermenting cell to cell masses in diagnosable form. Cancer latency period has been estimated to be four times longer than its diagnosable or clinical stage. Only when the tumor becomes recognized does orthodox medicine commence its crisis treatment of surgery, poisoning or burning.

Mainstream medicine warns us to avoid one substance or environment after another. Almost every day we read about yet another cancer irritant exposed by the FDA, the NCI or the ACS. One tongue-in-cheek story circulated about these stalwart guardians of our health is that they have now determined saliva causes cancer when swallowed in small amounts over a prolonged period of time.

All we are offered, after billions of tax and contributed research dollars, are negative solutions; things to avoid like environments, food additives, smoking and a continually lengthening list of carcinogens. But never one positive action that we can take by way of preparing our bodies to prevent cancer, or to provide immunity to contact with these substances, which, in truth, only trigger the cancer or determine the location where it will strike, as no doubt cigarettes do in the case of lung cancer.

The cancer establishment (the whole alphabet of governmental and contribution-supported agencies) professes to see light at the end of the tunnel. Yet all the while they admit they haven't found the cause of cancer. Most often for the affected, the light at the end of the tunnel is "an oncoming train" of surgeries, and debilitating and demoralizing therapies.

Immunity Through Biological Experience

The holistic- or metabolically-oriented physician recognizes the natural intrinsic immune system designed into the human body and the extrinsic backup system provided in our natural food supply. The resistance of the body to disease must be maintained and any inherited weakness of the natural immune system within our body strengthened or overcome.

I believe that the body can stand up to any disease if it is fed foods natural to its biological experience and if we eliminate from our diet the many non-foods that fill the shelves of our supermarkets.

As you will note in the next chapter when I discuss my Bio-X Diet, I love to repeat my rule of thumb: EAT GOD-MADE FOODS AS CLOSE TO THE WAY GOD MADE THEM AS IS POSSIBLE IN A MODERN WORLD. People are often amazed at my lectures when I tell them that there has been no discovered incidence of cancer among any wild animals killed in the hunt. Yet these same species, when domesticated or placed in zoos where they must eat food prepared for them by humans, suffer from the same epidemiological cancer found in homo sapiens. Cultivated carbohydrates and domesticated meat products prepared by animal food companies and zoo keepers do not contain the nitrilosides available to animals in their natural habitats. This simple empirical observation alone should stimulate the investigation of nutrition as it affects the incidence of cancer.

Those few in the medical profession who exhibit interest in cancer and nutrition are thwarted by either inadequate information or none at all. Medical schools traditionally include no required courses in nutrition, and the U. S. Health and Human Services Department is influenced by large and affluent food industries. Agriculture is the cornerstone of our nation's economy. We cannot expect government education to reflect negatively on a section of this national resource.

The nation's agricultural schools do not include courses on human nutrition, even though they are inextricably linked through animal husbandry (raising animals for consumption) or crop science (again, food for our tables).

By contrast, schools of veterinary medicine recognize the value of nutrition in animal health maintenance. This awareness is demonstrated during each visit with your dog or cat to a small-animal clinic. Invariably the veterinarian will ask, "What have you been feeding this animal?" I sincerely doubt your personal physician has ever considered your diet as a primary source of any symptom, other than acne or a stomachache. Certainly his medical school never trained him to do so.

The Alteration of Our Foods

The scientific study of animal nutrition is researched not only in our large veterinary schools, but also by such giant food conglomerates as Ralston Purina and General Foods. These companies maintain flocks and herds of "laboratory" meat animals with the sole purpose of altering their basic biology to achieve certain profitable ends. Disregarding the possible detrimental effect their experiments might have on the nutritional aspect of these food sources, scientists attempt to hasten reproduction, accelerate growth rate, and increase production of butterfat, eggs and other farm products through variation in feed and chemical supplementation. Animals are also genetically altered by selectively breeding to produce progeny that reach market earlier or in a more advanced state of maturation.

Since the days of Luther Burbank, horticultural experts have hybridized our food supply until many grains cannot even reproduce themselves. All efforts are bent at increasing per-acre yield, earlier ripening and a longer shelf-life. Present-day tomatoes, corn, wheat and rice bear scant resemblance to their original form. If the crops of this artificial selection and cultivation system provide complete nutrition, it is purely by accident. Usually the opposite is true. The desire for earlier maturity in animals and plants has resulted in diminished nutritional value.

The introduction of chemical fertilizers and pesticides has not only resulted in lower natural nutritive quality but has introduced harmful substances into our food chain. The succulent flavor and satisfying appearance of home-grown vegetables is often the result of a most fortunate ignorance on the part of the gardener, unindoctrinated in the various harmful chemicals available, who is satisfied with the naturally-selected and ripened harvest provided by a more natural horticulture.

Our government tells us half the world exists on a deficient food supply. Doesn't it seem logical, then, that some of these minimum-subsistence populations (already supported with food shipped through the generosity and concern of the United States) might serve as ideal experimental and control groups for the determination of human nutritional needs? Such research would not take advantage of an impoverished people, but would be conducted to predetermine and program true nutritional requirements for future generations of stronger, more disease-resistant societies.

Unfortunately, nutritional research in animal husbandry does not extend to the selection and development of proper nutritional plants and animals for human consumption, only for progressively earlier production of those plants and animals. Our United States

Departments of Health and of Agriculture have never proposed or underwritten such basic nutritional research in the available world laboratory. This fact, I believe, indicates their lack of desire to support studies that might discover weaknesses in current agricultural production techniques.

Agricultural science continues its efforts to transform our natural food supply into just the right size to pick, package or can, or to make it more resistant to storage and shipping damage. Every genetic change results in lowered food values. These nutritional changes, like it or not, have been the unfortunate aftermath of the mechanization and urbanization of modern Euro-American civilization.

What We Don't Eat Causes Cancer

Cancer has often been called a disease of civilization. Nutritional authors regularly cite research that tends to prove that whenever man, because of deprivation, geographical necessity or cultural preferences, exists on a diet high in one particular type of food, the result is degenerative disease. The orthodox researchers follow a progression of logic that leads to a simplistic conclusion: excessive food is a causative factor of disease. Seldom do they consider that what is left out of the diet may be the true culprit. In the few cases where cancer is mentioned in passing by these authorities, it is usually to cite populations of heavy meat or fat eaters who have a high incidence of cancer.

Cultures that exhibit the lowest cancer rates have varied dietary habits and preferences. It is true, for example, that cultures with the consistently lowest cancer rates are mainly vegetarian and embrace diets high in complex carbohydrates. Yet, in cultures like the Northern Eskimo, with negligible vegetable intake and a cultural preference for blubber and similar animal fats, cancer is virtually unknown. Or consider the Bantu or Masai of Africa, whose diet is almost exclusively red meat or blood and milk. These natives are also cancer-free. The one thing common to all diets of cancer-free cultures is they daily eat over 500 times the amount of foods high in nitrilo-sides than the diets of modern Europeans and Americans.

In the case of the Eskimo, large residual amounts of nitrilosides (amygdalin) are obtained from the staple meat of the caribou that feeds itself on the nitriloside-rich salmon berries abundant in northern latitudes. African tribesmen commonly consider the rumen contents (first stomach) of grazing animals a delicacy. These animals regular-ly forage on high nitriloside plants.

Anyone studying these cancer-free cultures will come to a speedy conclusion that it is not what we eat but what we do not eat that results in cancer. Incidentally, it should be pointed out while the aforemen-tioned Eskimos, Bantu and Masai have no cancer because of their high intake of nitrilosides, they do suffer the extremely high incidence of other degenerative diseases you would expect from high-fat meat diets. This is, in itself, indicative of the specific extrinsic cancer pre-vention we receive by including nitriloside-containing plants in our diet. No matter how otherwise unhealthful a diet is, the inclusion of high-nitriloside, amygdalin food seems to prevent the incidence of cancer.

In the next chapter you will see how my Bio-X Diet restores the nitriloside foods that our modern culture, agricultural economy, and eating habits have virtually eliminated over the last 50 years.

CHAPTER 11:

The Bio-X Diet

"Therefore the place was named Kibroth Hattaavah, because there they buried the people who had craved other food."
                                                            —Numbers 11:34

The foundation of my Bio-X Diet is built upon the natural extrinsic immune system that God designed into the human body. As I mentioned in the previous chapter, this remarkable immune system, along with an extrinsic backup system provided in our natural food supply, is capable of resisting any disease – and cancer is no exception. The function of the Bio-X Diet is to keep the immune and the backup systems fully operational. To achieve this, Bio-X simply returns to our bodies the food substances natural to our biological experience. At the same time, Bio-X includes no non-foods that place stresses on our metabolic systems.

It is interesting to note that in all chronic metabolic diseases – scurvy, pellagra, and among others, rickets – the cause and the cure is nutritional. At many medical symposiums where I have lectured, I have asked the audience to name one chronic metabolic disease where the eventual control was not found to be dietary. I have never been challenged. Cancer is no exception.

As we saw in Chapter 9, a non-definitive model protocol was presented for the patient to whom the knowledge of prevention has come too late. After detoxification of the body, the treatment consists of attempting to rebuild metabolic balance or homeostasis with vitamins, minerals and enzymes, the goal being to reactivate the immune system for a massive resistance to an entrenched enemy. How much better it would be if the body's forces of resistance had been nurtured and maintained throughout life!

The bad news is that one out of every three Americans alive today will contract cancer. The good news is that by following a simple nutritional program, such as the Bio-X Diet, you will never be that one, and you are going to feel better and live better than ever before.

You are going to feel better because Bio-X will return your body to the nutritional environment originally designed by God.

The human body is a superb engineering feat, an unmatchable machine. And like any other fine piece of machinery, it leaves the factory with directions for care and maintenance, as specified by its designer. It is very much like a new automobile. We all know that when your new car is delivered it comes with a maintenance manual. This manual specifies the octane rating of gasoline to be used, the viscosity of the lubricating oil, the type of air cleaner and oil filter, the grade of coolant required in the radiator. Your car will operate at maximum efficiency and last longer if you use the lubricants and fuels specified.

I believe that the many references to nutrition in the Bible, beginning with Genesis 1:29, can be considered the maintenance book from our designer and manufacturer. The Biblical references to diet are exacting and, incidentally, correlate to the cancer prevention program outlined in this book. I like to think of the human body as an intricately designed and balanced machine. Each metabolic system within the whole is integrated and matched for total life-support. When all systems are functioning properly, the body is remarkably resilient to trauma. Like any other fine piece of machinery, the body has safety margins and tolerances included in its design which allow it to temporarily continue functioning even though not fueled properly.

Referring again to our analogous automobile, we see that although all fuels and lubricants have been definitively specified, the machinery can tolerate, for limited periods, low-octane gasoline, impure air and contaminated lubricants. The machinery will continue to operate. Built into the machinery are safety factors that allow the equipment to function above or below factory-specified norms. In addition, the engine is equipped with various filters and cleaners that eliminate many harmful contaminants.

Eventually, however, improper maintenance will have its deleterious effect. Perhaps starting will be a little difficult, pick-up will be sluggish, vibration will occur in idle or there may be a cloudy exhaust. Some or all of these minor symptoms of inadequate lubrication and fueling will sooner or later appear. Though the symptoms are irritating, the automobile will continue to provide transportation. At this stage, returning the machine to optimum performance can be accomplished by resuming the use of proper fuels and lubricants. The alternative is eventual major breakdowns, staggering repair bills, and finally total loss of function.

Similarly, the human body has intrinsic protective mechanisms and tolerance factors that allow it to continue to function under abusive conditions. Modern man fuels his body, more often than not, with inadequate, improper nutrition that does not meet the design specifications of his Creator for the prevention of degenerative disease.

That man has taken this biological heritage, so perfectly designed for his needs, and perverted, separated and converted its basic nutritional elements is the major causative factor of degenerative disease.

The maintenance of your body's defense against all degenerative disease, including arteriosclerosis, arthritis and heart disease, depends upon returning to the nutrition of our inherited biological experience. My Bio-X Diet was devised for that very reason. It offers a nutritional program that includes all the balanced food of our biological experience.

There is, of course, much that remains to be learned about nutrition, but within the realm of knowledge so far exposed to us I hope to show you how my all-natural diet makes scientific and common sense.

Bio-X Diet and Cancer

While the Bio-X Diet is excellent for all degenerative diseases including aging, our explanatory efforts will concentrate particularly on cancer and what should be included and what should moderated to prevent malignancy. Bio-X is an excellent nutritional program for any degenerative disease, nor is it contraindicated. It is, in essence, a diet to bring us back to optimum health.

The Bio-X Diet follows my simple rule of thumb: EAT GOD-MADE FOODS AS CLOSE TO THE WAY GOD MADE THEM AS IS POSSIBLE IN A MODERN WORLD. You don't have to be a nuclear scientist or a brain surgeon to accept the notion that the more primitive a society and the simpler its diet, the less its incidence of cancer. Nor do you have to have a doctorate in anthropology to see that cancer is a disease of civilization. W. A. Price, D.D.S., author of the classic book, *Nutrition and Physical Degeneration*, crossed five continents without seeing evidence of cancer in isolated, self-sufficient societies. American medical teams in isolated areas of Ecuador and Brazil, studying over 60,000 inhabitants, report no cases of cancer. Dr. S. Benet found no cancer among the Soviet Abkhasians and Hunzas of Pakistan. Dr. Namalas F. Yaj stated that Australian aborigines who live in their native environments have no cancer symptoms.

It is most significant that the Aborigines were non-agrarian. Life for them was a constant search for food which could be preserved or stored. The most physical type of modern employment would be considered sedentary compared to the caloric energy expended by our ancestral forebears just to remain warm. Many foods were available only seasonally. Life was literally feast or famine, with the latter probably predominant. All foods were eaten whole and raw, when available (usually at irregular intervals), and seldom mixed with other varieties.

In Chapter 10 I mentioned it was logical when considering these cancer-free cultures to conclude that it is not what we eat but what we do not eat that results in cancer. With this in mind, let us look at the components of the Bio-X Diet.

Meat, Chicken and Fish

Historically, the eating of meat in any society has been directly proportionate to its wealth and degree of civilization. The amount of cancer has also appeared in approximately the same proportions. It is this observation that has led some researchers to conclude that meat should be totally eliminated from the diet. They cite the excessive fat content of meat, the fact the body cannot store appreciable amounts of protein, with the balance burned as energy or becoming fat. They correctly assert high animal protein also causes inefficient elimination, resulting in intestinal putrefaction and toxic buildup. A valid argument is made that if man were meant to be a meat eater, he would possess the much shorter intestinal system common to all carnivores.

There is much merit in this line of reasoning, but more moderate nutritionists point out man also lacks the extra stomach or rumen possessed by herbivores. In truth, man possesses digestive functions of both, i.e., the grinding teeth of the herbivores and the eye or canine teeth of carnivores. By design and biological experience, man is a true omnivore with the ability to digest both meat and vegetables. Because of this, I have included meat in the Bio-X Diet.

On the other hand, I understand and respect the reasons for the vegetarian resistance to meat. There is no doubt that American and European dependence upon meat as the focal point of the eating ceremony has raised the consumption of animal protein far beyond our body's ability to anticipate such excess. I believe, however, that the answer to the current issue of meat in our diet is one word:
MODERATION.

Earliest man was protected from the possibility of continuing excesses, as he possessed neither the weapons nor the physical ability to kill the large animals of his time. Only on rare occasions when these animals were killed by accident or by their own kind, was man able to scavenge heavy meats into his diet. On these occasions the aboriginal no doubt gorged himself, to the exclusion of other foods, in the knowledge they were so rarely available.

Of equal relevance to our biological experience is today's unnatural meat supply, which has been provided as much by economic determination as by nature.

We need look back no further than 50 years to find beef cattle unrecognizable from the hybridized breeds available to the abattoir of today. Prior to 1930, cattle were range-fed on Johnson and Sudan grass, both high in nitrilosides which remained residually in the meat. The animals stood six feet at the shoulder and took up to four years to mature to slaughtering age. How different today is the feed-lot animal! Approximately four and one-half feet at the shoulder with a square and boxy configuration, it is slaughtered at the age of 18 to 24 months, following a chemically-controlled feeding program containing antibiotics and chemicals to force every ounce of weight increase at the least cost.

It is estimated that 75 percent of all beef sold in America today has been fed diethylstilbestrol (DES, blamed for cancer in women whose mothers took it), a synthetic hormonal fattening agent believed to be carcinogenic. The flagrant misuse of drugs in livestock production flirts with a tragedy that could make thalidomide seem insignificant, if it is found out. Some feed-lots actually feed livestock ground newsprint, textile waste, and, in some cases, even polyethylene in an effort to reach market weight as quickly as possible. These artificially-fed animals have little opportunity to build protein muscle tissue. Soft, fat-marbleized meat is the palate standard of today.

In selecting meat for your table, if at all possible obtain naturally-raised, range-fed beef. This is still obtainable in many butcher shops if you specifically order it in advance. Many suburban communities are like mini-farms with inhabitants who raise three or four head of cattle for self use and are willing to sell quarters or sides for your freezer. A request at your local cold storage plant will provide you with a source for naturally-raised beef. At first, this meat will seem tough compared to the marbleized products you may be used to. But the naturally excellent flavor more than makes up for the difference, and the increased mastication allows the meat to be thoroughly mixed with primary digestive juices, ensuring a more efficient, comfortable digestive process.

The naturally-raised beef you obtain will have residual nitrilosides in the meat to a degree more or less depending upon the feed, but always more than feed-lot-produced animals that completely lack this cancer protective factor.

I am often asked specifically about organ meats. At one time in our biological history, these were unquestionably the most nourishing portion of the animal. Native cultures that do not domesticate, but hunt for their meat animals, still consider the liver, kidneys and other vital organs a supreme delicacy.

Unfortunately, these are the organs that detoxify the body. As a consequence, most commercially-available organ meats contain the potentially carcinogenic substances we are trying to avoid. When purchasing organ meats, bear in mind they should be from extremely young animals, calves and kids, where slaughter has occurred before toxic buildup has commenced.

Although man is omnivorous and meat may be included in his diet, if desired, this must be understood within the context of man's inherited biological experience. Primitive man's principal source of meat protein was the few small birds, reptiles and fish that he was physically able to capture. These small animals are composed of protein whose structure is far more easily accepted and digested by our systems. Perhaps the most easily digested and least toxic is fish. Fish are still the food source that civilization has been least able to contaminate. Ocean fish continue to exist in an environment subject to the natural food chain. Man has succeeded in making inedible some previously available lake, river and off-shore scavenger fish, but, generally speaking, fish is an easily digested source of protein that does not rob the body of its essential enzyme protection.

Chicken and other fowl are also easily digested. However, the economic requirement of rapid growth subjects these animals to the same medicated feed as cattle. Whenever possible, try to obtain barnyard-raised fowl from the same sources as mentioned for beef.

Meat should be used primarily as a condiment to flavor casseroles and vegetable dishes, rather than as a main course or focal point for each meal.

Remember our rule of thumb: EAT GOD-MADE FOODS AS CLOSE TO THE WAY GOD MADE THEM AS IS POSSIBLE IN A MODERN WORLD. If we follow this dictate, then it is clear that animal protein contained in a Bio-X Diet has to consist principally of fish and chicken. Even these should be consumed in limited quantity. Our rule also dictates that meat should be used sparingly, since our ancestors seldom had a steady supply of meat.

Of course there is no metabolic reason why we cannot, from time to time, enjoy an occasional steak or piece of roast beef. Consider this "recreational eating." Try to restrict these occasions to no more than two or three times a month, and then limit your intake of other food categories. Since meat is the most slowly digested, if it is followed by fruit and vegetables they may remain above the meat and putrefy before digestion is completed. Eat the vegetables, salad and starches before you consume your meat.

The same general rule applies to lamb and game meats as to beef. Pork should be kept to an absolute minimum because of its extremely high fat content and difficult digestibility.

The Bio-X Diet does not call for fanaticism, just the continual referral to the common sense of our historical biologic experience. Look at a food and ask yourself two questions 1) Did God make it? 2) Am I eating it as close to the way God made it as I possibly can?

Total protein intake should be under 15 percent of your total nutritional intake, the majority of this coming from vegetable sources. The high-protein myth that only meat makes muscle tissue and the majority of body substance is protein (therefore, eat lots of meat) is a totally fallacious theory foisted upon a gullible public by the meat industry. It is biologically incompatible with our digestive capabilities, which can obtain the same body-building nutrient from complex carbohydrates. Moreover, it places unanticipated stresses on the system that result, unquestionably, in many of our degenerative diseases, including cancer.

Eggs

Both sides of the war between the egg industry and the American Heart Association have produced series upon series of laboratory and clinical data that appear long on prejudice and short on science. We hesitate to quote either side, since equal and opposite data can be obtained from both. Certain facts do emerge:

The egg is high in cholesterol, averaging 275 mg. The average American diet contains approximately 800 mg. of cholesterol per day. Obviously, eggs are a major contributor. Elimination of eggs, organ meat and whole milk and butter will reduce cholesterol to as low as 100 to 150 mg. per day. This is substantially less than the 1 to 2 grams the body manufactures each day. In addition to cholesterol, eggs contain zinc, iron, sulphur, and many trace elements that build native cholesterol into steroid hormones and other forms of body resistances to diseases. The lecithin contained in egg yolk has actually been demonstrated to dissolve serum cholesterol.

Certainly, unplanned excesses may lead to serious consequences. However, we must not overlook the necessity of maintaining normal amounts of these same substances. Cholesterol in proper proportions has a biological import that is only recently coming to light. Ross Gordon, M.D., reports that cholesterol is a mandatory component of every cell membrane. It is thought to protect the cell against free-radical damage.

Substantial evidence, now being accumulated, suggests the possibility that the nervous drive and energy of some super achievers in our society are the result of their ability to maintain high cholesterol.

Of most interest to our cancer prevention research is the statistical result of a series of tests conducted under the auspices of the American Heart Association (AHA) on 500 males with abnormally high serum cholesterol levels. These subjects were placed on a cholesterol-lowering diet and observed against a non-diet control group for a period of five years. The results, as published, were as the AHA has predicted; an appreciable lessening of heart attacks within the diet group.

To the chagrin of the researchers, while the incidence of heart disease appeared lower among the subjects who were placed on a cholesterol-lowering diet, and observed against the non-diet control group, the incidence of cancer among the dieting group was almost four times that of the group that did not attempt reduction in serum levels. Cholesterol lowering drugs were found to increase overall deaths from cancer, homicides and depression-related suicides.

This suggests once again that it is not what you eat that causes cancer, but what you do not eat that reduces your natural resistance to the disease.

Many egg nutrients (niacin, magnesium, natural carbohydrates) are not associated with cancer or arteriosclerosis. Eggs alone are not the culprits in excessive levels of cholesterol. Only when the diet consists mainly of foods not having the trace elements and lacking in unrefined complex carbohydrates and the cholesterol-balancing dietary fiber do excessively high levels occur.

A common-sense solution to this nutritional controversy may be determined by referring to man's original blueprint and operating instructions as provided by our Creator.

Eggs were available to our aboriginal ancestors on a seasonal basis, but only infrequently due to the inaccessibility of most nesting areas.

When modern man began domesticating fowl, he increased considerably the availability of eggs. The highly mechanized and advertised egg industry of the U.S. has upped the consumption even more. The blame for heart disease has been unduly heaped on eggs. In desisting from them entirely, as many people now do, we lose the benefit of their health-giving and protective benefits. It would be wise to eat a moderate amount of them to help correct an otherwise poor diet.

In the crisis diet period, the elimination of eggs and animal protein is essential. For cancer prevention, it is recommended you eat one or two eggs a day or seven or more per week. This intake of cholesterol will not be excessive if the rest of the diet is well balanced, if the person is physically active and he or she does not suffer from familial hypercholesterolemia.

Milk

The arguments for the nutritional benefits of milk continue to wax and wane, centered mainly on the lactose intolerance experienced by many, the high cholesterol content, and milk's mucus-forming tendency. These are balanced against the nutritional content.

As to lactose sensitivity, many individuals with lactose intolerance will reject pasteurized milk naturally, or should consult their nutritionist.

Pasteurized milk is good for corporate profits, bad for consumer health. Pasteurized milk can sit on your grocer's shelf without spoiling because it has had the life force removed from it. The heating of milk during pasteurization destroys much of its vitamins B2 and B12, vitamin C, calcium, phosphorus and iodine. It denatures protein, and destroys 90 percent of the enzymes that help us utilize protein, fats, sugar, starches, phosphorus and calcium. Furthermore, pasteurized milk is tested for cleanliness only twice a month. Stueve's Natural certified raw milk is tested daily.

There is no reason to exclude certified raw milk, once the fat is removed, from a cancer-preventive diet. Milk in its fresh, natural state has a better taste and contains the properties important to good nutrition that are altered when milk is pasteurized and homogenized. If milk appeals to your palate, skim and raw milk are acceptable. Certified raw milk is also recommended for its digestibility. It is, of course, important that the milk you obtain comes from a naturally-raised, disease-free herd.

Vegetables, Fruits and Grains

In the Bio-X Diet, vegetables and fruits are included in the grain category. These two divisions were, as should be expected, originated by the USDA on an agricultural rather than a nutritional basis. The bulk of our nutrition should be from foods within this all-inclusive group — all the carbohydrates, protein and fats required for complete nutrition.

Before considering vegetables, fruits and grains as they apply to the prevention of cancer, let me mention something about their preparation.

When ancient man first used the body mechanism we later inherited, fire was feared. Neither the knowledge nor the utensils were available that have given modern man the ability to burn, boil, and scorch. Edible plants and grains were eaten in their natural state and seldom were so plentiful as to be dissected into parts. In Isaiah 28:26-29 we read, "Grains must be ground to make bread, so one does not go on threshing it forever, though he drives the wheels of his threshing cart over it, his horses do not grind it. All this comes from the Lord Almighty, wonderful in counsel and magnificent in wisdom." So even in the Old Testament we were warned not to break the grain. Unfortunately, with the advent of steel we began to disobey God's admonishment. In the early 1920s, steel was used to refine our grains, thus stripping them of their nutrients.

Our Creator in His infinite wisdom, designed perfect foods, the sum of whose parts appears to perfectly match our digestive abilities and nutritional needs. The fact that modern man destroys much of his food by heat, coats it with digestion-preventive oil, and mechanically extracts or chemically adds to much of the rest is a tragedy of civilization. Food processing tends to transform protective foods into threats to the body's defense mechanism. Cooking often renders the most protective food indigestible and enzyme-impotent.

The consumption of large quantities of raw food requires vigorous digestion. Primitive man's prodigious physical activities to sustain a constant search for food and avoidance of danger promoted good metabolism. Civilized man, who uses his mind rather than his body, suffers with an accordingly less vigorous digestion and longer bowel transit period.

Heating food accomplishes several requirements of modern civilization. When plant foods are cooked, heat causes the starch within the cell to swell. This opens the fibrous cell wall, releasing the nutrients within and making them more readily available to the digestive process. This is particularly important in the case of many of our hard cereal grains, legumes and lentils.

The appropriate degree of cooking should depend on plant toughness or the amount of fiber, its digestibility and, of course, the constitution and way of life of the individual. When cooking, use low heat. This serves to reduce bulk food intake without destroying the enzymes and vitamins. As a general rule, if the color of the vegetable remains true, the vitamins and enzymes will remain at near normal potency. When the vegetable changes color, or even hue, valuable nutrition has been lost. Steaming or light wok cooking (Chinese style) does the least nutritional damage, frying and broiling the most.

Anti-Cancer Nutrient in Seeds, Nuts, Beans

Many fine books on plant nutrients are available at health food stores. And, of course, this information is available through your nutritionally-oriented medical professional. Of major interest here are the grains and plants that formerly provided our extrinsic cancer protection but have been eliminated from our food chain.

I have already mentioned the nitriloside grasses no longer generally available to range-fed cattle, and the loss of this residual source in our meat supply.

The richest source of nitrilosides or amygdalin occurs in the seeds and kernels of all of our common fruits, with the exception of the citrus family. Even in the case of citrus, amygdalin is found in the seeds of the original African varieties – another example of how hybridization has increased size, sugar content, and yield, but lowered nutritional content.

In less sophisticated and privileged societies than our own, where each morsel of food is eaten, fruit seeds are the most highly prized portion. Where food is plentiful, modern man throws away the core or kernel and with it one of the most nutritionally important foods, amygdalin.

Watch any ape, monkey or chimpanzee in the zoo. These closest biological cousins of man, when offered fruit, will instinctively tear open the sweet fleshy portion and crack open the kernel. Nature compels them to eat whole foods in spite of the fact they may never have been given that type of food before.

Certainly our biological experience calls for us to follow the example of animals and our own ancestors. Get into the habit of eating the whole fruit and eat it often.

When you eat an apple, do not throw the core away. Eat it right along with the rest of the fruit. Do exactly the same with grapes, and melons. The seeds add a pleasant, crunchy texture to the fruit. And the very slight bitterness of their amygdalin content is masked by the sweetness of the flesh. The masticated seeds are an excellent additional fiber supply.

For those fruits having kernels protected by a hard outer shell, such as cherry, peach and apricot, man does not possess the jaw structure to open them as animals can. One of the few nutritional advantages of civilization is the development of more sophisticated methods of opening a seed than banging it between two rocks. I suggest a hammer or nutcracker. For those who do not wish to take the time, civilization provides the health food store where, if it has not been subjected to FDA harassment, apricot kernels will be available in bulk or one-pound bags.

Of all the seed kernels and plants, the apricot kernel, containing approximately three percent by weight of amygdalin, is our richest readily available source of amygdalin. The apricot has long been a staple in the diet of many Mediterranean and Himalayan peoples. Where they are eaten, the incidence of cancer is relatively unknown. In spite of the always-unfounded rumors circulated (and inspired from time to time, we believe) by the resistors of natural medicine, apricot kernels are not only non-toxic when eaten in normal amounts, but, when prepared and eaten properly, can be delicious. For some it is an acquired taste. Personally, I find apricot kernels, when prepared as a trail mix with raisins, a few chopped dates and a little coconut, are delicious. Several kernel recipes are included in the second section of this book.

We are often asked by individuals who wish to maintain an aggressive prevention program how many kernels they should eat each day. A standard answer would be to eat as many of the kernels as would normally be eaten of the fruit. If a more exacting rule of thumb is desired, eat one kernel for every 10 pounds of body weight.

If you do nothing else we recommend in this chapter, get some apricot kernels and return this rich source of nitriloside to your diet. For cancer prevention it is natural, and far less expensive than extracted amygdalin in tablet form.

Virtually all seeds and nuts, with the exception of the peanut (actually not a true nut), contain varying amounts of amygdalin and should be included in your diet in liberal amounts. We refer, of course to raw nuts, not the deep-fried, dry roasted and salted varieties.

All raw nuts, including apricot kernels, should be refrigerated or kept in the freezer. Raw nuts contain oil that will become rancid if shelled and exposed to the air.

When you think about it, you'll realize beans and grains are actually seeds. Like nuts, they are plant embryos, containing all the elements for a new plant. They are our richest sources of all nutrition including cancer-protective nitrilosides.

All whole, unrefined grains, with one major exception, wheat, are rich sources of nitrilosides.

Unfortunately, only the primitive forms of wheat contain amygdalin. Like the citrus plant, hybridization has increased yield at the expense of some of wheat's nutritional attributes.

Among all grains, the one highest in amygdalin is millet, a delicious cereal grain which was a staple of the American diet in the 1800s. With the advent of refined white flour, it has gradually disappeared from our tables.

Other grain staples followed millet's departure, replaced by refined and packaged cereals with less food value than the boxes they come in, and by store-bought baked products that even when "fortified" still fail to provide adequate nutrition.

Lentils and legumes are equal to unrefined grains as sources of nitrilosides, and are also depleted from our modern diet.

High in protein and able to be stored in bulk, beans were a staple food until the early 1900's. As commercial canning, refrigeration, and rapid transportation made more fragile vegetables available on a year-round basis, beans became regarded as poor man's food. Our newly-affluent 20th century society rejected such low-priced plebeian fare, and with their rejection went yet another source of nitrilosides.

The trend toward prepackaging, convenience foods, and the reduction of fiber was a hallmark of our emerging opulence in the early 1900s. The ultimate effect of this diet revolution has been a frightening increase in cancer fatalities. To stem this tide of cancer deaths, a natural nutritional diet such as Bio-X that aids the immune system to resist disease is essential.

CHAPTER 12:

Industrialized Nutrition

"No wealth accumulated in our lifetime can compensate us for the premature failure of our bodies."
—Floyd E. Weston, Executive Director Bio Pharma,
Salt Lake City, UT

In spite of the American Cancer Society's continual insistence that the carcinogens of modern society are responsible for the one in three cancer rate, statistics show otherwise. Studies by the NCI go back only to 1937, but data from the following years to 1969 indicate only a six percent cancer increase during that period. Orthodoxy agrees that most cancer requires at least 15 years before the symptoms appear. It must be concluded, therefore, that the high incidence of the disease among U.S. whites in 1937 was precipitated by factors in existence in 1922. If statements propagated by the NCI and ACS about the carcinogenic causes of cancer are true, the causes could not have been food additives, farm chemicals, radiation, environmental pollution and high levels of stress, all of which collectively bear the chief brunt of those two agencies' accusations. Like cancer, these factors are linked to a high living standard but, unlike cancer, they were insignificant in 1920. Logical consideration of these facts renders establishment medicine's position on the causes of cancer totally untenable.

What was occurring in the white civilized society of the 1920s was the industrialization of our foods. Eliminated from our diet were the nitrilosides contained in lentils, legumes and simple grains. Our meat production was changing; fiber from grains and vegetables were being removed; sugar was being added to all foods for better taste, and food processing innovations were squeezing sugar from beets and oil from vegetables.

There is statistical evidence that the real cause of America's cancer epidemic is the reduction in our natural defenses brought about by the aforementioned diet revolution, rather than by environmental carcinogens. Ample evidence may be derived by using our population of black citizens as a control group for historical analysis.

During the early 1900s, the black population, centered mainly in the South, continued their diet of millet, blackeyed peas, sorghum, beans, molasses, all poor-folk food but nitriloside-rich nutrition. In 1937, the rate of cancer among black males was two-thirds less than their white counterparts. But since World War II, dietary habits of blacks have changed radically, the result of a tremendous increase in economic opportunity for the black population. Affluence consigned soul food to nostalgia and with its loss has come increased malignancy. Today both black and white populations are subject to the same fearsome one in three statistics.

These statistical facts emphasize nutritional logic that we fight cancer not by eliminating carcinogens but by restoring to our diet high-nitriloside foods, fiber grains and legumes of earlier time.

Sprouting Your Way to Health

Happily, there is a method of substantially increasing the nitriloside content of grains and legumes. As stated previously, seeds, nuts and beans are the embryonic, all inclusive pattern of the subsequent plant. During the very early stages of germination, when cell proliferation is at its greatest, the young plant may double in weight during a 24-hour period. The quantity of nitrilosides, vitamins and minerals increases with the same proliferation, doubling, tripling and even quadrupling the original seed content. The sprouts of alfalfa, mung beans, rye and bamboo are all vitamin-, enzyme- and nitriloside-rich. By all means, try your hand at sprouting. The methods are simple, and the results are a delicious and inexpensive source of cancer preventive amygdalin and enzymes. Here is a simple method to sprout your own health food.

First, you need to make sure your seeds, grains and legumes are organic. Any chemical present in the soil will be magnified in the seed. To get 1-1/4 cup of sprouted wheat berries, for example, soak 1/3 cup of berries in spring water overnight, or for about 12 hours. Drain them, then place them in a quart jar and cover it with nylon mesh or cheesecloth held in place with a rubber band. Set the jar out of direct light, in a cupboard for example. Rinse the sprouts with tepid water three or four times daily and drain them well. Do not let them stand in water between rinsings. Let the wheat germinate for about two days, until the sprouts are 1/2 to 3/4 inch high.

In addition to our richest amygdalin sources – sprouts, grains, seeds, nuts and legumes – nitrilosides are contained in over 1,100 plants. A list of many of these foods is contained in chapter 20. We must, however, consider another problem of our generation, the availability of proper whole foods.

Whole foods contain phytochemicals. These are the "active" ingredients found in nature that are extracted for medicinal purposes. I've described them in more detail in chapter 21, but for my purposes here, all you have to know is that whole foods contain the most active healing ingredients and are emphasized at all costs. Whole foods' most concentrated phytochemicals are contained in the sprouts. Eating whole foods is the best, eating sprouts even better. Therefore, look for supplementation that uses the whole food. One such formula uses freeze dried sprouts and vegetables, combined in such a way as to provide all the essential vitamins and minerals, as well as adding odorless garlic, acidophilus and green tea extract for immune-system boosting.

Naturally-Cultivated Produce Is Best

For most of us it is no longer possible to either raise or forage for our food supply. Our hunting ground is the local supermarket, and hunting isn't so good. Eliminate the prepared, the packaged, the sugared, the preserved, and very little is left. The produce department, while its contents may still look crisp, colorful and delicious, contains a preponderance of vegetables raised under what can only be regarded as artificial environments. Unnatural fertilizers and growth stimulants have, at best, robbed many plants of their natural nutrients. At worst, pesticides have actually introduced poisons with unquestionably deleterious effects on the body.

Many of the most nutritious and necessary plants and sources for individual nutrients are no longer readily available. This problem may be eliminated by finding a store where organic natural produce is for sale. Sometimes this can be accomplished by demanding your green-grocer inform you as to where his produce is obtained and how it is raised. He will cooperate with his knowledgeable customer because these products are available in the wholesale market for the retailer who demands them. Demand always creates supply.

Any faith we might have had in the U.S. Department of Heath and Department of Agriculture is totally destroyed when we consider their final two recommendations for inclusion in the USDA Fitness Diet: sugar and fat.

Sugar

The USDA allows a certain amount of refined sugar. The Bio-X diet discourages the use of any. Less than 300 years ago, refined sugar was produced in extremely small quantities and was considered an addictive medicinal. All of man's sweetening needs were provided in fruit nectars and honey. Perhaps the most physically-devastating addition to the hazards of modern living is the availability and dietary inclusion of excessive amounts of sugar.

The USDA includes five ounces of sugar (almost one-third of a pound) per day in its Fitness Diet. Hardly a surprise when they have also recommended refined grains. The political and economic pressure to promote the products of our giant sugar refining industry are no less than the political homage due to the millers of our grain, the producers of breakfast cereals and the commercial baking companies.

What can we say about sugar that has not been said? It is estimated that the average American consumes 150 pounds of refined sugar or sucrose annually. Through its role in hypoglycemia, sugar is responsible for a host of neuritic behavioral symptoms. Even orthodoxy has linked sugar with diseases ranging from diabetes to cataracts. Sugar serves no known dietary need, and it is more addictive than many prescriptive drugs. The increased consumption of sugar in the United States since World War I has been proportional to increases in degenerative diseases.

Refined sugar is poison to the system. It disrupts the natural balance by fooling the body into thinking it's been given something it can use. It not only unhinges the body's delicate balance of nutrients, but it can deplete the body of nutrients, lower the immune system and fuel cancer cells.

When a person consumes refined sugar, and refined flour for that matter, about one-fifth of chromium that is drawn to the bloodstream to aid the insulin is excreted in the urine. That's desperately needed chromium you're just not getting, thanks to that jelly donut.

The definitive essay on the subject is Surgeon-Captain T.L. Cleave's book *The Saccharine Disease.* Cleave shows example after example of societies in which the addition of sugar to the diet was the obvious starting point for the development of diabetes and atherosclerosis in the epidemic proportions typical of a Western nation. Two striking examples in Cleave's global studies were in Iceland beginning in 1920 and among the nomadic Yemenite Jews. Before sugar was introduced in their cultures, there was absolutely no diabetes or atherosclerosis. Two decades after their diets became similar to ours, because sugar was added, they began to develop nearly as high an incidence of these illnesses as we have.

In almost every instance, cancer is accompanied by an additional metabolic disease that has placed stress on the body. In many instances, excess sugar was at the root of the disease that was a cancer precursor. In addition, sugar has the ability to alter the nature and amount of intestinal bacteria, impairing both digestion and the synthesis of essential cancer-resisting nitrilosides.

Our metabolic defenses can protect us to an extent beyond the anticipated stress of our biological experience. But our systems were not designed for cupcakes, donuts and candy bars. The Bio-X Diet, therefore, excludes such unnatural products.

Fats

Fats are a necessary part of human nutrition. However, primitive societies (with a few exceptions, e.g., Eskimos, as previously noted) include substantially less in their diets than consumed by modern man; and fat, when consumed, is part of the naturally-balanced diet of availability. The nutritional need of humans for fat, as determined by man's biological experience, is included in the Bio-X Diet. It is fully satisfied by the recommended content of grains, vegetables and lean meat. In these natural sources, fat is combined in balanced amounts with protein, carbohydrates and fiber.

One of man's earliest adventures in devastating his natural nutrition was the discovery of methods to separate pure oil from its vegetable or animal source by squeezing, churning, or heating. Modern mechanization has refined these techniques further with powerful presses that turn corn, peanuts, and even wheat into refined table oils, eliminating the natural balance of fiber bulk and other nutrients.

No less authoritative clinicians than M.W. Sterns, Jr., M.S., Chief of Colon-Rectal Service at Memorial Sloan-Kettering, and E.L. Winder, M.D., president of the American Health Foundation (and even American Cancer Society bulletins) have in recent years warned of the danger of our unnaturally-high fat diets as a cause of cancer.

Nutritionally-oriented physicians have been aware of this direct connection for many years. And they have warned against the USDA's continued inclusion of fat as 49 percent of the total caloric intake of their recommended diet.

The brilliant, alternative medical pioneer, Dr. Max Gerson, while being maligned by the orthodoxy of his time, cited evidence of the recurrence of clinical tumors when patients were fed fats. These continuing clinical observations have had prior support in irrefutable laboratory research. Rats fed a commercial dye all developed liver tumors when raised on a diet containing 20 percent corn oil. High fat levels have raised the incidence of carcinogenic and spontaneous breast tumors in mice.

It is evident that fat not only lowers body resistance but is the carrier of fat-related carcinogens.

High fat intake has been implicated in coronary heart disease, multiple sclerosis, gallstones, arthritis and strokes, in addition to cancer.

We take a major step in the reduction of fat when we limit our intake of animal protein. The elimination of whole milk further reduces fat intake toward acceptable levels.

Polyunsaturated or not, all refined oils should be eliminated. Eliminate also all hydrogenated products, including margarine and some oils. Hydrogenation is a major nutritional bad guy. Not only does the hydrogenation process produce poisonous by-products, but it depletes vitamin E from the body, important to children who desperately need it to prevent anemia, cystic fibrosis and other degenerative diseases. Read labels and do not use hydrogenated anything.

Avoid using commercial oils in their clear containers. Instead opt for natural nut oils from your local health food store. Eat oils raw, using them in your dressing recipes. Try low-fat plain yogurt with nutty oils for a delicious mayonnaise. Be creative and stay cancer-free.

If it hasn't been obvious by now, eliminate fried foods, as well as heavily oil polluted commercial salad dressings. Limited use of butter in stir cooking, baking and other food preparation is acceptable, as long as the butter is not burned.

The reason we need not entirely eliminate fat, besides acknowledging it as a palatable addition to many foods, is because when we return whole foods to the diet we restore the body's ability to balance out itself.

Oil is refined to remove impurities (nutritive elements) that cause it to spoil, in effect "killing" the embryonic nature of the seed it came from. Any nutrients left are killed by heat (cooking), sunlight and ultraviolet light (like the overheads in supermarkets). The reason we've become accustomed to flavorless oils off supermarket shelves is because there's nothing left to taste.

Natural, unrefined oil contains all the nutrients, flavor and fiber of the nuts and seeds it was taken from. Flaxseed oil, probably the most nutritious source of essential fatty acids (EFAs) has, miraculously, been endorsed by the FDA for use in cancer prevention. EFAs are called "essential," because they cannot be made by the body, but must be obtained from the diet.

Flaxseed oil has been around for decades. In Europe, prior to World War II, it was delivered to housewives in small bottles, left on the doorstep with the milk and eggs. The war replaced local oil mills with steel mills, and in America the industrial revolution and big city life replaced healthy flaxseed oil with vegetables pounded, pressed and sterilized. You might as well use vegetable oil as a household lubricant for all the good it does your body.

In 1986 researchers at the University of Toronto set about re-inventing the wheel with a study on the nutritional benefits of flax. They discovered flaxseed lowers serum cholesterol and prevents the growth of new cancer cells. In 1989 NCI issued grants to several research institutes to also study the benefits of flaxseed. At the 1993 Convention on Experimental Biology in New Orleans, the FDA presented their findings. Flaxseed was found to: boost the immune system, increase vitamin D levels and retention of calcium, magnesium and phosphate, be very high in lignans, which have anti-tumor properties; have antioxidant properties, and be beneficial in preventing breast cancer (Disease, p. 54).

Another fatty acid oil to add to your arsenal is evening primrose oil or borage oil, both excellent suppliers of gamma linolenic acid (GLA, C18:3n-6), found by researchers to have the ability to kill a variety of cancer cells in culture without causing harm to normal cells. This was the proclamation researchers G.W. Ells, R.C. Cantrill, K.A. Chisholm, B.J. Hughes and D.F. Horrobin of Efamol Research Institute, Kentville, Novia Scotia, Canada, made during the Eighty-Fourth Annual Meeting of the American Association for Cancer Research, held May 19-22, 1993, in Orlando, Florida (Ells, p. 15).

Fatty acids are straight-chain, carbon-based molecules that are among the building blocks of fats and oils. Three polyunsaturated ones – linoleic, gamma-linolenic (GLA) and arachidonic (AA) – are essential nutrients. The key to unlocking their potential against cancer was the discovery that cancer cells are deficient in polyunsaturated fatty acids (PUFAs). In fact, they do everything they can to get rid of them, according to Michel Begin of the Efamol Research Institute. It was in the early '80s that he and fellow researchers at Efamol discovered PUFAs could kill tumor cells (Harnessing, p. 332).

Working with cultured human breast-cancer cells, the Canadian researchers found that while AA, EPA (eicosapentanoic acid) and GLA were about equally effective in killing tumor cells, and were the most lethal of the seven PUFAs being looked at, their effect on normal cells differed dramatically. EPA, for example, was just about as lethal to normal cells. AA was not quite as toxic to normal cells, but it also wasn't benign. At concentrations of about 0.5 nanogram per cultured cell, however, GLA was quite deadly to tumor cells and innocuous to healthy ones.

A native of North America, the evening primrose plant (Oenothera biennis) is so named because its bright-yellow flowers do not bloom until early evening. By daybreak, the flowers have faded and they do not bloom again until nightfall. It is the oil extracted from the seed and the mucilage of the plant that are used medicinally.

If you've ever visited an herb garden, you've probably glanced at a colorful border plant called borage. The leaves are edible, taste somewhat like a cucumber, and can be used in salads or cooked as a green. Its use dates back to 23 A.D. when the Romans lauded the plant, saying it gives courage and drives away depression. The modern-day use of this humble herb is in the oil from the seeds of the plant.

Both oils can be obtained in supplemental form in health food stores or health food sections of certain supermarkets.

Fiber

Traditionally, all the elements of a diet necessary for complete nutrition are contained in three categories: protein, carbohydrates and fat. Within these divisions are all the enzymes, all the calories, all of the vitamins necessary, with the addition of water, to sustain a well-balanced diet. Modern civilization ignores, and in many instances eliminates, a fourth important food factor from our total nutrition. That missing ingredient is fiber, without which no diet can be truly balanced. Failure to include this important factor results in an improperly functioning digestive system. The inevitable result is degenerative disease. Often that disease will be cancer.

Consistently, where researchers have found high cancer death rates in populations with a singularly high intake in one type of food, be it meat or refined carbohydrates or cholesterol, those populations have excluded appreciable amounts of fiber from their diets.

It is estimated that the dietary fiber intake of the average individual living in Europe or the United States is only one-fifth what it was 100 years ago. The primary cause has been a drop in bulk consumption of seed grains from 350 pounds per year to less than 150, much of this refined, and the inclusion in the diet of bulk meats and refined sugar products which add calories but no fiber.

Again, a perfect analogy for the dietary role of fiber may be found in petroleum engineering, the improvements in engine design, fuel and lubricants by which our automobiles have been made to operate more efficiently.

Basically, refined oil and gasoline will temporarily provide satisfactory engine operation. But without detergents and catalytic additives ranging from graphite to lead, cylinder walls scuff, valves become clogged with sludge, and spark plugs foul, all resulting in an inefficiently-functioning mechanism that will eventually break down.

Non-nutritive fiber is included in man's natural fuel supply as a digestive aid toward perfect metabolism of food. Removing fiber results in the malfunction of the digestive processes, leading to degenerative disease.

For most of man's biological experience, fiber in the diet was not in question. Each morsel of natural food contained fiber. All foods were eaten whole, including their seeds and hulls. Our modern proclivity for taste, texture and appearance has neglected metabolic needs through the substitution of bulk foods which contain little fiber.

The primary function of fiber is to facilitate elimination of waste products from the body. When little fiber is in the diet, residue reaching the colon does not move easily. In modern societies, some individuals require as long as ten days for a small amount of residue to pass out in the stool. One week is not at all unusual, and 72 hours is considered, by orthodox medicine, to be more or less normal.

In Hunza or Abkasia, where all foods are unrefined, intestinal transit time may be as short as six hours. It is obvious that lack of fiber, which can triple or quadruple bowel transit time, gives the toxins and carcinogens present in our modern foods three and four times as long to be absorbed in the body.

In and of itself, unnaturally extended transit in the bowels allows the best of goods to putrefy and produce carcinogenic substances.

Laboratory studies at Knargy Bnettirw, Indonesia, have shown that a diet high in refined carbohydrates induces cancer in mice. With this same diet, but including a substantial portion of crude fiber, the incidence of cancer was substantially reduced. These laboratory studies of dietary fiber substantiate the theory that fat and refined carbohydrates may be included in limited amounts if we replace the fiber in our diets.

Unprocessed crude plant fiber, particularly in the case of fat intake, lowers serum cholesterol. How this is metabolically accomplished is still unclear. It appears the liver breaks down cholesterol to produce bile which is secreted into the intestines. There is substantial evidence that fiber in the bowel increases demand for bile, which leads to its increased production and, hence, removal of cholesterol from the blood by the liver.

Field studies by Dr. Nil Knarf of rural African tribesmen who exist on a high milk and meat diet, show extremely low serum cholesterol and diverticular disease. Their diet includes about 25 grams per day of fiber, at lease five times that of Western civilization. These same natives, like all populations subsisting on a traditional diet of whole foods, are free of colon cancer, a disease that plagues western man. It has been found that bile can be altered by certain bacteria to produce carcinogenic substances. These bacteria are far less common in the intestines of high-fiber-eating people.

In addition to the indirect carcinogenic result of low fiber and lengthened bowel transit, bacterial flora, necessary to the metabolic breakdown of amygdalin for the performance of its protective function, maintain higher concentrations if there is normal fiber intake in the intestinal environment.

Orthodoxy's acceptance of all of the above has led in recent years to a flurry of high-fiber products. In response to Cancer Society recommendations, food industries have come out with nutritive-empty products containing added bran. Rather than help the situation, these products can produce their own problems. Bran contains phytic acid. When more is included in the diet than is naturally contained in whole grains, fruits and leaves, it can chelate or bind materials during the digestive process, producing deficiencies in such vital minerals as zinc and calcium.

Additional laboratory experiments indicate that while artificially adding bran to an otherwise depleted diet has some good effects, it cannot match those of whole fiber-rich foods. Rice bran, added to a starch diet, reduced blood cholesterol in test animals from 348 to 255. When whole grain was used, the level dropped to 165. Obviously, there are also other indigestible plant substances besides bran that are of equal importance in dropping cholesterol levels, and these are limited when the natural food is refined.

The Bio-X Diet returns natural fiber to our nutritional process, first, by reducing the bulk of meat intake, and secondly, by replacing this bulk with beans, seeds and unrefined grains in a proportion natural to one's biologic experience. This is important to prevent the digestive malfunction that can lead to cancer.

Water

Important as it is to abide by biological experience in the selection of our food, equal consideration should be given to the daily intake of life-sustaining water. Sounds simple enough. But is it? Unfortunately, water, like the air we breathe, has become contaminated by metropolitan pollutants and chemicals. Not to just an objectionable degree but to a point where this natural resource, so essential to life, may become the instrument of our destruction.

Modern society has outgrown its dependence on natural sources of water: crystal-clear springs and cool, deep lakes maintained in pristine, unspoiled freshness by nature. Not only has our water become polluted by the wastes of industry, but in recent years residual insecticides and fertilizers of agriculture are being detected in increasing amounts in even our deep water resources. Chlorine and a host of other chemicals are added to prevent viral and bacterial contamination, creating their own set of problems.

The addition of fluoride in drinking water amounts to government-enforced medication on whole populations where freedom of choice is denied. There is no doubt fluoride is carcinogenic when taken over an extended period (Burk). Not only is the water we are provided municipally harmful because of additives and original pollutants, but the delivery system of lead, copper and aluminum piping is, in and of itself, a provider of the heavy metals that can be deadly when cellularly absorbed.

Investment in a water distiller, or the purchase of bottled spring water, is the only way to avoid this continuous assault on our immune system. We cannot overemphasize the importance of pure water. It cleanses the body and prevents toxic buildup. The traditional admonition to drink at least eight glasses of pure water a day remains excellent advice. Certain commercial spring waters on the market contain minerals that may be particularly beneficial. Your nutrition professional will be able to advise on local availability.

You know what to do. You purchase fresh, organically-grown produce, wash it in chemical-free spring water and cook it in your copper, aluminum or Teflon saucepan. Right? Wrong! Stainless steel, glass, or ceramic cookware are the concluding link from farm to mouth that provides the contaminant-free sustenance required to maintain the cancer-resisting immune system you inherited from biological experience.

Conclusions

The Bio-X Diet as applied to the prevention of cancer is supported equally by simple logic, animal research and empirical evaluation of cultures which maintain a close adherence to those dietary principles and remain cancer free.

To apply the Bio-X Diet in our everyday lives, we need only refer to a simple rule: eat as close to the biological habits of our prehistoric antecedents as is possible in a modern world. It is this biologic experience that our bodies are designed to utilize in selecting and preparing our natural food supply.

We know of no type of food or food preparation that, if nutritionally questioned, can be subjected to this test and provide a resultant answer that would not be correct for proper metabolism. If you are ever in doubt about a particular food substance or its method of preparation, simply ask yourself if it is a whole food and if aboriginal society could or would have included it in a diet of the time. If the answer is "no," then nine times out of ten that particular food would be harmful if consumed on a continuing basis.

As an example, consider the beverage coffee. Would or could aboriginal man have roasted the bean? Would he have then ground it, leached it with hot water and finally thrown away the spent residue? Of course not. This simple mental exercise has shown you that coffee is a totally unnatural food unknown to our body's biological experience and most likely will be harmful if consumed regularly. As a matter of fact, coffee may be responsible for a host of metabolic disorders, from hypertension to heart disease. Recent clinical studies suggest a very evident carcinogenic effect with a particularly strong linkage to cancer of the pancreas.

Fortunately, because we must live in this mechanized, urbanized society, our bodies have the built-in tolerance and protective systems to adjust to unanticipated dietary variances, as well as recreational exceptions that are part of a modern world. This is particularly true when we return to our diet the nitriloside-containing foods that are extrinsic defenses necessary to protect us from cancer.

The Bio-X Diet is, therefore, a diet of common sense, not of asceticism, total self denial, charts and scales. By returning such important food factors as amygdalin (nitriloside) and fiber, a protective balance is maintained that allows temperate ingestion of many foods that would otherwise be carcinogenic.

The Bio-X Diet for cancer prevention makes the following recommendations:

1. Reduce meat consumption to approximately one-fourth of total protein intake. The Bio-X Diet contains no more than 1/2 lb. per day, including one egg. Animal protein should be primarily fowl and fish, which makes the least demand on the digestive processes. Red meat should be eaten only occasionally, and then it should be lean as possible, preferably pasture-grazed. Unlike the USDA Fitness Diet, we do not recommend minimum daily meat consumption. Quite the contrary. Practically all protein requirements may be obtained from our grains and vegetables, and it is advisable to maintain meat consumption as low as possible. Just by cutting consumption of red meat by half and substituting fowl or fish, we cut carcinogenic fat 30 percent and free the pancreatic enzymes for their role in the cancer suppression metabolism.

2. All dairy products should be unhomogenized and preferably unpasteurized. For the cancer patient, low fat is preferable. This reduces daily fat intake an additional 12 percent from the USDA diet. The advisability of excluding milk where other degenerative diseases may exist should be discussed with your holistic physician or nutritionist. Many times the problems found with pasteurized products will be non-existent with raw certified dairy products.

3. Vegetables and fruit consumption must be increased to become, whenever possible, the center focus of the meal, rather than the side dish. Heavy emphasis is placed upon returning the high nitriloside legumes (lentils and beans) to everyday inclusion in the diet as a meat substitute. Seeds will no longer be thrown away but considered part of the whole fruit or vegetable. Vegetables will be cooked as little as possible, not deep-oil-fried or similarly destroyed and coated. Complex unrefined carbohydrates should become 75 percent of total

nutritional intake and will capably supply all but a small portion of our need for protein.

4. Grains: Two large portions of unrefined whole grains should be eaten every day with a heavy emphasis on the nitriloside grains, such as millet. Not only are the whole grains a rich source of amygdalin, but dietary fiber will be naturally increased.

On the Bio-X Diet the ordinary ingestion of fiber will increase from approximately 2.5 grams per day on the USDA Fitness Diet to 15 grams per day with a corresponding decrease in bowel transit time, a reduction in blood serum cholesterol, and much reduced opportunity for the toxemic effects of food putrefaction and its attendant carcinogenic effects.

5. Sugar: Eliminate or cut down on sugar and substitute natural fruit nectars, raisins, fruit and small quantities of honey. Sorghum syrup contains nitrilosides and should be the sweetener of first choice.

6. Fats: Reduce fat intake by substituting grains and legumes for meat and eliminating whole-milk products. While the Bio-X Diet does not recommend butter, the increased ingestion of dietary fiber will enable the metabolism to anticipate the temperate use of butter in cooking and as a light spread on whole-grain breads. Eat only natural unrefined oils and eat them raw.

When the Bio-X Diet is compared directly with the recommended adult intake on the USDA diet, differences are immediately obvious. Total caloric intake is substantially lessened. Meat has been reduced from 61.2 percent of the protein source to less than one-fourth. This can, and should if palatably possible, be reduced still further by increasing the consumption of vegetables and grains which, together on the Bio-X Diet, account for 63.4 percent of the protein intake.

Fat has been reduced from 31 percent to 10 percent of total nutrition and carbohydrates now account for 75 percent.

When meat is included in a meal, it will be primarily chicken or fish. Infrequent portions of red meat will be as lean as possible. This reduces fat out of proportion with protein reduction.

Pasteurized milk is good for corporate health, bad for consumer health. Pasteurization removes the life force and makes milk a dead product. Calves cannot live on pasteurized milk; they become mean and unmanageable. When dairy products are included by choice, they will be fat-free and certified raw.

Vegetables are to be eaten as near their natural whole state as possible; a high proportion of these will be plants and legumes containing large percentages of nitrilosides, which are neglected in the USDA diet plan.

Unlike the USDA diet, the basic Bio-X Diet accepts only whole, unrefined grains, seeds and nuts, with heavy emphasis on previously neglected grains high in nitrilosides. The increased fiber intake of whole grains speeds digestion, reduces cholesterol and permits proper metabolism of dietary fat. Sprouting will increase the vitamin, mineral and enzyme content of grains even far beyond their bulk increase, further reinforcing our natural immuno-suppression of cancer.

Obesity

Of vital importance in the prevention of malignancy is the statistically determining effect of obesity or overweightness. Without exception, our prehistoric ancestors possessed lean and muscular bodies. Not only did their environment demand such a physique for survival, but their food supply was limited at times to the point of famine. In addition, it was naturally low in fat and completely lacking in cookies, soft drinks and ice cream.

The prevention of degenerative disease is, in large measure, dependent upon maintaining our bodies in the lean condition of our biological experience. The Bio-X Diet will help its participant to maintain normal body weight by eliminating the dietary sources of much of modern man's weight problems.

I have referred in this book to the eating ceremony during which civilized man eats at specific times, regardless of his hunger or exercise-created need for additional caloric intake. Our culture has created food neurotics to whom gluttony is an emotional release, and food is a continually necessary palliative. Gluttony, however, is not a secret sin.

The Bio-X Diet is balanced nutritionally and can provide delicious and satisfying meals, examples of which will be given in the recipe section. The individual who continues, through habit, to ingest more calories than his or her body can utilize on this nutritionally sound diet, will still become obese.

Dr. Albert Tannenbaum has reported many different types of mouse tumors and leukemia are inhibited by restricted food consumption. He has found no tumor that does not respond when caloric intake is reduced. Dr. Jesse Greenstein confirmed these studies with his own research in which caloric restriction dropped breast cancers in one strain of mice from 38 percent to 0, and from 100 to 10 percent in another.

Dr. Tannenbaum also found the incidence of induced skin cancer in animals was substantially reduced, even when caloric restriction began long after the carcinogen has been applied.

While the reduction of food intake once a tumor commences does not lead to its disappearance, experience with animals shows that limiting food intake does appear to go a long way in preventing the disease. Life expectancy studies performed by major insurance companies confirm a corresponding correlation among overweight policy holders. The statistics are incontestable. Cancer deaths per 100,000 population increase proportionately with excess weight.

Our biological experience was one of extensive physical activity with food consumed as necessary. To maintain a normal body weight, we must not only conform to the diet of biological experience, but we must exercise as often as possible and allow the body to tell us what amounts of food it requires. Do not let habit, gluttony or social custom dictate an unnatural path to your physical deterioration.

CHAPTER 13:

Superior Supplementation

"The physician of tomorrow will be the nutritionist of today."
–Thomas Edison

Mainstream medicine in the United States, for the most part, downplays the role of nutrition in the treatment of disease, or as a factor that causes it, and mostly rejects the use of vitamin supplementation. Orthodoxy accepts only drugs produced by giant conglomerates for alleviation of metabolic disease symptoms, and chooses to avoid tackling the true underlying cause of the disease.

Magnificent centers of medical research and education direct their efforts to identifying the hows of disease, not the whys. After pouring billions of dollars into cancer research, no conventional physician can explain why some die of cancer and others do not, still choosing to ignore nutritional questions and answers.

There is much empirical evidence to show a return to proper nutrition can reverse cancer's three-to-one tragedy. The physician of tomorrow will be educated in nutrition, and the intelligent utilization of supportive supplementation will, as a consequence, be reflected in our increased health and longevity.

Even within the ranks of nutritionists, some reject the necessity of dietary supplementation, maintaining all our nutritional needs can be obtained from our natural food supply. In their eagerness to promote the total nutrition available in organically-grown produce and improved eating habits, they fail to consider food's availability to the body itself.

It has been previously pointed out we are not what we eat, but rather what we can absorb, digest and deliver to our cells. The ability to metabolize and utilize what is available is the final determining factor in human nutrition. It varies greatly between individuals. Even when nutritional foods are eaten, not everyone has the same ability to properly digest and metabolize them. Modern civilized man, in his urbanized, mechanized environment, is weak, compared to his ancient ancestors. No longer do only the physically strong and swift, who logically best convert food to energy, survive. In today's world, mental acumen may well prove even more contributory to longevity than physical ability.

How do these dieticians explain population groups that eat the same foods in the same way, yet have different levels of metabolism, stamina, resistance and disease? Individuals with poor digestive and metabolic processes are no longer eliminated by environmental selection from passing their weaknesses on to succeeding generations, and therefore must learn to compensate. Fortunately, nutritional science has given us methods and products to supplement the body processes that nature made weak.

The Bio-X Diet presents total availability of all nutritional needs. There may be individuals, however, who lack the ability to obtain complete nutritional value from their food. This may be due to poor intestinal structure, too few or too much intestinal flora, inadequate stomach acid, too few pancreatic enzymes, or organs which have been damaged due to injury, malnutrition or inadequate nutrition. For those with diagnosed weaknesses, tablets and liquid supplements help get the body back on track. This is best accomplished with the help of a competent professional nutritionist or alternative physician who can diagnostically evaluate individual dietary needs. Numerous techniques and testing procedures are available to help determine what supplementation may be required.

As a general rule, if nutritional availability is adequate as outlined in the Bio-X Diet, most normal, healthy individuals will require little supplementation during their prime, from approximately 15 to 40 years of age. At the end of this period, if longevity and vibrant health are to be maintained, we must work against nature. Of course, even during prime years there are circumstances in which supplementation may be required. Lifestyle and situational factors such as pregnancy, high stress levels, excessive drinking, smoking or injury may require special supplementation for maintenance or getting back to health.

In each living plant, animal and human being, there is established at birth a metabolic time clock that guides the individual's growth through infancy and establishes a period of reproduction and maturity. Once the species has procreated itself, nature prepares to eliminate the aging organism to make room for the next generation. Degenerative diseases are a result.

If we intend to lengthen the normal life cycle beyond the reproductive years, there comes a time when we must work against the natural metabolic slowdown which is preparing us for our final recycling.

It has been proven in various races and cultures that proper nutrition, exercise, and freedom from environmental stress can prevent degeneration, and even extend the reproductive years decades beyond what is considered normal in our Euro-American culture. Many experienced nutritionists believe dietary supplementation, applied as necessary, can play a vital part in increasing the reproductive period.

Dietary supplementation in no way implies ingestion of unnatural substances. It simply normalizes digestive fluids, enzymes, vitamins and minerals the various body mechanisms or organs depend upon but may not be producing or metabolizing adequately.

The Bio-X Diet assumes a natural and plentiful supply of vegetables, grains and fruits. There are geographic areas in Western civilization where grains and lentils are not available on a year-round basis. Where such is the case, supplementation becomes vitally necessary; for example, during certain seasons devoid of fresh produce, or when what is available has been cultivated in mineral-depleted soil (devoid of selenium, for instance).

Megavitamin dosages have stimulated considerable discussion in recent years. The theory seems to be that if a few vitamins are good, a lot of vitamins are better. This doesn't work any better for nutrients than it does for pain killers. Under normal health conditions, with a few exceptions, such a belief is erroneous; it can even be dangerous if, in individual or extreme circumstances, it is applied without professional guidance. Oil-soluble vitamins, unbuffered by the balanced ingredients and fiber present in their natural food sources, can potentially be absorbed when taken in excessive amounts and build to highly toxic levels in the liver and fatty tissues. Too much of one vitamin or mineral can create a dangerous deficiency of another. Zinc without copper, for example, is as good as no zinc at all. Balance and moderation in all things, including nutritional supplementation, is essential.

The majority of vitamins, however, are water-soluble. The body will use what it needs, with excesses excreted. Critics will point to our recommendation of bowel tolerance levels of vitamin C as megadoses. Not so. It is only recently that nutritionists, not blinded by orthodoxy, have determined our body's large vitamin C requirements. In previous ages (and even in some present-day primitive cultures) vitamin C was adequately supplied in diets high in green leafy vegetables. In present day northern latitudes it is no longer true.

We need to return to our inherited metabolic requirements. Certain diseases may place extra vitamin or enzyme demand on nutrition. Requirements for vitamin A are increased by cancer. Preventive supplementation is needed to bolster an aging or malfunctioning metabolism. Vitamins, enzymes, and other supplements are extremely important additions to dietary intake. However, when synthesized or extracted by man, supplements are, like fiber, second best to their true food source (assuming the source is available and that sufficient amounts of it can be eaten to fulfill nutritional demand). The next best thing to whole foods are supplements that are derived from whole foods. One supplement formula takes the most nutritious and immune-boosting food and freeze-dries it, packing it into pellets that can be taken when whole foods are not available.

It may be wise, however, to provide additional nutritional cancer insurance beyond the natural protection provided by the nitriloside foods that are part of the Bio-X Diet. For example, during periods of extended mental or physical stress, or where there is the symptomatic presence of some other metabolic disease, or a family history of cancer.

As stated previously, one apricot kernel per each ten pounds of body weight per day should adequately support the body's intrinsic defense system. The addition of antioxidants or other specifics required for a good cancer preventive profile should be determined by your nutritional professional.

Everyone interested in good health should become acquainted with the facilities, products and services provided by local health food stores. Most owners are extremely knowledgeable about nutrition and can be helpful in recommending holistic medical professionals in the community. This is one field of expertise in which these specialty stores are indispensable – and why they must survive. Not only do they carry a broad selection of superior quality health products, but they are also fully informed about their usage and benefits. All of the products mentioned in this book are available from your holistic physician or health food store.

PART 2:
Foreword

The Gourmet Guide to Cancer Prevention

The recipes in this Gourmet Guide to Cancer Prevention have been selected primarily for the purpose of returning cancer-preventive, Bio-X foods to the diet.

I do not feel it is necessary to include chicken and fish dishes. Recommendations for their preparation abound in the myriad of cookbooks already available. We leave these to the talent and imagination of the cook as we do the preparation of meat dishes, with the reminder that meat should be as lean as possible and when on the menu preferably used as a condiment, casseroled and extended by the inclusion of vegetables or grains.

The emphasis is palate-perfect prevention through the pleasing preparation of the high nitriloside foods that have been culturally eliminated from our diets and neglected even in many of the excellent vegetarian cookbooks.

Each sample daily menu contains between 300 and 600 milligrams of therapeutic amygdalin which, in most cases, is fifty times the present average adult intake in the United States.

Although many cancer-free populations consume larger daily amounts, knowledgeable nutritionists believe 50-250 mg. per day of amygdalin should adequately support the body's natural defenses when included with proper enzymes and dietary fiber.

Both enzymes and fiber are presented in abundance by the whole grains and lentils in these recipes. They provide the dietary balance which allows inclusion of temperate amounts of processed fats and oils in cooking and for salads and spreads.

Grains and legumes may be purchased in bulk at substantial savings. The Bio-X Diet will save you money while providing a substantial increase in health maintenance.

Search out a greengrocer who can provide fresh organically-grown vegetables. While he will, no doubt, include sprouts in his produce, I have included in this section directions on how to sprout. It is fun, nutritionally enhancing, and as close to having a garden as many urban dwellers can come.

It is vital you purchase vegetables as fresh and young as possible. To this end, I have enlisted the aid of my dear and trusted friend, Karl Rolfes, to whom I entrust my gastrointestinal health. He is an excellent chef and judge of produce.

Leafy Greens

Choose brightly colored, crisp leaves. Avoid plants with bruised or excessively dirty leaves; they have been improperly handled. Spotted, yellow or wilting plants are old and have lost vital nutrients. The only exception to this rule are beet greens, which turn red at the tips when they age. Kale, mustard greens and collard greens, if left in the field too long, have woody stems and leaves webbed with thick, coarse veins. Coarse-stemmed, straggly spinach should also be avoided. Buy leaf vegetables that are displayed on refrigerated racks, where low temperatures discourage decay.

Karl says it's best to use greens the same day you buy them. If you must store them, keep them for no longer than two days. After that, much of the vegetables' rich supply of vitamins and minerals have disappeared. Do not cleanse leaves before storage. Too much moisture encourages bacteria. Store them in a perforated plastic bag so air can circulate.

The Cabbage Family

Look for cabbage heads and Brussels sprouts that are tightly curled, and feel hard and heavy. Outer leaves should be opaque and cores white, not yellow. Chinese cabbages should be long and straight, pale green and very crisp. Broccoli buds should be tightly closed. The tips may be tinged with blue or purple but not yellow. A cauliflower should be an unblemished snow-or cream-white, with florets tightly pressed together. Kohlrabi is young and tender when the bulb diameter is less than three inches. To store, put unwashed cabbage vegetables in a plastic bag poked with holes.

Roots and Tubers

Any potato you buy should be firm. They should not have sprouting eyes, soft black spots or green areas. Turnips and greens should be small – no larger than two inches in diameter. Older carrots have a woody core that should be removed before cooking. Parsnips are young and tender only when about eight inches in length. They should be free of gashes and wet, soft spots. Look for smooth, heavy rutabagas without punctures. Buy only Jerusalem artichokes which are hard. Salsify should be smoothly tapered, firm and about six inches long. Celeriac, or celery root, shouldn't be larger than a man's fist or it is old and woody.

Store roots and tubers unwashed. Cut off beet, turnip, carrot and parsnip leaves so they won't take moisture from the roots. Be sure to leave stems at least two inches long on beets, lest color ooze out as they cook. Jerusalem artichokes, refrigerated in perforated plastic bags, will keep for two days. Beets, carrots, celeriac, parsnips and turnips will last one week. Salsify will keep for three or four days, but its oyster-like flavor diminishes daily. Sweet potatoes, potatoes and rutabagas should be stored outside the refrigerator, ideally at 50 degrees Fahrenheit, where they will keep for up to two months. At normal room temperature, potatoes will last a week. Keep white potatoes in the dark; direct light develops chlorophyll, which turns them green and bitter.

Pods and Seeds

Choose the smallest and brightest-colored seeds and pods you can find. Those that are wrinkled, dry, flabby or yellowed are average. Ones with thick, fibrous pods are old. The most tender green beans and yellow wax beans are only 1/4 inch wide and four inches long. Crisp, fresh beans will snap when bent. Lima beans are available as the small, so-called "butter limas," or as the larger "potato"-type beans – plump, flat and oval with green or greenish-white skins. Good limas and broad beans are encased in velvety, dark green pods, which should be tightly closed and bulging. Good peas are round, shiny and come in smooth, bright green pods. The best are bright green and so thin you can see the outline of the immature peas within.

For the best corn, buy ears that were picked that morning and are displayed on ice. The cobs should be at least six inches long under green husks. Dry or yellowed husks indicate the corn is old or damaged. The stem ends should be moist and the silk a pale greenish-white. The silk tassel at the tip should be brown and brittle. The kernels should be plump and firm. When you pierce a kernel, it should spurt thick white liquid.

Bean sprouts, whether they come from alfalfa or from mung beans, should be cream-colored or white and crisp with moist tips. Alfalfa sprouts are best when they are approximately one inch long. Mung sprouts ideally should be three inches in length.

Keep lima and broad beans, as well as peas, unwashed and in their pods. Refrigerated in perforated plastic bags, they will keep for two days. Cook corn as soon as you buy it.

Mushrooms

Pick out mushrooms with smooth, unblemished skins. The caps should be closed so no gills show around the stems. Store mushrooms refrigerated, unwashed and loosely covered. They will last one to two days. Mushrooms are grown in sterilized soil so they require little cleaning. To prepare for cooking, cut off the bottom of the mushroom stems and wipe off the dirt with a damp cloth. Do not buy mushrooms that have been washed or sprayed with water.

Vegetable Fruits

In botanical terms, a tomato, eggplant or pepper is a fruit; a cucumber is a squash and an okra is a pod. For shopping and cooking purposes, however, they form one group. All are warm-weather plants that reach their peak of flavor and availability in the summer.

Choose tomatoes labeled "greenhouse" or "hothouse" – they have been picked when almost ripe. Most tomatoes are picked green and artificially ripened without sunlight. Buy hard, green cucumbers. Wrinkled or rubbery cucumbers are old and may be bitter. The best size for cucumbers is six to seven inches. The best eggplants are a glossy, uniform purple. When eggplants grow old their skins turn dull and have brown spots.

Peppers, including the frying varieties, change from green to red as they ripen. The red peppers you see in the store are a separate variety. Any pepper should have a shiny skin, free from holes or punctures and from soft or black decaying spots. Buy okra when it is so young and firm a pod will snap when you bend it. The green pods should be two to four inches long.

The best storage temperature for these quickly-decaying vegetables is 50 degrees Fahrenheit. Ideally, tomatoes shouldn't be refrigerated. Chilling diminishes the flavor. Underripe tomatoes will ripen best when they are wrapped in newspaper or a brown paper bag and kept at room temperature.

The Squashes

Zucchini and yellow squashes should be three to six inches long, scalloped squash no more than four inches in diameter. The rind should be easy to pierce and the squash should feel firm and heavy. Winter squashes should feel hard and have no cracks or blemishes.

Hubbard or acorn squash should be blue-gray or green; buttercup squash should be dark green with lighter stripes or flecks. All three will develop orange patches as they ripen. Butternut squash should be entirely tan and pumpkins bright orange. Refrigerated in plastic bags, summer squashes and chayotes will keep three or four days. The thick rinds of winter squashes make it possible to store them for up to three months in net bags hung in a cool, dry place.

Stalk Vegetables

In general, stalk vegetables should be firm, clean and crisp. Vegetables with coarsely striated stalks are old; those with limp, rubbery stalks and wilted, yellowed or browned leaves have dried out and lost nutrients. Slippery brown spots indicate the vegetables have become overchilled.

Choose young asparagus with tightly closed buds. Reject spears with open or seedy tips. The stalks should be round, not flattened or ridged. Celery should always be green, with fresh leaves and brittle stalks that snap crisply. Fennel should have a compact, greenish-white, bulbous base, green upper stalks and grass-green, ferny shoots. Bok choy should have very white stalks and shiny, dark green leaves.

Do not wash stalks before storing. Remove any limp outer leaves, wrap the stalks in a perforated plastic bag and refrigerate. Celery and fennel will last a week kept this way, bok choy and asparagus three days, and chard two days.

The Onion Family

Vegetables in the onion or allium family are garlic, onions, shallots, leeks and scallions. Look for alliums that feel firm and dry. Those with green shoots growing from the root ends have been stored at too high a temperature and humidity, and have lost much of their nutrients. Those with soft or discolored spots are rotting.

Garlic bulbs and their cloves should be tightly closed, with unwrinkled skins of white, pink to purple, or white with purple streaks. Buy leeks and scallions with crisp, green, unwithered tops and clean white bottoms. Leeks should be straight and cylindrical. Those with bulbous ends will be tough and woody inside. Some varieties of scallions develop bulbous ends naturally.

Do not store alliums in the refrigerator; the damp air encourages rot. Hang them in baskets or in net bags in a cool, dark place. Direct light causes them to produce chlorophyll, which turns their flesh green and their flavor bitter. After cutting off any brown or limp tops, refrigerate leeks and scallions in perforated plastic bags and use them within three to five days.

Emphasizing fresh vegetables will put you on the road to a cancer-free life. Eating according to your biological experience need not be dull or monotonous. Try these recipes and when you find one you like, share it with others. Get plenty of exercise and, whenever possible, eliminate stress and enjoy your good health. I know these sample menus and recipes will guide you to a long, active life. Bon appetit!

CHAPTER 14:

A Seven Day Cancer-Free Diet

LEGEND

T = tablespoon   t = teaspoon   c = cup

DAY ONE

Breakfast

- MENU -

Enzyme Cocktail

Millet Crunch

Cashew Nut Milk or Raw Skim Milk

Fruit - Cantaloupe if in Season

- RECIPE -

Enzyme Cocktail

2 c. papaya or pineapple juice   1 T. 500 brewers yeast

Add small amount of juice to yeast. When well absorbed, add to rest of juice. Mix well.

-RECIPE-

Millet Crunch

1 c. millet	1 t. salt or kelp
1/2 c. wheat germ	2 c. spring water
1/2 c. bran	1/2 c. raisins
1 T. cinnamon	1/3 c. flaxseed

Soak millet in spring water overnight, or 3-4 hours. Add wheat germ, bran, salt, cinnamon, raisins and flaxseed, and mix thoroughly. Place mixture in a baking dish and barely cover with spring water (approximately 1 cup). Place in the oven on pilot light until the water has evaporated, leaving cereal moist. Eat while still warm with cashew cream, almond milk or coconut-pineapple juice and unpasteurized tupelo honey.

Cashew Nut Milk or Cashew Cream

1 c. spring water	1 t. real vanilla
1 t. raw (unpasteurized) honey	3 T. sesame seeds
1/2 c. raw cashews or	
blanched almonds	

Wash the unsalted, unroasted raw cashews or almonds thoroughly. In blender, liquify nuts with water. Add sesame seeds and blend. Add honey and vanilla slowly until a creamy texture is achieved.

Lunch

- MENU -

Complete Meal Salad with Herb Dressing

Bible Bread (available at health food store)

Almond Spread

Fresh Carrot Juice

-RECIPE-

Complete Meal Salad

Has 542.6 calories, all 8 essential amino acids, 15 grams of protein, rich in vitamins, minerals and enzymes.

1/2 c. dark leafy greens	2 T. sunflower seeds
1/8 c. fresh flaxseed oil	1 T. ground apricot kernels
1/2 c. summer squash	red pepper to taste
1/2 cucumber, sliced	kelp to taste
1/2 tomato, sliced	1/2 ripe avocado
1 c. mung sprouts	

Toss greens with oil until lightly coated. Add rest of ingredients except avocado, toss well. Just before eating, slice avocado and put on top. Freshly-squeezed lemon juice can top the avocado to avoid browning. Serves One.

Herb Dressing

1/2 c. fresh flaxseed oil	1/2 t. ground tarragon
3 T. apple cider vinegar	1 t. kelp
1/2 t. ground thyme	1/2 t. ground basil
1 t. marjoram	1 T. ground apricot kernels
1 T. finely chopped parsley	

Put in jar and mix together. Pour on your complete salad.

Dinner

- MENU -

Lentil Millet Patties

Tossed Salad with Herb Dressing

Tropical Cooler Drink

Papaya Leaf Tea

- RECIPE -

Lentil Millet Patties

1 c. chopped onion
1/4 c. water
1 c. cooked lentils
1 c. cooked whole millet

pinch of nutmeg
pinch of black pepper
1/4 c. pure sorghum syrup

Saute chopped onion in water. Mash lentils, millet and onion well with pepper and nutmeg. Form patties. Place in lightly-greased baking pan and bake at 350 degree oven for 20 minutes. Serve with syrup.

-RECIPE-

Tossed Salad

1 head green leafy lettuce
1/4 c. alfalfa sprouts
1/4 c. chopped beet tops
1/4 c. raw grated beets

1/2 c. sunflower seed sprouts
2 sliced tomatoes
1/2 thinly sliced cauliflower
1 T. slivered apricot kernels

Lightly toss ingredients together and top with dressing. Garnish with sliced radishes and raw mushrooms. Serves four.

Lemon Herb Dressing

2 T. chopped fresh parsley
1 small green onion & top, chopped
1/2 t. dried sweet basil chopped very fine
2/3 c. flaxseed oil
1 t. vegetable broth

pinch marjoram
juice of one lemon
1 t. kelp
celery seed to taste

Shake vigorously in covered jar until blended. Allow to stand in refrigerator until flavors are blended.

Tropical Cooler Drink

1 banana
1/2 c. spring water

1 papaya, cut-up
1 mango, cut-up

Pour water in blender; add banana, mango and papaya while blender is in motion. Blend until smooth. Add water, if needed, for desired consistency. Serve in clear glasses or bowls.

DAY TWO

Breakfast

- MENU -

Glass of Fresh Carrot and Beet Juice
Slenderizing Pancakes with Apricot Sauce
Raw Fruit in Season
Rose Hips Tea with Lemon Juice and Raw Honey

- RECIPE -

Slenderizing Pancakes

1/4 c. millet	1 t. kelp
1/4 c. oats	1 t. date spread
1/4 c. barley	lecithin oil
3/4 c. raw skim milk	

Soak grains overnight in 3/4 c. cold water. Drain water and place grains in blender with raw skim milk. Blend three to five minutes. Add kelp, date spread and blend another minute. Continue blending until fluffy and filled with air. In hot skillet add small amount of lecithin oil. Pour mixture in pool to form desired size pancakes. Top with apricot sauce.

Apricot Sauce

4 T. dried apricots	2 c. non-fluoridated water
2 oranges	3/4 c. unsweetened pineapple juice

Soak apricots in water overnight. Put apricots, oranges and water in which they were soaked in blender. Whiz briefly. Add pineapple juice slowly while blending.

Lunch

- MENU -

Nitriloside Salad with B17 Dressing
Raisin Muffin with Apple Date Spread
Papaya Mint Tea with Raw Honey & Lemon

- RECIPE -

Nitriloside Salad

1/2 medium head red leaf lettuce	1 c. cabbage, finely chopped
1 small red onion, minced	1 stalk celery, sliced
1 c. chopped spinach, pressed firm	1 c. sesame seeds
1 medium tomato, cubed	4 stalks watercress, chopped
4 broccoli tops	2 T. slivered apricot kernels
1 large carrot, grated	1/2 c. each mung sprouts,
4 cauliflower tops	lentil sprouts, alfalfa sprouts

Combine ingredients and toss gently. Top with dressing.

B17 Dressing

2 T. sesame oil	1/2 t. cayenne pepper
2 T. freshly-squeezed lemon juice	1/2 t. basil
1 heaping t. brewers yeast	1 large clove garlic, pressed
1/2 t. celery seed	

Combine oil and lemon juice in a jar. Add yeast, herbs and garlic.
Shake well.

Raisin Muffins

3 c. whole oats	1 c. wheat germ
1/2 c. millet flour	1/2 T. ground apricot kernels
1 c. bran	1/2 c. raisins
1/2 t. kelp	1/2 c. sesame seed butter

Mix together oats, flour, bran, kelp and wheat germ. Add kernels and raisins. Set aside. Put sesame butter (sold as Tahini) in one cup hot water and stir well. Add to flour mixture and mix well. Let stand five to 10 minutes. Pour into greased 12-cup muffin tin. Bake 350 degrees until lightly browned, about 30 minutes. Or drop by the spoonful on a cookie sheet lightly greased with lecithin oil. Serve warm topped with apple date spread.

Apple Date Spread

2 apples, chopped   1/2 c. date spread

Mix in blender until smooth.

Dinner

- MENU -

Fresh Carrot Juice

California Tostada

Guacamole Dip

Tahini's Purple Surprise Salad

Fresh Pineapple or Papaya

Mint Tea or Papaya Juice

- RECIPE -

California Tostada

(from *How I Conquered Cancer Nutritionally* by Edie May Hunsburger)

4 corn tortillas   parsley
grated lettuce   cherry tomatoes
cooked pinto beans   guacamole
alfalfa sprouts or mung bean sprouts   red chili taco sauce
radishes

Lightly fry corn tortilla in 1 t. olive oil. Add a layer of grated lettuce. Top with cooked pinto beans. On top of that in a circle add a layer of alfalfa sprouts or mung bean sprouts. Garnish with radishes cut into florets, parsley and cherry tomatoes. Top with a large mound of guacamole and red salsa taco sauce.

Guacamole

4 medium avocados, mashed	2 green scallions, finely diced
juice of 1/2 lemon	Pinch of cayenne
2 small tomatoes, finely diced	1 to 2 t. tamari
1 clove garlic, pressed	1 t. olive oil

Mash avocados. Gently blend in lemon juice. Add tomatoes, garlic, scallions, cayenne, tamari and olive oil, mixing lightly.

Red Salsa Taco Sauce

2 c. fresh tomatoes, coarsely chopped	2 steamed fresh green chilies,
juice of 2 lemons	seeded & minced
1 very ripe avocado, finely diced	1 sweet onion, finely chopped
2 cloves garlic, pressed	

In blender, mix tomatoes and chilies until finely chopped. In bowl, mix together avocado and lemon. Add tomato-chili mixture, then onion and garlic. Refrigerate overnight.

Purple Surprise Salad
(Tahini Salsbury)

1 medium red cabbage, grated	1 medium purple bermuda onion,
1/2 c. Fenugreek sprouts	sliced thinly

Mix ingredients and toss with lemon herb dressing (recipe above).

DAY THREE

Breakfast

- MENU -

Fresh Squeezed Orange Juice

Millet Cereal, Soft and Moist, with

Raw Skim Milk (or try apple cider) and

Sorghum Syrup (an excellent source of B17)

- RECIPE -

Millet Cereal, Soft and Moist

1 c. whole hulled millet	1 c. raisins
1 qt. spring water	1/2 c. sesame seeds
1 t. kelp	1/2 c. flax seeds
1 c. chopped apple	sorghum syrup

Put millet, water and kelp in a saucepan. Bring to a boil, cover and simmer on low heat for 45 minutes or until soft. Remember, never cook on high heat. Add apples, raisins and seeds. Serve with raw skim milk and sorghum syrup to taste.

Lunch

- MENU -

Lentil Millet Soup

Sesame Crackers

Karl's Millet Raspberry Birds Nest

- RECIPE -

Lentil Millet Soup

5 c. spring water	1/8 t. oregano
1 c. millet	1 onion, chopped
1 c. dry lentils	2 tomatoes, chopped
2 t. kelp	1 carrot, grated
1/4 t. thyme	1/4 c. chopped parsley

In water, cook millet, lentils, kelp, thyme and oregano in a covered saucepan for 15 minutes. Add onion, tomatoes, carrot and parsley. Simmer all ingredients together 45 minutes or until lentils and millet are tender. Add more water if needed.

Sesame Crackers

1/3 c. macadamia nuts	1/2 c. wheat germ
(an excellent source of B17)	1/2 c. barley flour
1/3 c. sesame seeds	1/4 c. rye flour
2/3 c. spring water	1/3 c. full fat soy flour, sifted
1/2 c. millet	1/2 t. kelp

Grind macadamia nuts and sesame seeds separately until slightly pasty. Put into blender and add 2/3 cup water. Blend until smooth. In a bowl, mix together millet, wheat germ, flours and kelp. Add blended mixture to dry ingredients. Mix well and knead lightly. Dough should not be sticky when all dry ingredients are kneaded. If sticky, add a bit more flour as needed. Roll between waxed paper until very thin; 1/8" or less. Put on a cookie sheet that has been prepared with a thin film of lecithin oil. Cut in squares and prick with a fork. Bake at 400 degrees until lightly brown and crisp. Crackers at edges of pan will brown first. Remove these and continue the rest until done.

Karl's Millet Raspberry Birds Nest

2 c. cooked millet	2 c. raspberries
4 bunches spinach, chopped	1/4 c. raspberry vinegar
2 med. turnips, chopped	pinch cayenne pepper
1/4 c. raw honey	1 pear, sliced

Steam together spinach and turnips. Mix with millet. In saucepan heat honey, raspberries, vinegar and cayenne together on low heat for two minutes. On serving platter, mound millet mixture and pour raspberry sauce on top. Decorate with pear slices. Serves four.

Dinner

- MENU -

Liver Tasty (for liver haters)
Karl's Brussels Sprouts Barley Soup
Strawberry Watercress Salad
Uncooked Applesauce
Cinnamon Orange Tea with Lemon and Raw Honey

- RECIPE -

Liver Tasty

4 large onions, thinly sliced	1/2 t. kelp
1 lb. calves liver	pinch cayenne pepper
1/2 c. wheat germ	1 t. sesame oil
1/2 c. whole wheat flour	2 c. fresh mushrooms

Sauté onions until transparent. Slice liver into small strips 2" by 1/4" thick. In dish or plastic bag, combine wheat germ, whole-wheat flour, kelp and cayenne. Heat oil in skillet. Coat strips of liver in flour mixture and sauté lightly, rotating until all surfaces of liver are lightly browned. Do not overcook. After cooking liver, sauté mushrooms lightly in same pan. Combine mushrooms in pan with liver; sauté lightly. Serves six.

Karl's Brussels Sprouts Barley Soup

1 lb. fresh Brussels sprouts, cleaned and trimmed	1/2 t. black pepper
	1/2 t. white pepper
8 c. vegetable stock	1/4 t. grated nutmeg
1 c. barley	1/4 t. tarragon
1 large potato, cubed	1/2 lemon, sliced
1/4 c. cilantro	

After cleaning, freeze Brussels sprouts overnight to remove bitterness. Slice base of sprouts before cooking to encourage cooking through. Put stock in large saucepan and add sprouts, barley and potato. Let simmer on low heat 30 minutes. Add rest of ingredients and let simmer 10 minutes more. Serves four.

Strawberry Watercress Salad

1/4 c. honey	pinch cayenne pepper
juice of one lime	2 c. cottage cheese
1/4 c. pine nuts	2 c. chopped watercress
5 fresh mint leaves, crushed	2 c. strawberries, sliced

Mix together honey, lime juice, nuts, crushed mint leaves and pepper. On serving platter mound the cottage cheese. Create an indentation in the middle, or make a ring, and fill with watercress and strawberries. Top with honey sauce and sprinkle with sesame seeds. Serves four.

Uncooked Applesauce

3 organic sweet apples	1/8 tsp. nutmeg
1/2 c. water	1/8 tsp. cinnamon
1 T. lemon juice	Sorghum syrup

Cut up the apples (peels, cores, seeds and all). Put water and lemon juice in blender. Blend while dropping in cut-up apples. Blend just until smooth. Pour mixture in bowl. Add nutmeg, cinnamon and syrup to taste.

DAY FOUR

Breakfast

- MENU -

Fresh Carrot Juice

Fruit in Season

Millet Soy Waffles Topped with

Berry Sauce or Apple Marmalade

Brigham or Mormon Tea

- RECIPE -

Millet Soy Waffles

1 c. soaked soy beans	1 c.(equivalent of 1/2 c. dry) millet seeds
2-1/4 c. spring water	1/2 t. salt
1-1/4 c. millet flour or	flaxseed oil

Soak beans several hours or overnight covered in water. Drain. Discard water. (Soaked, drained soy beans may be kept in the refrigerator for a week or freezer for longer periods. Keep on hand for immediate use.) Combine all ingredients and blend until light and foamy, about 1/2 minute. Let stand while waffle iron is heating. The batter thickens on standing. Mix briefly. Bake in hot iron for 8 minutes or until brown. If you do not wish to use the oil, you may put sesame seeds in the waffle iron - the oil from the sesame seeds will grease the waffle iron and keep it from sticking. Set timer for 8 minutes and do not open before time is up. Cook a few seconds longer if the iron sticks. When serving a large number bake waffles ahead. Cook, stack and cover with wax paper. Just before serving, reheat in waffle iron, oven or toaster briefly. These can be frozen nicely.

Berry Sauce

2 c. sliced strawberries
1 c. raspberries, mashed
1/4 c. raw honey

1/2 t. mint extract or 2 crushed mint leaves
pinch cayenne pepper

In frying pan, melt honey on low heat. Add pepper and mint, then fruit. Heat and stir on low heat until desired consistency.

Apple Marmalade

5 med. apples, cored and sliced
1 T. butter
1/2 c. raw honey
1/4 c. spring water

1 strip lemon peel
1 cinnamon stick
1 mint leaf, crushed

In saucepan, combine all ingredients. Simmer on low heat until desired consistency. Add water if needed.

Lunch

- MENU -

Sweet Potato Kale Soup

Wheat Germ Millet Bread

Sprout Salad

Chamomile Tea with Raw Honey & Lemon

Sweet Potato Kale Soup

8 c. vegetable stock
2 bunch kale, stripped
3 large sweet potatoes, chopped
2 cloves garlic, sliced
1/2 t. black pepper

1/2 t. white pepper
1/4 t. nutmeg
2 bay leaves
1 onion, sliced

Put kale in freezer overnight to bring out the taste. Prior to cooking, strip leaves from stem. Put stock in cooking pot, add kale and potato, and let cook on low heat 30 minutes. Add rest of ingredients except onion. In skillet, sauté onion in a little oil until brown. Add to pot and simmer ten minutes. Serves four.

Wheat Germ Millet Bread

1 c. millet
1/2 c. wheat germ
1-1/2 c. boiling spring water
1 pkg. active dry yeast
1/4 c. tepid spring water

1/4 c. raw honey
2 T. flaxseed oil
2 t. cayenne pepper
4 c. whole wheat flour

Combine millet and wheat germ in large bowl; pour 1-1/2 c. boiling water over them and set aside. Mix the yeast in 1/4 c. tepid water and set aside 10 minutes until mixture is foamy. To millet/wheat germ mixture add honey, pepper and oil. When this mixture has cooled, add yeast and 1-1/2 c. wheat flour. Beat vigorously, adding enough flour to make dough smooth and pliable. Knead well. Set the dough aside in an oiled bowl, covered with a damp cloth, to rise for one hour, or until doubled in bulk.

Punch down dough, shape it into two loaves, and place the loaves in two 9" x 5" loaf pans or on a baking sheet. Let the dough rise once more, for about an hour. Bake in preheated 375 degree oven for 50 minutes. Remove the loaves from the pans or baking sheet immediately, and let them cool on a wire rack before slicing them.

Sprout Salad

2 c. bean sprouts
1/2 c. raw fresh peas
2 c. alfalfa sprouts

8 dates, pitted and chopped
1 c. raw mushrooms, sliced

Mix all ingredients in large bowl and top with avocado dressing. Or, for individual salads serve on lettuce leaf with dressing, or cupped in red cabbage leaves.

Avocado Dressing

2 large ripe avocados
1/2 t. salt
2 T. lemon juice
2 T. plain yogurt

2 small onions, minced
2 T. chopped red bell pepper
pinch of sea salt or kelp

Mash avocado with fork. Add rest of ingredients and blend together.

Dinner

- MENU -

Vegetable Pizza

Orange Salad

Sparkling Cider

- RECIPE -

Entree
Vegetable Pizza

Crust:

4 c. spring water	1/3 c. raw sesame seeds, ground
1/2 c. buckwheat	1 T. sesame tahini
1/2 c. millet	2 T. tamari

Bring water to boil, adding grains. Drain if there is water after cooking. Moisten grains with tahini and tamari. Add sesame seeds and mix with hands until dough is soft. Press in greased pizza pan.

Topping:

2 med. yams, cooked and mashed	1/4 c. raw honey
1/2 med. cauliflower, chopped	juice of one lime
2 med. turnips, chopped	1/2 apple, sliced
2 bunch spinach, chopped	1/4 c. raisins
2 carrots, sliced	1 T. lemon pepper

Over crust, press the mashed yam, covering pizza pan. Top with vegetables. In small saucepan on low heat, combine honey, juice, raisins and apples, just until raisins are plump. Pour mixture over top and sprinkle with lemon pepper. Bake for 15-20 minutes at 375 degrees. Serves four.

Orange Salad

6 oranges, sectioned	juice of two lemons
1/2 c. crushed pine nuts	2 T. raw honey
1/4 c. cilantro, chopped	

To orange segments, nuts and cilantro, add blended lemon juice and honey. Serves four.

DAY FIVE

Breakfast

- MENU -

Fresh Carrot Juice

Old Fashioned Buckwheat Cakes

Fruit in Season

Split Peameal (a legume oatmeal)

- RECIPE -

Old Fashioned Buckwheat Cakes

1-1/2 c. buckwheat flour	1 T. raw sesame oil
1 t. baking powder	1-1/2 c. spring water
1/2 c. whole wheat flour	1 egg white, beaten
1 t. sea salt	

In a large bowl, stir dry ingredients. Add oil and water, then beaten egg white, a little at a time as you mix. Pour small amount onto a hot oiled griddle or skillet. Turn cakes when bubbles appear. Serve hot with sorghum maple syrup.

Sorghum Maple Syrup

1/4 c. pure maple syrup	1/4 c. water
2 T. sorghum	

Combine ingredients and heat over low flame. Serve hot over buckwheat cakes.

Split Peameal

1 lb. split peas	2 stalks celery, chopped
2 carrots, diced	1 t. celery salt
1 onion, chopped	

In large saucepan or crock pot, cover peas with two inches of spring water. Add carrots, onion, celery and salt. Cook at low heat until tender. Prior to serving, blenderize half or all for a smooth consistency. May be made the night before and gently heated in the morning.

Lunch

- MENU -
Stuffed Red Peppers
Potato Salad
Millet Chews (a sweet treat)

- RECIPE -

Stuffed Red Peppers

6 small red peppers	1 tomato, finely chopped
1/4 c. finely chopped cabbage	4 t. chopped parsley
1/4 c. cooked barley	3 t. chopped fresh dillweed
2 green onions, chopped	pinch cayenne pepper

Cut off top of red peppers and scoop out seeds. Combine rest of ingredients in bowl, mixing together well. Place peppers in baking pan with a enough spring water on the bottom to prevent scorching (peppers will steam while filling heats). Stuff peppers with filling and bake at 325 degrees 25-30 minutes. Warm tomato sauce may be added after baking.

Potato Salad

2 qts. cooked potatoes	1/4 c. chopped onion
1 t. sea salt	1/2 c. chopped celery
1 c. plain yogurt	2 T. chopped pimento
1/4 c. mustard	1/2 c. shredded carrot
1/4 c. lemon juice	1/2 c. chopped green bell pepper
1/2 t. paprika	

Dice and salt cold potatoes. Set aside. In large bowl mix together yogurt, mustard, lemon juice and paprika. Add onion, celery, pimento, carrot and bell pepper. Add potatoes and gently stir until evenly coated. Refrigerate several hours or overnight for flavors to blend. Serve on fresh mustard greens.

Millet Chews

1 c. cooked millet	1/2 c. sesame seeds
1-1/2 c. finely chopped dates	1 t. vanilla
1/2 c. shredded coconut	2 T. orange rind
1 c. sesame butter	1 T. lemon rind
1/2 c. sorghum	1/2 t. sea salt

Be sure fruit is organically grown (without pesticides). Mix all ingredients well. Use a long wooden spoon and plenty of elbow grease. You may find it easier and preferable to roll the mixture with your hands. Shape into two inch long rolls the thickness of your thumb. Wrap in wax paper and chill until hard.

Dinner

- MENU -

Sweet Potato Bake

Garbanzo Lima Salad

Pumpkin Pie

Cereal Blend

- RECIPE -

Sweet Potato Bake

3 lbs. sweet potatoes	1 c. plain yogurt
3 egg yolks, beaten	3 egg whites, beaten
1 T. butter, melted	1 T. slivered apricot kernels
1 t. sea salt	

Boil and mash sweet potatoes. Add egg yolks, butter, sea salt and yogurt. Mix well. Fold in egg whites. Put in greased mold or dish and sprinkle top with kernels. Bake in 350 degree oven for 30 minutes or until firm.

Pumpkin Pie in Granola Crust

1-1/2 c. coarsely chopped pumpkin
1/2 c. soy milk
2 T. raw honey
1/2 t. vanilla
1/4 c. date sugar

1/2 t. lemon rind
3 T. Arrowroot powder
1 t. ground coriander seed
1/4 t. sea salt

Put ingredients in saucepan and cook until thick, stirring occasionally. Mix in blender until smooth. Pour into baked pie shell. Refrigerate until ready to serve.

Granola Pie Crust

1-1/2 c. fat-free granola
1/2 c. chopped almonds
1/2 c. chopped macadamia nuts
1-1/2 c. coconut

1/4 c. whole wheat flour
1/4 c. wheat germ
1/2 c. raw skim milk

Grind granola and nuts in a blender until fine. In bowl, stir together granola mixture, coconut, flour and wheat germ. Add milk and stir until wet. Press into pie pan using spoon. Bake at 350 degrees for about 8 to 10 minutes. Watch carefully to prevent burning.

DAY SIX

Breakfast

- MENU -

Fresh Carrot & Beet Juice

Pot of Lentils

Honeydew Melon or Fruit in Season

Mint Tea

- RECIPE -

Pot of Lentils

2 c. uncooked lentils	5 tomatoes, diced
2 c. chopped onion	1/2 t. oregano
1/2 c. diced carrot	1 t. cumin
1/2 c. diced celery	1 t. sea salt
1/2 c. chopped green bell pepper	2 T. vegetable seasoning

In four cups of spring water, place all ingredients except tomatoes. Simmer on low heat until almost done, then add tomatoes. Simmer until skin slides off tomatoes. Serves six.

Lunch

- MENU -

Karl's Legume Pepper Stew

Wild Cabbage Salad

Savory Garbanzos

- RECIPE -

Karl's Legume Pepper Stew

1 c. garbanzo beans, cooked	2 cloves garlic, sliced
6 c. vegetable stock	1/4 c. chopped fresh parsley
1 yellow onion, sliced	1 t. black pepper
1 green bell pepper, sliced	1/2 t. oregano
1 red bell pepper, sliced	1/4 t. nutmeg
1 c. barley	pinch cayenne pepper
1/2 lemon, sliced	

In large stew pot, combine all ingredients. Simmer on low heat 30-40 minutes, until barley is soft and peppers are crispy/tender. Serves four.

Wild Cabbage Salad

1 med. cabbage, cored and grated	1/2 c. raisins
2 carrots, grated	1/4 c. raw honey
1/2 apple, cored and grated	juice of 1 lime
1/4 c. chopped cashews	1 t. lemon pepper

In large bowl, combine cabbage, carrots, apple, nuts and raisins. In small bowl, combine honey, lime juice and lemon pepper. Pour honey mixture on top of vegetables and toss lightly. Chill overnight to blend flavors. Serves four.

Savory Garbanzos

3 c. garbanzos, cooked	1/2 bell pepper, minced
1/4 t. sweet basil	2 c. chopped tomatoes
1 onion, minced	

Combine all ingredients and pour into a casserole dish. Top with whole grain bread crumbs. Bake 350 degrees, 25 to 30 minutes, adding a little water if necessary. Serves 6 to 8.

Dinner

- MENU -

Spanakopita or Greek Spinach Pie

Tahini's Taboole

Cider Ale

- RECIPE -

Spanakopita

2 c. spinach, chopped, cooked and well-drained	2 T. chopped fresh dillweed
	4 eggs
1 c. chopped onion	4 T. soy butter
2 T. olive oil	1/2 c. olive oil
3 green onions, chopped	filo or strudel leaves
1-1/2 c. feta cheese, crumbled	2 c. whole grain bread crumbs
1/2 c. parsley, chopped	

Put spinach into large mixing bowl. Sauté onion in 2 tablespoons oil until tender. Add to spinach. Add green onions, feta cheese, parsley and dillweed. Mix well. Beat eggs slightly, add to spinach mixture. Mix well. Preheat oven to 350 degrees. Oil two 8" x 8" pans. Melt butter with 1/2 cup oil.

Cover bottom of pan with filo leaves. Edges may overlap sides. Brush lightly with oil mixture and sprinkle with bread crumbs. Fold over any overlapped edges neatly and add another filo leaf. Brush and sprinkle six layers. Top with half of spinach mixture and brush/sprinkle another six layers, same as the first. Do not brush and sprinkle the last layer. Repeat the process for the second pan. Bake pies one hour or until slightly brown and puffy. Cut into squares or wedges with sharp knife and serve hot or cold. Serves 12.

Tahini's Taboole

2 cucumbers, diced	6 tomatoes, diced
1 bunch parsley, chopped	4 green scallions, sliced
1 head curly leaf lettuce	2-1/2 c. sprouted wheat berries

If sprouted wheat berries aren't available in your health food store, sprout them yourself by keeping them covered with water for three to five days. Gently toss all ingredients together, reserving the sprouts for last. Serve with garlic lemon dressing. Serves four.

Garlic Lemon Dressing

2 cups olive oil	1 to 10 cloves pressed garlic
1 c. lemon juice	Vegasal to taste

Blend and serve over salad or use as a vegetable marinade.

DAY SEVEN

Breakfast

- MENU -

Fresh Carrot Juice

Scrambled Tofu

Lentil Millet Patties with Tomato Sauce

Juniper Berry Tea or Burdock Tea

(a good blood purifier)

- RECIPE -

Scrambled Tofu

1 pkg. tofu	1/8 t. turmeric
2 T. natural soy sauce	1 to 1-1/2 t. chicken-like seasoning
1 bunch green onions, chopped	(I recommend Loma Linda's Savorex)

Drain the tofu well, then cube it. Brown in hot skillet with a touch of oil. Add soy sauce, onions and seasonings. Continue cooking and scrambling until onions are cooked.

Lentil Millet Patties

Can be fixed the night before and heated at a very low heat in the oven with the tomato sauce.

1 c. dried lentils	cayenne pepper to taste
3/4 c. whole hulled millet	2 eggs lightly beaten
1 onion, chopped	2 c. wheat germ
kelp to taste	

Put lentils in a saucepan with spring water to cover. Bring to a boil and simmer on low heat until tender, about 45 minutes. Put millet and 1-1/2 cups water in a second saucepan. Cover and simmer 30 minutes or until tender and water is absorbed. Drain the lentils and mix with millet. Add onion, kelp and cayenne. Shape mixture into patties. Dip into beaten egg and coat with wheat germ. Heat sesame or olive oil in heavy skillet and fry patties until golden. Drain on paper towels and serve with tomato sauce. Serves 6.

Tomato Sauce

12 large ripe tomatoes, skinned	2 onions, chopped
6 stalks of celery	2 T. chopped fresh basil
2 T. chopped fresh chives	2 carrots, chopped
2 green peppers, seeded and chopped	2 cloves garlic finely chopped
2 T. chopped fresh parsley	

Combine all ingredients in a stainless steel or porcelain steel pan or casserole. Bring to a boil and simmer uncovered for 45 minutes. Puree in a blender if desired. Refrigerate overnight or freeze for future use if desired. Makes about 2 quarts.

Lunch

- MENU -
Meatless Burgers with Energy Sauce on
Whole Grain Pita Bread

- RECIPE -

Meatless Burgers

1 t. Savorex or Vegex
1/4 c. hot water
1 c. grated raw potatoes
1 c. oatmeal
1/2 c. finely chopped onion
1/4 c. finely chopped macadamia nuts
1/3 c. finely chopped celery
1 bunch parsley, chopped

1 c. cooked millet
2 T. chopped black olives
1 T. wheat germ
1/8 t. sage
1 t. garlic salt
1 t. no-MSG soy sauce
1/4 t. sea salt or to taste

In large bowl, dissolve Savorex in hot water. Mix with rest of ingredients and form patties. If batter is too thick, add more water. Sauté in hot oil or broil until both sides are browned. Serve with energy spread on whole wheat pita bread.

Energy Sauce

1 cup yogurt
1/4 tsp. cayenne
1 small tomato, chopped

1/2 cucumber, chopped
2 T. lemon juice
sea salt to taste

To make sauce, combine all ingredients. Serve in whole wheat pita bread topped with sauce.

Dinner

- MENU -
Ratatouilli
Karl's Fennel Salad
Bible Bread (health food store)
Apricot Sorbet

- RECIPE -

Ratatouilli

1 T. olive oil	2 c. stewed tomatoes
1 medium onion, chopped	1 t. dried basil
1 glove garlic, minced	1 T. chopped fresh parsley
2 zucchini squash, thinly sliced	1 t. kelp
1 small eggplant peeled and cubed	1 t. Worcestershire
1 bell pepper cut into 1" pieces	

Sauté onions and garlic in olive oil for five minutes. Add squash, eggplant and bell pepper and cook for 10 minutes more, stirring gently. Add small amount of water if needed. Stir in tomatoes and seasoning. Reduce heat to low, cover skillet tightly and cook 15 minutes more. Serve immediately over a mixture of one-half cooked millet and one-half cooked brown rice.

Karl's Fennel Salad

4 med. fennel roots, steamed and diced	1 apple, sliced
1 c. blue cheese	1 c. chopped cashews
1 onion, diced	4 c. low-fat cottage cheese
1 endive, sliced	

Combine all ingredients and serve with cottage cheese. Serves four.

Apricot Sorbet

5 c. chopped fresh apricots	1-1/2 c. fresh squeezed orange juice, strained
1 c. raw honey	3/4 c. fresh squeezed lemon juice, strained

In a bowl, combine all ingredients, stir gently, and let stand at room temperature two to three hours. Pureé mixture in a blender and pour into two large ice cube trays. Freeze until one inch of the mixture is frozen on all sides of the trays. Remove and beat until mushy. Return mixture to the trays and freeze until firm. For a more delicate sorbet, beat the mixture twice, freezing slightly in between.

CHAPTER 15:

The Children's Lunchbox

Among children ages 1-14, cancer causes more deaths in the U.S. than any other disease (*Cancer Facts & Figures 1993*). There is nothing sadder than when a child's life and energy is taken by this voracious and truly preventable killer. Life comes from life, so we want to include in our loved ones' lunches as much live food as possible. We want well-balanced meals for growing children for whom optimum nutrition is so important.

Many B17 enzyme foods can be made at home and included in school lunches such as hearty millet soup, apricot kernels wrapped in dried fruit, baked beans, raw vegetable sticks, nuts, seeds and granola. A plastic thermos is a necessity for many of these variations. As your child gets used to eating healthy lunches, his or her tastes will beg for more. In the meantime, institute a strict policy against trading lunches and losing thermoses. Make a habit of including a "prize inside" every lunch to preclude trading.

Lunch box surprises
1. A complimentary note – even if it was the way his or her arm hung from its socket.
2. A new pencil or eraser.
3. A small toy.
4. A surprise apple. Remove core. Stuff with raisins, dates and a rolled up note with a funny line such as "Dear Teacher: please do not let Johnny be blue – it stains his clothes."

5. A greeting card. A Christmas card in April imploring him not to open until Christmas.
6. Short questionnaire requesting feedback on a new recipe.

SOUPS

Lentil Soup

4 c. stock or water	1 bay leaf
1 c. dried lentils, washed	1/2 green bell pepper, diced
1 t. cayenne pepper	few sprigs of parsley
1 t. celery seed	2 medium carrots, diced
1 large white onion, diced	1 t. sweet basil
2 stalks celery plus tops, chopped	1 t. nutmeg
1 t. thyme	1 T. tamari soy sauce

Bring liquid to a boil and add lentils. Reduce heat and simmer for 30 minutes, partially covered. Add remaining ingredients and simmer for 20 minutes more. Add tamari last (more or less to taste) to preserve its nutritional content. Remove half of soup from pan to blender and whiz for a few seconds to obtain a thick, warm lentil puree. Mix back into the remaining soup in the pot, stir to desired consistency. Top with minced parsley. Eat whatever's left for your lunch and compare notes when your child gets home. An older child can help adjust the recipe to his or her tastes.

Magical Millet Soup

2 qt. stock, liquid or water	2 c. zucchini squash, sliced
1/2 c. uncooked millet	1 t. basil
1 large red onion, diced	1 t. dried mint
2 stalks celery & tops, chopped	1/2 c. parsley, finely chopped
1 c. small mushrooms	juice of 1 lemon

Bring stock or water to boil in a large pot. Then add millet, onion and celery. Simmer gently in covered pot 30 to 40 minutes. During the last 10 minutes of cooking add remaining ingredients.

Black-eyed Pea Soup

4 leeks & tops, chopped
2 stalks celery, chopped
4 T. flaxseed oil
2 c. black-eyed peas, cooked
3 c. vegetable stock

1 c. raw skim milk
1 T. sorghum
1/2 t. cayenne pepper
2 T. Vegasal or other

In a soup pot, sauté leeks and celery in the oil. Cook 10 minutes stirring occasionally. Add black-eyed peas, stock and vegetable seasoning. Stir, cover, and simmer on low heat 15 minutes. Add milk, sorghum, cayenne and other seasoning to taste. Stir and simmer 10 more minutes. Include sesame crackers (recipe in chapter 14) for variety.

Hearty Vegetable Soup

2 qts. spring water
1/2 c. barley
1/2 c. chopped cabbage
1/2 c. chopped kale
4 T. vegetable seasoning
2 large tomatoes, chopped
1 large beet, grated
1 c. cooked garbanzos
1 large red onion, chopped

2 to 3 diced carrots
1 large potato, cubed
3 bay leaves
1 pkg. frozen green beans
2 cups garden peas
1 c. fresh zucchini, sliced
pinch dill weed, thyme, sweet basil,
rosemary, marjoram, garlic powder

Cook barley 30 minutes in 2 quarts water. Add rest of ingredients and simmer slowly on low heat until tender. Can vary vegetables and seasonings to suit taste.

Minestrone Soup

3 qts. spring water
2 c. millet
1/2 c. chopped carrot
1/2 c. chopped cabbage
1/2 c. chopped Swiss chard
1/2 c. chopped red onion
1/2 c. chopped celery

2 fresh tomatoes, chopped
1 clove garlic, mashed
kelp to taste
Spike or Vegasal to taste
1 c. uncooked vegetable or amino acid pasta
1 c. lima beans cooked or soaked overnight

Bring water to a boil in large pot. Add millet, chopped vegetables, garlic and seasoning. Cook for at least one hour. For last 1/2 hour of cooking time, add the pasta. Stir in lima beans last, only until warm, if not already cooked.

Black Bean Soup

1 red onion, sliced	3 T. vegetable seasoning
1 clove garlic, minced	5 tomatoes, chopped
2 cups black beans,	1 qt. tomato sauce (see chapter 13 for recipe)
soaked overnight	2 cups sliced zucchini
1 bay leaf	1-1/2 c. green bell pepper cut in med. pieces
1 T. oregano	1/2 freshly-squeezed lemon
4 T. Dr. Bronner's bouillon	1/2 c. minced parsley

In large soup pot, sauté onion and garlic in 1/2 cup spring water. Add black beans. Cover with water and cook for 1/2 hour. Add more water as needed. Add rest of ingredients and finish cooking until pepper is tender but still crisp. Add 1/2 cup minced parsley near end of cooking period. Add more water if needed, to make soupy consistency.

Cream of Carrot Soup

1 large red onion, sliced thin	1/4 c. millet flour
1 T. fresh minced garlic	1/2 t. chervil
1 c. fresh whole mushrooms	1 T. Magi
6 carrots, cut into pieces	1 T. Dr. Bronner's
1/3 c. cornstarch	2 t. freshly squeezed lemon juice
1 T. sweet basil	1/2 c. white grape juice
1/2 t. tarragon	2 c. raw skim milk
3 T. Savorex	

In large soup pot, sauté onion and garlic in 1/4 cup spring water. Add mushrooms and carrots. Cover with hot water about three inches above vegetables and cook until tender. Remove from heat and cool slightly. Pour mixture into blender and add next eight ingredients. Blend until smooth. Return to pot and add lemon and grape juice. Bring just to a boil and let simmer on low heat 15 minutes. Stir, turn off heat and add milk, stirring until blended.

SANDWICHES AND
SANDWICH FILLINGS

Bean (Burrito) Sandwiches

Are your children fond of burritos? Most bean burritos contain artery-clogging, brain-fogging animal lard, both in the bean mixture and the tortilla. Many beans contain vitamin B17, and without the additives are very healthy. You can control what goes into your child by making bean burritos yourself.

Start off by cooking or soaking any number of delicious B17 beans. (One cup of dry beans cooks up to three cups.) Garbanzos, kidney, sprouted lentils, limas, mung, navy or scarlet runners can be used. Then follow this recipe:

2 lb. beans, soaked	1 T. sorghum
2 T. sesame oil	2 T. plain yogurt (optional)
1/2 c. raw skim milk	whole wheat bread or pita
1 sprig fresh savory	1 tomato, sliced
sea salt to taste	

In skillet, sauté beans in oil for a few minutes. Moisten with the milk; add savory, salt and sorghum. Cover and cook over low heat 20 minutes. Mash and puree in a food processor or blender. If mixture is too dry, add yogurt. Serve on bread topped with tomato slice and pimento cashew sauce, if desired.

Pimento Cashew Sauce

4 c. water	1-1/4 t. sea salt
4 c. cashews	3/4 c. brewer's yeast flakes
1-1/4 T. garlic powder	16 oz. pimento
1-1/4 T. onion powder	1-1/3 c. freshly-squeezed lemon juice

In blender or food processor blend water and cashews until smooth. Add rest of ingredients, blending between, saving lemon juice for last.

Falafel (Greek Garbanzo Burgers)

1/4 c. bulgur	1/2 t. cumin
2 c. cooked garbanzos, mashed	1/4 t. black pepper
2 garlic cloves, pressed	1/4 t. turmeric
3 T. whole grain bread crumbs	1/4 t. coriander
1 egg, beaten	1 T. minced parsley
1/2 t. kelp	1/8 t. cayenne pepper

Blend all ingredients well. Refrigerate until cold. Shape into patties and fry in olive oil until brown. Serve hot or cold in whole wheat pita bread with tahini dressing.

Tahini Dressing

1/4 c. freshly-squeezed lemon juice	1/2 c. chopped parsley
1 c. plain yogurt	cayenne pepper to taste
1/4 c. cubed cucumber	sea salt to taste
1/4 c. cubed tomato	black pepper to taste

Fold mixture together and serve with falafel.

Lima Bean Filling

2 c. cooked lima beans	3/4 c. plain yogurt
1 c. finely chopped onion	1 T. soy sauce
2 cloves garlic, minced	1 T. wheat germ
1 T. olive oil	sea salt to taste
1 t. oregano	

Mash the lima beans until smooth. Sauté onion and garlic in olive oil until onion is soft, then add to lima beans. Mix together rest of ingredients and add to lima bean mixture. Blend well. Refrigerate overnight to blend flavors.

Carrot Macadamia Nut Filling

1 c. finely grated carrots	1 t. sea salt
1/4 c. plain yogurt	1 t. lemon juice
1/2 c. chopped macadamia nuts	

Combine all ingredients. Chill. Cashews may be substituted for macadamia nuts.

Sweet Potato Sandwich Filling

2 sweet potatoes, baked   1 t. grated nutmeg
1/2 c. plain yogurt   1 t. ground allspice
2 green onions, chopped (optional)   whole grain bread slices

Skin and mash sweet potato. Add yogurt and beat with electric mixer until smooth. Add rest of ingredients. Spread over bread or rolls. Can add pureed applesauce, a little honey and cinnamon or raisins for variety.

Basic Nut Butter

Place 1-1/2 cups whole or broken nuts in blender or food processor. Blend until fine and then add water in the amounts listed below depending on the type of nuts used. Add a small amount of water at a time, blending after each addition. Start and stop as necessary. Use a spatula to keep butter in motion. Mixture is thick – to avoid overtaxing the motor, make nut butter in small batches. Add sea salt to taste. Blend until very smooth. Makes about 1 cup.

Almonds, blanched- 2 to 3 T.   Pecans- 1-1/2 T.
Cashews, toasted- 4 to 6 T.   Pine nuts- 1 to 2 T.
Peanuts, toasted- 2 to 4 T.

Spread whole wheat bread with any one of your basic nut butters. Serve topped with sliced bananas and raisins.

Olive Sandwich Filling

1 c. chopped ripe olives   1/4 c. celery, finely chopped
1/4 c. sesame or sunflower seeds   1/4 c. almonds, finely chopped
1/2 c. chopped macadamia nuts

Mix with enough plain yogurt to moisten.

Eggless Burgers

1 t. Savorex or Vegasal	1 c. oatmeal
1 c. millet	1/8 t. sage
1/4 c. hot water	1/2 c. onion, finely chopped
2 T. chopped olives	1 t. garlic salt
1 c. grated raw potatoes	1/4 c. chopped macadamia nuts
1 T. wheat germ	1 t. soy sauce
1 sprig parsley, chopped	1/4 t. sea salt or to taste

Dissolve Savorex in hot water. Mix all ingredients together and form into patties. If batter is too thick, add more water. Cook over low heat in skillet or broil.

Bean Burgers

2 cups cooked B17 beans	1 t. Vegasal, Spike or sea salt
2/3 c. ground sunflower seeds	3 to 4 T. tomato sauce
1/4 c. chopped onion	1/2 c. wheat germ
1/4 t. cumin	

Combine all ingredients, adding enough wheat germ so mixture will hold its shape. Form eight patties and bake at 200° for 45 minutes, or broil 5 minutes on each side until lightly browned and crusty.

Tofu Mint Dressing

1 pkg. tofu	1 T. coarsely chopped fresh mint
1/2 to 1 c. raw skim milk	1 small garlic clove, pressed
3 T. freshly-squeezed lemon juice	sea salt to taste

In blender or food processor, blend tofu, adding milk until smooth. Add rest of ingredients and blend until smooth.

California Mission Sandwich

avocado	hot chili peppers
kelp	green bell peppers
vegetable seasoning	sliced mushrooms
1 T. lemon juice	sunflower seeds
corn tortilla or Bible Bread	alfalfa sprouts
eggless mayonnaise	

Mash or slice avocado and season with kelp, vegetable seasoning and lemon juice. Warm tortilla or bread. If using Bible bread, split the loaf and spread each side with eggless mayonnaise. Spread with avocado. Add hot chili peppers or sweet bell peppers or both, depending on your taste. Add raw mushroom slices and sprinkle with sunflower seeds. Top with alfalfa sprouts, a good covering. Serve them open face at home or put a second piece on top for a lunch box or brown bag lunch.

Nut Loaf

1 c. grated carrots	1 clove garlic, minced
1 c. chopped tomatoes	2 T. flaxseed oil
1/2 c. chopped parsley	1 c. chopped macadamia nuts
1/2 c. bell pepper pieces	1/2 t. dill

In blender or food processor, blend all ingredients. To form, pack into loaf pan. Cut in slices or mold into patties.

Avocado Filling

2 avocados, mashed	1/2 t. sea salt, or to taste
1 T. grated onion	1/2 t. sea salt, or to taste
2 T. lemon juice	

Mix all ingredients well. Chill.

CHAPTER 16:

Salads, Salad Dressings, Spreads and Sauces

SALADS

Karl's Spinach Salad

1 c. raspberry vinegar	4 cloves garlic, chopped
1/4 c. raspberries	2 med. onions, sliced
2 oz. small mushroom	6 bunch spinach, cleaned and de-stemmed
1/4 t. black pepper	1/2 c. chopped fresh cilantro
1/4 t. white pepper	1/4 c. sliced green onions

In saucepan, combine vinegar, raspberries, mushrooms, pepper, garlic and onions. Simmer on low heat five minutes. Pour over spinach and sprinkle with cilantro and green onions. Serves four.

Hawaiian Carrot Salad

1/4 c. grated carrots	1/4 c. cashews or macadamia nuts
1/4 c. grated coconut	1/4 c. apricot juice
1/3 c. grated red apples	1/8 tsp. nutmeg
1/3 c. pineapple tidbits	1 T. ground apricot kernels
1/4 c. raisins or currants	

Mix all ingredients and refrigerate overnight to blend flavors.

Cucumber Salad

1 c. plain yogurt	pinch of fresh dill
1/4 c. apple cider vinegar	sea salt to taste
1 garlic clove, pressed	2-3 cucumbers, peeled and thinly sliced

In medium bowl, combine all ingredients except cucumbers. Add cucumber and stir gently. Cover and refrigerate overnight to blend flavors.

Stuffed Tomato Salad

Core tomatoes and cut diagonally into 6 to 8 sections almost through, leaving sections connected at base. Spread to look like flowers and place on crisp greens. Stuff with tofu cottage cheese. Or in tiny tomatoes individually stuffed as an hors d'oeuvre.

Tofu Cottage Cheese

1/2 c. tofu	1/4 t. no-MSG soy sauce
1/4 t. celery salt	pinch cayenne pepper
1/8 t. onion powder	

Mix together with fork to medium curd. One serving.

Stuffed Avocado Salad

1 c. plain yogurt	1/4 c. chopped cauliflower
1 T. fresh lemon juice	1/4 c. chopped onion
1 T. minced fresh parsley	2 stalks celery, diced
1/4 t. ground cumin	1/4 c. diced beets
1/4 t. garlic powder	4 ripe avocados
sea salt to taste	lemon juice
1/4 c. green peas	

In small bowl, mix together yogurt, lemon juice, parsley and seasonings. Add vegetables (except avocados) and stir gently until they are thoroughly covered. Slice avocados in half and remove pit. Remove skin by gently sliding slotted spoon between fruit and flesh and carving the avocado out. Drizzle small amount of lemon juice over top and bottom and spoon in filling, garnishing with sprigs of parsley.

Stuffed Tomatoes

4 fresh, organic tomatoes
1 c. plain yogurt
1/4 c. lemon juice
3 T. fresh, chopped parsley

1 garlic clove, minced
1 t. kelp or sea salt
1/4 c. ground macadamia nuts
1/4 c. lentil sprouts

Scoop the pulp from the inside of four tomatoes. Drain off juice and put pulp in bowl. Add rest of ingredients. Spoon mixture into tomato shell and refrigerate two hours for flavors to blend.

Liquid Salad in a Glass

3/4 c. finely chopped onion
3/4 t. pressed garlic
1-1/2 c. chopped green bell pepper
3-1/2 c. diced tomato
1 t. paprika

1 t. olive oil
1/2 c. lemon juice
1 c. spring water
1 t. kelp
1/2 c. thinly sliced cucumber

Blend all ingredients together except cucumber in blender or food processor. Chill two to three hours. Blend in cucumber just before serving. Serves two.

Sprout Salad

1/2 c. alfalfa
1/2 c. mung bean sprouts
1/2 c. grated celery
1/2 c. diced onions
1/2 c. grated onions

1 diced red pepper
1/2 c. lemon juice
1 t. kelp
1 t. vegetable seasoning

Combine the sprouts, celery, onions and red pepper. Mix thoroughly in a large bowl. Toss with lemon juice, kelp and seasoning.

Cauliflower Salad

1 c. plain yogurt
1/4 c. lemon juice
1/4 c. olive oil
3 T. fresh chopped parsley
1 garlic clove, minced

kelp to taste
1/4 c. sliced cauliflorets
1/4 c. chopped red bell pepper
1/4 c. chopped carrots

Combine yogurt, lemon juice, olive oil, parsley, garlic and kelp. Add vegetables and toss lightly. Serve on a bed of greens.

Super Supper Salad

2 medium potatoes, cooked
1 t. chopped parsley
1 t. chopped green onion
1 t. olive oil
1/2 t. apple cider vinegar
kelp
vegetable seasoning
3 T. eggless mayonnaise
   (see recipe page 193)

1/4 bunch watercress, chopped
2 c. salad greens
1 large tomato, cut in wedges
1/2 avocado, sliced
1/2 cucumber, cut into spears
1/2 red or green bell pepper,
sliced into rings
1/2 bunch radishes, sliced
1/4 red onion, thinly sliced

Slice potatoes, toss with parsley, green onion, oil, vinegar, kelp and vegetable seasoning to taste. Add eggless mayonnaise. Chill until ready to serve. Arrange bed of watercress and greens on serving platter. Mound potato mixture in center and arrange tomato wedges, avocado, cucumber, bell pepper and radishes on greens.

Rejuvenation Salad

4 large tomatoes, cubed
2 cucumbers, diced
2 stalks celery, diced
1/2 c. finely chopped red onion
1/2 bunch watercress, rinsed,
drained and chopped
1/4 c. chopped parsley

pinch basil
1/2 t. dried mint or 1 tsp. fresh mint
1/4 c. lemon juice
2 T. olive oil
2 t. sea salt
kelp

Combine vegetables, parsley, basil and mint. Toss. Sprinkle with lemon juice, oil, salt and kelp to taste.

Golden Cole Slaw

1 c. yogurt
1/4 c. lemon juice
1/4 c. flaxseed oil
1 T. sesame seeds
1/2 t. celery seed

1 c. shredded carrots
1 c. shredded cabbage
1 c. shredded rutabaga
Unsweetened shredded coconut

In large bowl, combine yogurt, lemon juice, oil and seeds. Add shredded vegetables. Toss together lightly. Sprinkle with coconut. These vegetables make a delightful flavor combination.

B17 Cole Slaw

2 c. finely shredded cabbage
1/2 green pepper, diced
1/2 carrot, grated
1/2 peeled cucumber, chopped
1 sweet onion, finely sliced
2 T. red wine vinegar
1/2 green pepper, diced

1 T. cold spring water
1 T. apple cider vinegar
1 T. sesame oil
1 T. kelp
1 clove garlic, finely chopped
1-1/2 T. sorghum

Combine cabbage, pepper, carrot, cucumber and onion in ceramic or glass bowl. Mix together the remaining ingredients and pour over the vegetables. Allow to marinate in the refrigerator a few hours or overnight. Serves 6.

Cashew Dressed Slaw

1 small head green cabbage, finely chopped
1 c. fresh pineapple, crushed
1/4 c. spring water
1 c. cashews

1/4 c. raw honey
2 T. cider vinegar
kelp to taste

Place cabbage and pineapple in a salad bowl. Toss. In blender, food processor or mortar, blend cashews with water to make a stiff paste. To cashew mixture, add honey, vinegar and kelp. Pour over cabbage mixture and toss. Serve 6-8.

Chinese Salad Fit for a Mandarin

4 baked chicken breasts, shredded
1 t. olive oil
1/2 c. sesame seeds
1 T. ground apricot kernels

1 bunch Chinese parsley, chopped
1/4 c. chopped cilantro
Chinese spice
cinnamon salt

Saute shredded chicken in oil and sesame seeds. Turn off heat and add kernels, parsley and cilantro. Mix well and season to taste.

Chop Suey Salad

1 c. hoisin sauce
5 t. finely crushed cashews
1 T. dry mustard
pinch sea salt
1/4 c. grated cabbage

1/2 bunch watercress, chopped
1 bunch parsley, chopped
1 bunch green onions, chopped
1/2 head bok choy, chopped

Mix together hoisin sauce, cashews, mustard and salt. Set aside. In large bowl, combine chopped vegetables. Add dressing and toss to coat. Sprinkle with raisins and apricot kernels.

Mushroom Salad

1/3 c. clam juice	1/4 t. tarragon
2 T. vinegar	1/4 lb. mushrooms, sliced
1/3 c. flaxseed oil	1 red onion, thinly sliced
1/2 t. kelp	1 tomato, cut in wedges

1 to 1-1/2 qt. salad greens: Escarole, chicory,
Boston and green curly leaf, crisped

In a glass or ceramic bowl, combine clam juice, vinegar, oil, kelp and tarragon. Mix with a rotary beater until well blended. Add mushrooms and onion. Chill well. Place salad greens in a large bowl. Add mushroom-onion mixture and toss. Garnish with tomato wedges and serve immediately.

Zucchini Salad

3 small young zucchini (1 lb.)	1/4 t. oregano
3 scallions finely chopped	1 cup plain yogurt
2 T. chopped fresh dillweed	1 T. lemon juice
1 T. chopped fresh parsley	1 t. raw honey

Wash zucchini and dice very fine. Place in a salad bowl with scallions, dill, parsley and oregano. In separate bowl, combine yogurt, lemon juice and honey, and pour over the zucchini mixture. Toss. Refrigerate 30 minutes or longer before serving.

Raw Beet Salad

1 bunch small young beets and tops	1/4 c. raw honey
2 c. shredded red cabbage	1/4 c. sesame oil
1 c. grated carrots	Vegasal or Spike to taste
1/2 c. freshly-squeezed lemon juice	

Finely grate the beets into a salad bowl. Add the cabbage and carrots. In separate bowl, mix together lemon juice, honey, oil and seasoning, and pour over beet mixture. Toss and chill well.

Apple Slaw

1 small head cabbage, shredded	1 T. honey
1 carrot, grated	1/2 t. sea salt
2 T. chopped celery	dash cayenne
1 T. chopped green bell pepper	1 T. vinegar
1 large apple, chopped	1 T. eggless mayonnaise
1 T. grated onion	

Combine cabbage, carrot, celery, bell pepper, apple and onion in a salad bowl. Mix together honey, sea salt, cayenne, vinegar and mayonnaise. Pour over cabbage mixture and toss well. Let stand at least 20 minutes in refrigerator before serving.

Apple Banana Salad

3 lbs. sweet apples, red and yellow	2 or 3 bananas
1 c. chopped macadamia nuts	Boston lettuce cups
2 to 3 T. eggless mayonnaise	

Wash and core the apples but do not peel. Cut into bite size pieces and place in a salad bowl. Slice bananas and add to apple. Sprinkle with the nuts and toss with mayonnaise. Serve in lettuce cups. About 6 servings.

California Fruit Salad

1 large cantaloupe cubed or balled	2 c. seedless grapes
8 bananas, sliced	1 c. orange segments
1/2 lb. fresh cherries, halved and pitted	8 oz. papaya juice or nectar
1 pt. strawberries, halved	1 qt. guava juice
4 fresh peaches, pitted and sliced	12 oz. low fat cottage cheese
1 fresh pineapple, peeled, cored and cubed	3 T. wheat germ

Combine all ingredients except cottage cheese in a large salad bowl. Toss with ambrosia dressing. Chill at least 3 hours. Suggested serving: fruit mixture topped with scoop of cottage cheese sprinkled with wheat germ.

Ambrosia Dressing
optional for California Fruit Salad

1 c. plain yogurt   2 T. honey or to taste
1 T. vanilla   pinch nutmeg

Blend ingredients in food processor or blender.   Fold into fruit mixture.

Waldorf Cabbage Salad

1-1/4 c. eggless mayonnaise   1 small onion, sliced
1 t. raw honey   1 tart apple, cored and sliced
1 t. cider vinegar   1/8 c. wheat sprouts
kelp to taste   1/4 c. alfalfa sprouts
1/4 head fresh cabbage, grated or shredded   1/4 c. cashews, chopped
4 oz. fresh mushrooms, sliced

Combine mayonnaise, honey, vinegar and kelp in small bowl. In large bowl, combine rest of ingredients, tossing until well-mixed. Add mayonnaise mixture and blend well. Top portions with fresh tarragon and paprika.

Taiwan Fuit Salad

6 medium carrots, grated   6 medium apples, cubed
1 fresh pineapple,   2/3 c. raw macadamia nuts or raw cashews
    cut in half lengthwise, cubed   1 cup grated coconut
1 cup raisins

Mix together and serve in pineapple shells.

Fruit and Nut Salad

2 c. plain yogurt   2 apples, cubed
1/4 c. raw honey or to taste   3 bananas, sliced
1 t. cinnamon   1/4 c. chopped cashews
1 pineapple, cubed   1/4 c. chopped macadamia nuts
2 oranges, cubed   1/2 c. raw wheat germ

In medium bowl combine yogurt, honey and cinnamon. Add fruit and nuts. Just before serving add wheat germ.

Marinated Broccoli Salad

1 bunch broccoli florets   1/2 c. flaxseed oil
1 clove garlic, chopped   1/2 c. lemon juice

Put broccoli in a skillet with small amount of spring water. Cover and simmer over low heat until broccoli is crisp-tender. Meanwhile, beat together remaining ingredients. Pour dressing over chilled broccoli.

Grated Salad

3 c. grated cabbage   1/4 c. chopped green pepper
2 c. grated carrots   1/4 c. chopped celery
1/2 c. broccoli stalks, finely chopped 1/2 c. chopped cucumber
1/3 c. sesame seeds, ground   1 tomato, diced
1/2 avocado, dipped in lemon juice

In a large bowl, combine cabbage, carrots, broccoli and sesame seeds. Use the avocado, green pepper, celery, cucumber and tomato to garnish the salad in an attractive pattern. Toss with favorite vegetable dressing.

SALAD DRESSINGS

Herb Dressing

1/2 c. flaxseed oil   1/4 t. ground tarragon
3 T. apple cider vinegar   1/2 t. ground basil
1/4 t. ground marjoram   1 t. kelp
1/4 t. ground thyme   1 T. finely chopped fresh parsley

Shake vigorously in covered jar until blended. Allow to stand in refrigerator until flavors are blended.

Lemon Herb Dressing

juice of one lemon   1/4 t. dried sweet basil
2/3 c. sesame oil   1 t. vegetable broth & seasoning
1/2 to 1 t. celery seed, to taste   1/16 t. marjoram
2 sprigs parsley, finely chopped   1/2 t. sea salt or kelp
1 green onion with tops, finely chopped

Shake vigorously in jar and cover. Allow to stand in refrigerator until flavors are blended.

Garlic Herb Dressing

2/3 c. apple cider vinegar
2/3 c. sesame oil
1/4 t. dry mustard
1 clove garlic, peeled and split
1/2 to 1 t. celery seed, to taste
2 sprigs parsley, finely chopped

1 green onion with tops, finely chopped
1/4 t. dried sweet basil
1 t. vegetable broth & seasoning
1/16 t. marjoram
1/2 t. sea salt or kelp

Shake vigorously in jar and cover. Allow to stand in refrigerator until flavors are blended. After the flavors are blended, the garlic may be discarded a day or two later.

Vegetable Salad Dressing

1 c. spring water
1/4 c. flour, unbleached or whole
   wheat pastry or millet flour
1/2 c. spring water
1/2 c. chopped carrot

1 T. chopped onion
1 T. raw honey
1 clove garlic, pressed
1 T. freshly-squeezed lemon juice

In blender or food processor, thoroughly mix water and flour. In saucepan, boil mixture five minutes stirring constantly. Cool and return to blender. Add rest of ingredients and blend until smooth. Refrigerate a couple hours or overnight.

Fruit Salad Dressing #1

1 c. spring water
1/4 c. flour, unbleached or whole
   wheat pastry or millet flour
1/2 c. papaya juice

1/2 c. chopped apple
1 T. raw honey
1 T. freshly-squeezed lemon juice

In blender or food processor, thoroughly mix water and flour. In saucepan, boil mixture five minutes stirring constantly. Cool and return to blender. Add rest of ingredients and blend until smooth. Refrigerate a couple hours or overnight.

Fruit Salad Dressing #2

1 c. orange juice   1 t. honey
1 T. sesame Tahini or almond butter

Stir together or blend in blender.

Golden Dressing for Fruit Salads

1/2 c. pineapple juice   2 to 3 T. honey
2 T. orange juice   1 T. grated orange peel (organic)
1-1/2 T. cornstarch   2 T. lemon juice

Put cornstarch in rounded-bottom cup and add very small amount of water. Stir until mixture is very thick and holds together when squeezed. In saucepan, on low, heat pineapple juice, orange juice and lemon juice. When hot, add cornstarch gradually, stirring until mixture has thickened. Add honey and orange peel. Continue heating until honey has melted. Remove from heat and put in covered heatproof container. Chill before serving.

Taste Tempting Dressing

1 quart plain yogurt   2 t. sweet basil
1/8 c. tomato sauce   1-1/2 t. dillweed
1/8 c. lemon juice   1/2 t. thyme
1/4 c. chopped green peppers   3/4 t. Maggi
1/4 c. chopped fresh parsley   1/2 t. marjoram
3/4 t. oregano   3/4 t. sea salt
1/8 t. garlic powder

Stir gently until well blended. Refrigerate a couple hours or overnight to meld flavors.

Thousand Island Dressing

2 c. plain yogurt   1/4 t. dillweed
1/2 c. lemon juice   1 T. finely chopped onion
2 T. tomato sauce   4 to 6 ripe olives, finely chopped
1 T. finely chopped green pepper   1 T. chopped pimento

Stir together until well blended. Refrigerate.

Low Calorie French Dressing

1 c. tomato juice
1/2 c. grapefruit juice

1/2 c. vegetable broth

Mix together well.

Healthy Eggless Mayonnaise

4 c. spring water
1 c. millet flour
2 T. honey
1-1/2 t. sea salt

1/2 t. garlic powder
1/2 t. onion powder
3/4 c. flaxseed oil
2 T. freshly-squeezed lemon juice

In blender or food processor, blend water and flour. In saucepan cook mixture until thick and bubbly, stirring constantly. Cool. In blender, measure two cups of the mixture and add honey, sea salt, garlic powder and onion powder. Blend well and add oil (until white and shiny) and lemon juice. Chill before using.

Cole Slaw Dressing

1/2 c. eggless mayonnaise
1/2 t. celery seed
1 T. honey

1/2 t. onion salt
1 t. lemon juice

Combine all ingredients and mix well.

Caesar Salad Dressing

1/4 c. lemon juice
1 clove garlic finely chopped
1/4 c. spring water
1 T. anchovy paste
1/4 c. cider vinegar

1 T. honey
1/4 to 1/2 t. vegetable salt
3 T. grated Romano cheese
1/4 t. fresh cayenne pepper
3/4 c. olive oil

Put all ingredients except oil in blender or food processor. Blend on medium speed until smooth. While blending, add the oil gradually until the mixture thickens. Chill well.

Russian Salad Dressing

1 c. low fat cottage cheese   1 T. apple cider vinegar
1/4 c. tomato juice   1 hard boiled egg, chopped

In blender or food processor blend together cottage cheese and vinegar. Add tomato juice and continue blending until very smooth, adding more tomato juice if necessary. Stir the egg into the dressing just before serving.

Parsley Dressing

2 cloves garlic, pressed   1 bunch parsley, chopped
1-1/2 c. sesame oil   1-1/2 c. lemon juice
1 t. dry mustard   kelp to taste

Put garlic, oil and mustard in blender or food processor. Blend briefly. Add parsley, lemon juice and kelp. Blend until just mixed.

Herb Dressing

1/4 c. apple cider vinegar   2 T. vegetable seasoning
1 t. sea salt or kelp   1 t. salad herbs to taste
2 T. spring water   2/3 c. sesame oil

Put all ingredients except oil in a jar. Shake well. Add oil and shake again. Chill several hours before using.

Sesame Salad Dressing

1/2 c. ground sesame seeds   juice of 1/2 lemon
1 c. spring water   1/2 clove garlic
1 t. kelp

Place seeds and 1 cup water in blender or food processor and blend until smooth. Add remaining ingredients and blend until smooth, adding more spring water if necessary to give thick consistency.

SAUCES AND SPREADS

Date Spread

1 cup chopped pitted dates   1 cup spring water

Cook dates and water on low heat, stirring often to prevent sticking until dates are very soft. Whiz in blender briefly. Refrigerate. Keeps well one week.

Mock Tuna Sandwich Spread

1/2 c. ground sesame seeds   1/2 clove garlic
1 c. spring water   1/2 c. chopped onions
1 t. kelp   1/2 c. chopped celery
juice of 1/2 lemon   1/2 c. mixed alfalfa, mung bean & lentil sprouts

Place seeds and 1 cup water in blender or food processor and blend until smooth. Add remaining ingredients and blend until desired consistency, adding more water if necessary.

Spicy Baked Potato Topping

1/4 c. spring water   1/2 chili pepper, chopped
1/4 c. apple cider vinegar   1/4 t. nutmeg
1 med. onion, chopped   1/4 t. oregano
3 garlic cloves, crushed   1/4 t. black pepper
4 med. tomatoes, chopped   1/8 c. cilantro, chopped

Combine all ingredients. Refrigerate overnight and serve over baked potatoes.

Berry Sauce

4 cups fresh frozen unsweetened berries, thawed   2 T. ground tapioca
berry juice and water to make 1-1/2 cups liquid   2 very ripe bananas

Pour juice off berries into a two-cup measure. Add water to make 1-1/2 cups. Put in blender or food processor. Add bananas and tapioca. Blend briefly. Pour mixture into saucepan, cook over medium heat until thickened. Add berries and heat through.

Serve over crepes, pancakes, waffles; in yogurt or over ice cream.

Date Syrup

1/4 lb. pitted dates   1/2 cup water

In saucepan, combine dates and water. Simmer over low heat until dates are soft. Mash dates and cook until thick syrup is formed. Refrigerate. Serve on crepes, pancakes or waffles.

Apricot Sauce

2 T. dried apricots   2 oranges, peeled and segmented
2 c. spring water   3/4 c. unsweetened pineapple juice

Soak apricots in spring water overnight. Put oranges, apricots, and water in which they were soaked in blender or food processor. Blend briefly. Add pineapple juice slowly while blending. Delicious on waffles, pancakes, hot cereal, etc.

Almond Fruit Milk

1-1/2 c. almonds   1/2 c. favorite dried fruit
4 c. spring water   1/8 t. sea salt

Grind almonds fine. Soak dried fruit in one cup of hot water five to 10 minutes to soften. In blender or food processor, blend almonds, fruit, soaking water, sea salt and rest of water until smooth. Use as cream on cereal.

Homestyle Mustard

1 cup eggless mayonnaise   1 T. fresh lemon juice
1 t. turmeric   dash paprika
2 t. onion juice   dash garlic salt
2 T. chopped parsley   dash onion salt

Mix all ingredients in a small bowl. Refrigerate until flavors are blended

Quick Tomato Catsup

1/2 c. chopped onion   1/4 c. lemon juice
1 garlic clove, minced   1/4 t. cumin
2 c. tomato puree   1/2 t. sweet basil
1 t. sea salt   1 c. tomato paste
1 t. paprika   1/4 cup spring water

In blender or food processor, blend onion and garlic with lemon juice and 1/2 cup tomato puree until smooth. Combine with rest of ingredients. Bring to a boil and let simmer a few minutes or until desired consistency. Makes 1 quart.

Lemon Juice Catsup

4 tomatoes, chopped	1/2 t. basil
6 oz. tomato paste	1 medium onion, chopped
1-1/2 t. sea salt	1 large stalk celery, diced
1 t. Savorex	2 sprigs parsley, chopped
1 clove garlic, minced	1/4 c. fresh lemon juice
1/2 pimento, diced	2 T. raw honey
1 bay leaf	

Simmer tomatoes, tomato paste, salt and Savorex in heavy saucepan while preparing vegetables. Add rest of ingredients except lemon juice and honey. Simmer until vegetables are crispy tender. Remove bay leaf. This makes a tomato relish. For catsup, whiz in blender or press through sieve. Cool. Add lemon juice and honey. Refrigerate.

Roasted Garlic Butter

The term butter is used loosely here, as there is no animal fat in this butter. I've devoted a whole chapter to the cancer benefits of garlic and now you may carry this one step further by substituting roasted garlic for margarine or butter on your bread.

To make it, peel off most of the outer husk of a whole head of garlic, but don't separate or peel the cloves. Place it in a small baking dish (or use a garlic roaster) and drizzle with a small amount of good-quality olive oil. Wrap tightly with foil and roast in a 325 degree oven until the cloves are completely soft, about 45 minutes. The result is sometimes known as "garlic toothpaste," because the pulp can be squeezed onto bread like toothpaste. The roasting mellows the flavor and aroma so your breath won't be as bad as if you'd eaten it raw.

Mushroom Gravy

2 T. minced onion
1/2 c. mushrooms
4 T. millet flour
2 cups vegetable stock

1/4 t. soy sauce
1/4 t. Savorex
1/4 t. salt

Combine onions and mushrooms in small saucepan over low heat. Add small amount of spring water to the flour to make a smooth paste. To saucepan add vegetable stock, then flour mixture, stirring until thickened. Add seasonings.

Basic Tomato Soup

12 large ripe tomatoes, skinned & chopped
2 green peppers seeded
2 onions, chopped
2 carrots, chopped
6 stalks celery, diced
2 T. chopped fresh chives

2 T. chopped fresh parsley
2 T. chopped fresh basil
2 cloves garlic, chopped fine
1/2 t. Worcestershire sauce
sea salt and pepper to taste

Combine all ingredients in a stainless steel or porcelain steel pan or casserole. Bring to a boil and simmer uncovered for 45 minutes. Puree in a blender if desired. Refrigerate overnight before using or freeze for future use. Makes about 2 quarts.

Barbecue Sauce

1/2 c. tomato sauce
juice of one lemon wedge
1 clove garlic, crushed

1/4 t. rosemary
1/4 t. sweet basil
dash of honegar (honey/vinegar)

To tomato sauce add lemon juice, garlic, herbs and honegar.

CHAPTER 17:

Breakfast Dishes

Millet Breakfast Cereal

1 c. whole hulled millet	1 c. chopped, unpeeled apples
1 qt. spring water	1 c. raisins
1 t. sea salt	1/2 c. sesame seeds

Put millet, water and salt in saucepan. Bring to a boil and simmer on low heat 45 minutes or until soft. Add apples, raisins, and sesame seeds. Add honey to sweeten, if desired. Serve with raw skim milk or omit apples and raisins and serve with hot fruit sauce. Serves 4 to 6.

Shop organic! Purchase grains which have been grown organically and are freshly-harvested. Three whole grain cereals all to be cooked the same:

Cereal #1

1/2 c. millet	5 c. spring water
1/2 c. buckwheat kernels (Kasha)	1 t. kelp
1/4 c. barley	

Cereal #2

1/2 c. whole wheat	3 c. spring water
1/2 c. millet	1 t. sea salt
1/4 c. whole rye	

Cereal #3

1/2 c. buckwheat groats   3 c. spring water
1/2 c. brown rice   1 t. kelp
1/4 c. whole wheat

Cook ingredients from one of the above groups overnight in a crock pot or steam on stove's lowest heat. Breakfast is ready when you get up. Serve with raisins, dates, nuts or with hot fruit sauce. Use other combinations of grains but keep selections to two or three grains.

Note: Of utmost importance is the change to low heat. Very slow cooking tenderizes the fibers without destroying the enzymes, vitamin B17, minerals or other nutrients.

Ground Whole Grain Cereal

1 c. grains   1 t. sea salt
2 c. cold spring water   Raisins, dates, other dried fruits (optional)

Use a combination of three different freshly-harvested, organically-grown grains. Put whole kernels of wheat, barley, rye, soy beans, corn or millet in blender or food processor and blend at high speed until they are as fine as you wish. Chopped dried fruit may be added to ground grains prior to cooking for added flavor and texture.

Cook in saucepan, double boiler or steamer. Boil 5 minutes, cover tightly and turn off heat. Let stand, without removing cover, for 20 minutes. Wheat germ may be added to cereal before serving. Serve with raw skim milk.

Whole Grain Cereal – Thermos Method

In the morning put one cup of chosen whole grains, whole or cut, in bowl. Cover with spring water to soak. In the evening add enough spring water to equal 3 cups (five cups for buckwheat groats). Bring to a boil with sea salt to taste. Pour into preheated thermos. Screw on cap and turn on its side until breakfast time the next morning. Serve as usual with raisins, dates, fruit sauce or raw skim milk. Note: save leftover cereal and mix with legumes, seeds or nuts and seasoning for tasty entrees. Mix while breakfast cereal is still warm. Pack into loaf pan or make into patties and bake.

Breakfast Beans

Pick from any one of the wide variety of B17 rich beans:

2 c. beans of your choice	1 large onion, chopped
6 c. boiling spring water	pinch basil
2 t. sea salt	slices whole wheat bread

Sort and wash beans. Add to boiling water and bring back to boiling point. Turn off heat and let stand for one hour, covered. Bring to boil and simmer until nearly done. Add salt and finish cooking. Sauté onion on low heat in its own juice. Add a little water if necessary. Add to beans with enough water to make a soupy consistency. Simmer until beans are very tender. Serve on toast.

El Rancho Breakfast Limas

2 medium white onions, diced	1 t. marjoram
2 stalks celery, finely chopped	2 T. brewer's yeast
2 T. sesame oil	2 c. cooked lima beans
1 c. tomato sauce	1-1/2 c. grated white cheddar cheese
1/4 t. celery seed	juice of 1/2 lemon
1 t. garlic powder	1 T. tamari soy sauce
1/4 t. cayenne pepper	sprigs Chinese parsley

In a Chinese wok or large frying pan, sauté onion and celery in the oil until golden. Add tomato sauce, spices, yeast and stir well over a low heat. Add limas, one cup grated cheese and continue to stir. Add lemon juice and tamari sauce. Heat through and serve, topping each portion with the remaining grated cheese and a garnish of parsley.

Triple Grain Cakes

1/4 c. millet whole grain	3/4 c. raw skim milk
1/4 c. barley whole grain	1 t. sea salt
1/4 c. oats whole grain	1 t. date spread

Soak grains overnight in cold water. Drain water from grains and place in blender with milk. Whiz three to five minutes. Add salt, date spread and blend another minute. Continue blending until fluffy and filled with air. Cook immediately on a pan that has been lightly greased with lecithin oil or cold pressed sesame oil.

Griddle Cakes

2 c. soaked soybeans
1 c. spring water
1 c. raw skim milk
1 t. raw honey

1 t. sea salt
2/3 c. whole wheat
2/3 c. millet flour

Blend all ingredients except flour and place in bowl. Stir in flour.
Spoon onto medium hot griddle. Cover and let brown; turn and
brown other side. Best if well cooked.

Sesame Millet Soy Waffles

1-1/2 c. soaked soybeans (1 c. dry)
2-1/4 c. spring water
1-1/4 c. millet flour

1/2 t. sea salt
1/2 c. raw sesame seeds

Soak beans several hours or overnight in sufficient water to cover.
Drain. Discard water. Soaked, drained soy beans may be kept in
refrigerator for a week or in freezer for longer periods. Keep on hand
for immediate use.

Combine all ingredients until light and foamy, about 1/2 minute.
Let stand while waffle iron is heating. The batter thickens upon standing. Stir. Bake in hot iron for eight minutes or until brown. Set timer
for eight minutes and do not open until time is up. Cook few seconds
longer if iron sticks. Sprinkle about a tablespoon of sesame seeds on
waffle iron prior to pouring the batter. The oil from the sesame seeds
will keep the waffles from sticking and give them added B17 punch.

Cashew Oat Waffles

2-1/2 c. spring water
1/3 c. raw cashews

1-3/4 c. old fashioned oats
1/2 t. sea salt

Blend all ingredients until smooth. Bake in preheated medium hot
waffle iron 10 to 12 minutes. Do not open before time is up.

Eggless French Toast

3/4 c. spring water
1/2 c. cashews
2-4 pitted dates

pinch sea salt
whole wheat toast

Whiz water, cashews and dates in blender. Dip bread in cashew mixture. Place on cookie sheet and under broiler to brown each side. Top with fruit sauce, sorghum, or sliced bananas.

Tahini French Toast

1 c. Tahini (sesame butter)
1-1/2 c. spring water

1/2 t. sea salt
slices of whole wheat bread

Mix until smooth. Dip bread into mixture - quick in, quick out. Let excess batter drip off. Brown on both sides in broiler.

Granola

3/4 c. spring water
3/4 c. pitted dates
1 T. pure vanilla
7 c. whole oats
1/2 c. soy flour

3/4 c. slivered almonds
1 c. millet flour
1 c. grated coconut
1 t. sea salt

In blender or food processor, combine water, dates and vanilla. Combine dry ingredients in a large bowl and add date mixture. Mix thoroughly. Put in large shallow pan and bake at 250°. Stir every 20 minutes to prevent burning and bake until golden brown and crisp, about 1-1/2 to 2 hours.

Barley Millet Muffins

1 c. barley flour
1 c. millet
1/2 t. sea salt
1 c. grated fresh apples

1 T. flaxseed oil
3/4 c. spring water
1/2 c. raisins

In large bowl, combine flour, millet and salt. In separate container, combine apples, oil, water and raisins. Stir. Add apple mixture to flour mixture and mix well. Let stand a few minutes to absorb. Stir and spoon into oiled muffin tins. Bake at 350° for 25 minutes.

Breakfast Cookies

3 bananas	1/2 t. sea salt
1 c. chopped dried apricots	1 T. vanilla
1/2 c. chopped cashews	2 c. quick oats

Mash bananas, leaving some chunks. Add dates and nuts. Beat well and add salt, vanilla and oats. Drop by spoonfuls onto ungreased cookie sheet. Bake 25 minutes or so in 400° oven. Loosen immediately. Some cookie sheets may need a little oil. The shiny ones need the least. If you need a bit of oil, lightly cover the pan either with lecithin oil or cold pressed sesame seed oil.

CHAPTER 18:

Homemade Breads

Common Defects in Bread and Their Possible Causes
(from *The Art of Making Bread* by Marian Dakin)

1. Sour taste – period of fermentation too long, or temperature too high while fermenting, causing formation of acid. Poor yeast or unstable yeast starter.

2. Dry or crumbly – too much flour in dough; overbaking.

3. Heaviness – unevenness of temperature while rising. Insufficient kneading.

4. Cracks in crust – cooling in a draft; baking before sufficiently light; oven too hot.

5. Too thick a crust – oven too slow, baked too long; too much salt.

6. Dark patches or streaks – poor starting material; shortening added to liquid before flour, thus allowing flour particles to become coated with fat before they had absorbed equal amounts of liquid.

7. Sogginess – too much liquid; insufficient baking.

8. Ill-shaped loaf – not molded well originally; too large a loaf for the pan; fermentation period too long; failure to rise to greatest size in oven.

9. Coarse grain – too high a temperature; fermented too long; too long rising in pan; oven too cool at first; pan too large for size of loaf.

Basic Bread Recipe

1 c. rolled oats	2 T. yeast or 2 pkgs. dried yeast
2 c. boiling spring water	5 c. whole wheat flour
1 large apple	3 c. millet flour
1/2 c. pitted dates	1-1/2 t. sea salt

Put oats into a large bowl and pour on boiling water. Let sit until water is absorbed, about 20 to 25 minutes. Wash and cut up apple. Put into blender with the dates and enough warm water to equal 1-1/2 cups liquid. Blend very well. Pour into a large bowl. Add the yeast and stir in. Let sit 10 minutes or until bubbly. Combine the salt with the flour. When yeast mixture is ready, add the special ingredients of the day (see variations below).

Stir in flour two cups at a time. Knead. Leave dough in bowl, scatter 1/2 cup flour on top of dough and with heel of hand press into the dough with one quick firm press. With the fingers, get hold of the dough and sift it around, sometimes turning it over. Repeat this process over and over with the rest of the flour. If dough is sticky, work in a little more flour. Shape dough into a mound in center of bowl and cover with damp towel. Let rise about two hours until double in bulk. Punch down. Divide and place into two lightly-oiled bread pans, shaping dough out to ends to cover sides of pans. Cover and let rise again until the top is well rounded, about one hour. Bake 50-60 minutes at 350° on rack about four inches from bottom of oven.

Special ingredients:

1 c. seedless raisins and	1/2 t. dried parsley
3/4 c. citron dried, fruits and peels	2 t. dried summer savory
2 t. leaf sage, crumbled	1 t. anise seed
1 t. leaf marjoram	1/2 t. caraway seed
1 t. dried basil	

These variations can be used singularly or together.

Orange Raisin Nut Bread

Use 2 cups near boiling orange juice instead of water. Add 1 t. grated orange ring, 1 cup seedless raisins, 1/2 cup chopped walnuts.

Dark Mixed Grain Bread

1/2 c. wheat germ	1-1/2 c. rye
1/2 c. buckwheat flour	4-1/2 c. whole wheat

Pumpernickel

1 T. caraway seeds	2-1/2 c. rye
1 c. bran flakes	3-1/2 c. whole wheat flour

CHAPTER 19:

Main Entrees

Eggplant Parmesan

1 large eggplant	oregano
6 large tomatoes, skinned	paprika
basil	1 lb. non-pasteurized, low-fat
thyme	Mozzarella cheese, thinly sliced
Italian seasoning	

Preheat oven to 400°. Peel the eggplant and slice crosswise into paper-thin slices. Blend the tomatoes in blender until smooth and add seasonings to taste. Oil a large casserole or baking dish and create alternating layers of eggplant, Mozzarella and tomato puree, topping with layer of cheese. Bake 1 hr. Serves 6.

Tofu Quiche

1 med. onion	2 pinches coriander
1 T. olive oil	1 light pinch cayenne pepper
3/4 c. mushrooms, sliced	1 t. kelp
1 med. zucchini, sliced	1 pkg. Tofu
1 pinch basil	1 T. tamari
1 pinch thyme	

Sauté onions in olive oil until translucent. Add mushrooms, zucchini, herbs and spices. Sauté until zucchini is crispy/tender. In blender or food processor, blend Tofu with tamari until creamy. Combine both mixtures in large bowl and stir well. Pour into whole grain pie crust and bake at 350° for approximately 30 to 45 minutes.

Whole Grain Pie Crust

4 c. spring water
1/2 c. buckwheat
1/2 c. millet

1/3 c. raw sesame seeds, ground
1 T. sesame tahini
2 T. tamari

Bring water to boil, adding grains. Drain if there is water after cooking. Moisten grains with tahini and tamari. Add sesame seeds and mix with hands until dough is soft. Press in greased pie plate.

Fritata

1 bunch spinach
1 bunch Swiss chard
4 zucchini, sliced
1 onion
1 clove garlic, minced
1/4 c. whole grain bread crumbs, minced

1/2 c. freshly grated parmesan cheese
3 eggs
1 t. Italian herb seasoning
Sea salt and cayenne pepper to taste
2 t. raw sesame seeds

Wash spinach, chard and zucchini. Drain. Steam swiss chard and spinach lightly. Chill. Sauté zucchini, onion and garlic in oil five minutes and cool. Combine bread crumbs, cheese, and Italian seasoning. Add beaten eggs to dry mixture. Add egg mixture to chilled vegetables. Grease square baking pan and sprinkle with sesame seeds. Shake off excess seeds. Bake in 300° oven 25 minutes or until firm.

French Lentil Loaf

1-3/4 c. chopped onion
1 clove garlic, minced
2 T. olive oil
1 c. grated carrots
1 c. shredded apples
2-1/2 c. cooked lentils

1 c. whole wheat bread crumbs
1/2 t. sea salt
1/2 t. ground rosemary
1/2 t. ground tarragon
2 beaten egg whites
1/3 c. vegetable broth

Sauté onions and garlic in oil until onions begin to soften. Add carrots and apples and sauté until soft. Allow to cool. In large bowl, combine lentils, bread crumbs, seasonings, egg whites and broth. Add cooled vegetables. Put mixture into lightly-oiled loaf pan. Bake 350° 45 minutes.

Lentil Loaf Sauce

1/3 c. sliced mushrooms　　　2 T. arrowroot
1 large onion, chopped　　　　2 T. vegetable seasoning
1 T. olive oil　　　　　　　　2 c. cold spring water

Sauté mushrooms and onions in oil over low heat. Cover for 10 minutes. Dissolve arrowroot and vegetable seasoning in the water. Pour mixture into sauté pan and slowly bring to a boil. Simmer on low heat until thickened. Serve over lentil loaf.

Karl's Bean Stew

2 c. assorted beans　　　　　1/4 t. nutmeg
2 c. vegetable broth　　　　　1/2 t. oregano
2 med. onions, chopped　　　　1/2 t. rosemary
2 cloves garlic, chopped　　　　1/2 c. chopped cilantro
1/2 t. black pepper　　　　　1 T. white vinegar
1/2 t. white pepper

Precook beans two times for about 10 minutes, each time. In large pot combine beans with broth, simmering on low heat 30 minutes. Add rest of ingredients except cilantro and vinegar. Let simmer five minutes. Serve with brown rice. Serves four.

Vegetable Chow Mein

1/2 c. spring water　　　　　　1/2 c. celery root, sliced
1 c. sliced celery　　　　　　　1 c. Chinese cabbage
1 c. sliced mushrooms　　　　　1 c. warm spring water
1 c. sliced onion　　　　　　　2 t. vegetable seasoning
1 c. broccoli florets　　　　　1 c. bean sprouts
1 c. broccoli stalks, peeled & sliced　2 T. arrowroot

In skillet, bring water to a boil, then cook vegetables over low heat 15 or 20 minutes. Combine warm water and vegetable seasoning. Pour over vegetables. Add sprouts. Mix arrowroot with a little cold water, and carefully add it to the vegetables. Cook and stir over low heat until thickened. Serve over cooked millet or brown rice.

Bulgur Burgers

1 t. garlic, pressed	3 c. cooked bulgur
10 mushrooms, chopped	1 beaten egg white
1 red onion, chopped	3 T. whole wheat flour
1/4 c. green bell pepper, chopped	2 T. tamari sauce

In saucepan, sauté vegetables, adding mushrooms last. Chill. Mix cold vegetables with the bulgur and add rest of ingredients. Form into patties. Place under broiler for about five minutes or until tops are golden brown. Can be topped with lentil loaf sauce or thickened vegetable stock.

Meatless Spaghetti Sauce

1/3 c. lentils	1 t. chives
2 c. red kidney beans, dried	1 t. parsley
2 bay leaves	1/2 t. sea salt
2 tomatoes, chopped	1 t. garlic powder
1/2 c. tomato juice	1 t. onion powder
2 whole onions, chopped	2 T. olive oil
1 c. sliced mushrooms	2 T. oregano
2 stalks celery with tops, chopped	1/4 t. cayenne pepper

Boil a quart of spring water and drop in lentils and kidney beans with two bay leaves. Turn off the heat. Allow the beans to sit one hour. Pour off and reserve the excess water for later. Put in remaining ingredients and simmer until celery is tender. Add reserved water as needed. Serve over spinach noodles.

Curried Pea Soup

2 c. dried split peas	1/2 t. celery seed
10 c. spring water	1/2 t. curry powder
1 carrot, grated	2 c. cooked brown rice
2 potatoes, grated	1 T. grated apricot kernels
1 onion, grated	

Place peas and water in large soup pot. Bring to a boil, cover and cook over low heat one hour. Add grated vegetables, celery seed and curry powder. Cover and cook 30 minutes. Add cooked rice and cook another 30 minutes. Sprinkle with apricot kernels before serving.

Vegetable Lasagna

1 bunch Swiss chard
4 med. carrots, sliced
2 turnips, chopped
1 zucchini, chopped
1 small cauliflower, chopped
4 c. tomato sauce
2 onions, sliced
3 cloves garlic, pressed

1 t. cilantro, chopped
1 c. olives, sliced
pinch of black pepper
pinch of oregano
pinch of nutmeg
spinach lasagna noodles
1 c. low-fat Mozzarella cheese, grated

Steam chard leaves, carrots, turnips, zucchini and cauliflower until crispy/tender. Boil lasagna noodles. In large bowl, combine tomato sauce with vegetables, olives and seasonings (omitting only chard and cheese). Pour 1 c. tomato/vegetable sauce in flat baking pan. Add 1 layer of lasagna noodles, then 1 layer of steamed chard leaves, then 1 layer of sauce. Continue layering, ending with sauce and cheese on top. Bake at 350° for 35 minutes and serve.

Bo's Spinach Potato Almond Casserole

1 c. chicken broth
1 med. onion, chopped
2 c. spinach, chopped
2 potatoes, cooked and diced
juice of 1/2 lime

pinch black pepper
1/2 t. basil
2 tomatoes, sliced
1/2 c. almonds, sliced

Sauté onion in chicken broth until clear. Pour in square cooking dish. Combine spinach, potatoes, lime juice, pepper and basil. Put on top of onion/broth. Top with tomato slices and sprinkle with almonds. Bake at 325° for about 25 minutes.

Lentil Turnip Stew

1 c. lentils
3 med. turnips, chopped
2 med. carrots, chopped
2 med. potatoes, chopped
1 bay leaf

pinch nutmeg
1 t. peppers
vegetable stock
1/4 c. apple cider vinegar

Cook lentils two times, starting with cold water each time, over low heat. Drain water. Add all ingredients except vinegar. Let simmer for about 90 minutes. Add vinegar and serve.

Vegetable Millet Souffle

3 c. whole millet, cooked
1 onion, chopped
1 carrot, sliced
1 bell pepper, sliced
1 c. chopped cabbage
1 zucchini, sliced

2 garlic cloves, chopped
1/4 t. oregano
1/4 t. pepper
1/4 t. nutmeg
1 c. vegetable broth

Spread millet evenly on bottom of oiled casserole dish. Combine vegetables, garlic and spices. Place on top of millet. Pour vegetable broth over top. Cover and bake 20 minutes at 350°. Take cover off and bake 10 more minutes and serve.

Lentil Potato Burger

2 c. cooked mashed potato
2 c. lentils, cooked
pinch nutmeg

pinch pepper
1 t. brewer's yeast
1 beaten egg yolk

In blender or food processor blend all ingredients until smooth. Form patties and cook in preheated oiled skillet or broil both sides until brown. Serve with apple or apricot sauce on side.

Lentil Souffle

1 c. vegetable stock
2 c. cooked lentils
1 c. chopped onion
1 c. chopped carrots

1 c. chopped celery
1 t. pepper salt
pinch nutmeg
pinch oregano

Pour vegetable stock in square baking pan. Add lentils, then add all other ingredients, spices last. Bake for 20 minutes at 350°.

Green Bean Salad

1 lb. small tender green beans
1/2 med. onion, diced
1 garlic clove, diced
pinch black pepper

2 T. freshly chopped tarragon
1/4 c. olive oil
3 T. tarragon vinegar

Wash and trim beans. Steam until crispy/tender. Chill. Add rest of ingredients and refrigerate several hours until flavors blend.

Millet Beans

1 lb. green beans
1-1/2 c. whole millet, cooked
1/2 med. onion, diced
1 garlic clove, diced

1 t. basil
pinch oregano
pinch black pepper
1/4 c. maple syrup

Wash and trim beans. Steam until crispy tender. Set aside. Spread millet on bottom of oiled casserole dish. Top with beans, onion, garlic. Sprinkle with seasoning. Pour maple syrup on top. Bake for about 20 minutes at 350°.

Variety Bean Millet Soup

1 c. beans of choice
1 c. whole millet
2 garlic cloves, pressed
2 onions, chopped
1 carrot, chopped

2 potatoes, chopped
1/4 c. cilantro, chopped
1/2 t. nutmeg
1/2 t. peppers
1/2 t. oregano

Cook beans twice in fresh water. The third time use vegetable stock. Let boil until beans are semi-soft. Add all ingredients including millet. Simmer on low heat until beans and millet are done.

Sweet Pea Stew

1 t. butter
1 lb. fresh sweet peas
1 onion, sliced
1 lb. combination bok choy leaves,
spinach and Swiss chard

1 t. chopped ginseng root
pinch pepper salt
1/2 c. chopped mushrooms
1/2 c. vegetable stock

Melt butter in saucepan. Add all ingredients and sauté for five minutes over medium heat. Add vegetable stock. Reheat and serve over brown rice or buckwheat groats.

Bo's Black Beans

1 c. black beans
1/2 c. maple syrup
1/4 c. raspberry vinegar

pinch lemon pepper
pinch cayenne pepper

Cook black beans slightly covered with water until soft, over low heat. Cook for 2-3 hours. Add all other ingredients. Simmer on low heat 30 more minutes and serve.

CREPES

Basic Whole Wheat Crepe Recipe

3 eggs	1-1/4 c. spring water
1-1/2 c. millet	1/2 c. whole wheat flour
1 c. soy milk	2 T. butter, melted
1 T. wheat germ	pinch sea salt

Place all ingredients in a blender or mixer and beat well. Stir periodically. Batter should be thin. In lightly-oiled hot skillet, pour about a tablespoon of batter. Roll skillet around until bottom is coated and pancake is thin. When first bubble forms, gently lift edge and flip to other side. Separate individual crepes with wax paper. Crepes can be frozen or refrigerated for future use.

Crepe Fillings:

Fresh Mushroom Sprout

2 T. olive oil	1 c. raw skim milk
2 c. fresh mushrooms, sliced	cayenne pepper to taste
3 green onions, chopped	sea salt to taste
3 T. millet flour	2 c. bean sprouts

Sauté onions and mushrooms in oil. Add flour and stir. Add milk gradually, cooking over low heat until thickened. Add salt and pepper. Wrap mixture in crepes, topping with bean sprouts just before serving.

Tofu and Cashew Crepes

4 pkgs. tofu, cut into small cubes	2 T. no-MSG soy sauce
1/2 c. coarsely chopped cashews	1 t. sesame oil
1/2 c. diced celery	1/2 t. black pepper
1/2 c. diced green pepper	1/2 t. white pepper
1/2 T. raw honey	

Place tofu, cashews, celery and green pepper in salad bowl. Combine honey, soy sauce and oil in small bowl. Combine two mixtures and toss with seasonings. Serve cold wrapped in crepes or as a salad with crepes on the side.

Karl's Gooseberry Sweet Potato Crepes

4 med. sweet potatoes,
cooked and mashed
2 c. gooseberries
1/2 c. pure maple syrup

1 t. cinnamon
juice of one lemon
pinch cayenne pepper

In saucepan combine berries, syrup, cinnamon, lemon juice and cayenne. Let simmer on low heat about seven minutes. Add to mashed sweet potato. Mixture may be served hot or cold, rolled in crepes.

CHAPTER 20:

Desserts

Basic Dessert Crepe

3/4 c. whole wheat flour	2 T. butter, melted
1-1/2 c. raw skim milk	1/2 t. lemon, rum or vanilla extract
3/4 c. millet flour	3 egg whites, beaten
2 T. raw honey	pinch sea salt

Place all ingredients in a blender or mixer and beat well. Stir periodically. Batter should be thin. Let stand while preheating iron skillet. In lightly-oiled hot skillet, pour about a tablespoon of batter. Roll skillet around until bottom is coated and pancake is thin. When first bubble forms, gently lift edge and flip to other side. Separate individual crepes with wax paper. Can be frozen or refrigerated for future use.

Apple-Filled Crepes

1/3 c. butter	1 t. ground cinnamon
3 lbs. tart cooking apples, chopped	2 T. chopped apricot kernels
1/2 c. honey	

Melt butter and honey over low heat. Add apples and cinnamon. Cook, stirring gently from time to time, until apples have softened and begin to change color. Fill crepes and fold. Sprinkle with chopped apricot kernels. Serve hot.

Gooseberry Crepes

2 c. gooseberries
1/4 c. raw honey

2 mint leaves, chopped
pinch cayenne

In saucepan, heat all ingredients on low until berries are heated through. Spoon over folded crepes.

Lemon Nut Crepes

1/2 c. raw honey
1/2 c. vanilla yogurt
juice of one lemon

1 c. macadamia nuts, crushed
1 t. dried mint

In small bowl, blend honey, lemon juice and yogurt. To each crepe pancake, spread with yogurt mixture and sprinkle with nuts. Crepes can be rolled or folded into fourths. Sprinkle with dried mint.

Carrot Cake

2 c. whole wheat flour
1/2 c. millet flour
5 t. baking powder
1/4 t. grated orange peel (organic)
1/4 t. grated lemon peel
1/2 t. cinnamon
3/4 c. raw honey

1 c. flaxseed oil
1 c. spring water
2 c. grated carrots
1 c. chopped cashews
1 c. raisins
3 egg whites

Sift flour and baking powder. Add orange peel, lemon peel and cinnamon. In a large bowl, beat honey and oil. Add water and mix well. Add flour mixture to honey/oil/water mixture. Add carrots, cashews and raisins, mixing in between. Beat egg whites until frothy. Fold in batter. Place in a 13" x 9" glass baking dish. Bake in 350° oven for 40-45 minutes.

Carob Cake

(The best I have ever tasted!)

2 eggs or egg whites
3/4 c. raw honey
1/2 c. carob
2 1/2 t. baking powder

1 c. and 2 T. barley flour
1/2 c. flaxseed oil
3/4 c. spring water
1 t. vanilla

Beat eggs, add honey. Beat. Mix carob, baking powder and flour. Add to mixture while adding oil and water alternately. Add vanilla. Place in a 13" x 9" glass baking dish. Bake at 350° for 20-25 minutes.

Note: If in doubt about doneness, remove from oven. Carob burns easily so care must be taken not to bake too long.

Carob Frosting

1 egg white   1/2 c. carob
1/2 c. honey

Beat egg white until stiff. While beating add honey. Add carob. Mix well.

Zucchini Cake

2 eggs or egg whites   1 c. flaxseed oil
1 c. raw honey   1 c. spring water
1/2 c. blackstrap molasses   2 c. grated zucchini
1 lemon, rind grated and juiced   1 c. chopped dried apricots
2-1/2 c. whole wheat flour   1 c. slivered almonds
2 t. baking powder

Beat eggs. Add honey and molasses while beating. Add lemon rind and juice. Sift together flour and baking powder. To honey mixture add flour mixture, water and oil alternately. Add zucchini and apricots. Place in a 13" x 9" baking dish. Sprinkle top with slivered almonds. Bake in 350° oven for 40 to 45 minutes.

Apple Brown Betty

10 apples   1/2 c. raisins
juice of one lemon   1/4 c. butter, hard
1 cup whole oats   1/2 c. chopped macadamia nuts
1/2 t. cinnamon   3 T. ground apricot kernels
1/2 c. date sugar

Peel and slice apples and sprinkle with lemon juice. Line bottom of 9" square baking dish with some of the oats. Sprinkle with cinnamon and a little date sugar. Dot with raisins and small pieces of butter. Repeat twice more. Place a layer of apples over the oats and sprinkle with a little cinnamon, date sugar and chopped macadamias. Dot with butter. Cover and place in a 250° oven until apples are tender. Green apples take about one hour. Delicious apples take about 30 minutes. Sprinkle with apricot kernels before serving.

Baklava

4 cups apricot kernels, finely chopped	1 cup melted butter
1 tsp. cinnamon	12 oz. (jar) raw honey
1 lb. filo or strudel leaves	

Make baklava at least 2-1/2 hours before serving.

Grease a 13" x 9" baking dish. In large bowl, combine apricot kernels and cinnamon. Blend well and set aside. In baking dish, place one sheet of filo or strudel leaf, extending it up the sides of the dish. Brush with melted butter. Repeat to make five more layers.

Sprinkle with one cup apricot and cinnamon mixture. Cut remaining filo into 13" x 9" rectangles. Place one sheet of filo in baking dish over apricot mixture. Brush with butter. Repeat to make at least six layers, overlapping small strips of filo to make rectangles, if necessary. Sprinkle one cup apricot/cinnamon mixture evenly over filo. Repeat procedure two more times, placing filo on top of last apricot/cinnamon layer. Trim any filo that extends over top of dish. With sharp knife, cut all layers in a diamond pattern to make 28 servings.

Bake in 300° oven 1 hour 25 minutes or until golden brown. While filo is cooking, in one-quart saucepan over medium low heat, heat honey until hot but not boiling. After filo is cooked, remove from oven and let warm. Spoon hot honey evenly over it. Cool on wire rack at least one hour, then cover and leave to cool at room temperature.

Barley Carob Cake

2 eggs, beaten	1 c. and 2 T. barley flour
3/4 c. honey	1/2 c. flaxseed oil
1/2 c. carob flour	3/4 c. spring water
2-1/2 t. baking powder	1 t. vanilla extract

Combine honey and eggs. Mix well. In separate bowl mix carob flour, baking powder and barley flour. Combine two mixtures. Add oil and water alternately. Add vanilla and blend thoroughly. Pour into an 8" x 8" oiled baking pan and bake 300° until toothpick inserted into center comes clean, about 40 minutes. Do not overbake as carob burns easily. Cool about five minutes then remove and cool on a rack.

Flourless Pie Shell

4 c. spring water	1/3 c. raw sesame seeds, ground
1/2 c. buckwheat	1 T. sesame tahini
1/2 c. millet	2 T. tamari

Bring water to boil, adding grains. Drain if there is water after cooking. Moisten grains with tahini and tamari. Add sesame seeds and mix with hands until dough is soft. Press in greased pie plate.

Apple Filling

1 whole apple, quartered	1/8 t. nutmeg
1/2 c. raw honey	1 T. fresh lemon juice
1 t. cinnamon	6 c. thinly sliced apple

Place whole apple, honey, cinnamon, nutmeg, butter and lemon juice into food processor or blender. Blend to liquid. Arrange the sliced apples in unbaked pie crust and top with liquid mixture. Place another pie crust or lattice work on top and cover with foil. Bake at 425° for 10 minutes and then 30 minutes at 350°. Uncover the last 10 minutes.

Mo's Avocado Pie

Pie Crust:

1 lb. dates, mashed   1/4 c. shredded fresh coconut
1/2 c. ground macadamia nuts   4 T. coconut juice

Mix with your hands until mixture is a soft dough. Lightly grease pie pan with soy margarine. Press mixture into pan.

Filling:

3 med. avocados, mashed   3 T. apple pectin
1/2 c. crushed pineapple   3 T. unsweetened pineapple juice
6 T. coconut juice   1 kiwi fruit, peeled and sliced
5 T. pure maple syrup

To avocados, add crushed pineapple, coconut juice and maple syrup. In saucepan, heat pineapple juice on low heat. When hot, add apple pectin, stirring until thickened. Add to avocado mixture and mix lightly. Spoon into pie crust, smoothing over. Decorate with sliced kiwifruit.

Cancer Fighting Food

We called her the garden lady. She was my childhood friend, and seemed like the oldest person in the world. Her eyes were deepest blue, set off by the solid brown skin that wrinkled when she smiled, which was all the time. I loved her the minute she introduced me to her backyard. She had the most spectacular garden. Her orchard boasted plump, juicy peaches, pears, plums and cherries; huge luscious vegetables burgeoned under her care; tantalizing herbs flourished; and flowers blossomed in an unbelievable array of color. She even coaxed almonds, walnuts and grapes to take root and offer their rewards.

Even the weeds were lovingly cultivated, though kept in one place. I used to love to sit on the marble bench in her backyard, taking in the fragrant jasmine blossoms of summer, watching her while she meticulously harvested her riches. She called her garden her "pharmacy." Everything there, she said, could cure every ailment known and unknown to man. She told me how she used the dandelions for her rheumatism, the daisies (chamomile) for her indigestion, and cabbage juice for her son's ulcer. Years later I would learn she was the last of the local "healers." When she was a child, neighbors far and wide came to her mother for extracts, dried herbs and plant combinations for various afflictions. Unfortunately for all of us, the garden lady's legacy of natural healing was lost as organized medicine took over.

Today, as we battle our civilized diseases, "uncivilized" populations grow old and thrive without benefit of organized medicine.
"Wise ones" among them have retained knowledge of nature's pharmacy, as we have lost it. The irony is that conventional medicine, as
it admits its failure to effectively treat illness without damaging side
effects, has prompted world scientists to go back to nature in search
of that lost knowledge.

The Healing Instinct

Michael A. Huffman of Kyoto University in Japan and Mohamedi
Seifu of the Mahale Mountains Wildlife Research Center, conducted
an observational study on the self-medication of primates at
Tanzania's Mahale Mountains National Park (Cowen, p. 280). They
observed a female Mahale chimpanzee whose symptoms read like a
classic hospital chart: lethargy, loss of appetite, darkened urine, bowel irregularity. No doubt about it, this was one sick chimp.

The patient, known simply as "CH" to her human observers, lay on
the ground or napped in a tree nest from time to time while her pri-
mate peers foraged for food. A few hours after her illness began, CH
started chomping on shoots of Vernonia amygdalina, a native shrub.
She sucked and swallowed the bitter juice from the macerated pit,
spitting out the fibrous remains.

By the next afternoon, though still fatigued, CH had begun eating,
defecating normally and foraging for longer periods without resting.

Mahale chimps rarely eat the plant, also known as "bitter leaf,"
strongly suggesting CH sought out the shrub for its medicinal quali-
ties. Moreover, studies have documented that African tribes use
extracts from the plant's bark, stems, roots, seeds and leaves to treat a
variety of human ailments including intestinal upset and appetite loss.
Based on its name and taste (apricot seeds or kernels, bitter in taste,
are high in cancer-fighting amygdalin), one could also assume it to be
helpful in treating cancer. Animals have an instinct we seem to have
either lost or ignore. They know what's good for them.

I had the opportunity to observe firsthand how animals heal themselves. At a speaking engagement in New Jersey, a woman greeted me shyly, her Siberian Husky in tow. "Maureen, in all your experience, has anyone ever asked you about alternative treatments for animals?", she asked. My gaze rested on the first thing about the poor creature that attracted my attention: a huge ugly tumor growing out of his forehead. I knelt down to comfort "Lucky," while examining the lump. I managed to keep my balance despite new heels too high for safety, when some apricot kernels dropped out of the bag I was holding.

Balance was out of the question as Lucky lunged at the kernels, gobbling them down. As I put my hand down to right myself, my canine friend spied the bag and lunged for it, spilling kernels and me all over the floor. Lucky's owner was aghast, apologizing profusely as I brushed dust from my suit. But I was more interested in Lucky's behavior. Apricot kernels are bitter and even for a human, an acquired taste. To see that dog woofing them down as if they were liver kibble was astounding! The only explanation was Lucky sensed, smelled or somehow instinctively knew the amygdalin contained in the kernels could help him. I told her how apricot pits contain high amounts of amygdalin, which could possibly help his tumor and suggested she give him more at home, which she did. We kept in touch and I'm happy to report Lucky's tumor went away, never to appear again.

Some years ago I had a beloved Siamese cat who was diagnosed with cancer. It was terminal, the veterinarian told me. Not content to accept the prognosis and give up on my loyal friend, I tried my own regimen. I began by crushing Laevalin (laetrile) tablets into his food. Then I fed him a diet of ground beef for taste, ground apricot seeds, garlic and millet. Within six months, the veterinarian declared my companion free of the life-threatening illness. I was overjoyed, and even threw a party to celebrate. He lived another five years, dying at the ripe old age of 19, but not from cancer.

The next time you see your pet eating plants from your garden or weeds from your yard, notice which he chooses. This simple process of observation has enabled scientists to track down plants and compounds confirmed as therapeutic.

The Search is On

About one quarter of U.S. prescription drugs contain at least one compound derived from plants. (Stix, p. 144). In recent years plants lost their appeal to pharmaceutical firms as synthetics proved cheaper to produce.

In 1986, The New York Botanical Garden received a five-year contract from the National Cancer Institute (NCI) to supply the Institute with flora that might prove useful in treating cancer and AIDS. Since 1986, 18,000 samples from 5,000 species have been gathered by the three participating institutions – the University of Illinois in Chicago, collecting in S⌐utheast Asia; the Missouri Botanical Garden in St. Louis, working in Africa; and the New York Botanical Garden, which is scouring the jungles of Central and South America (Selbert, pg.16).

Of 121 prescription drugs used widely around the world, "Seventy-four percent come from following up folklore claims," according to Norman Farnsworth, director of the program for collaborative research in the pharmaceutical sciences at the University of Illinois in Chicago (Stix, p. 143).

However, only a tiny fraction of today's discoveries are translated into medicine. What is developed will either be synthesized or include synthetic ingredients that can be patented for profit. The incredibly high cost of developing pharmaceuticals for market, coupled with FDA's persecution of alternative therapy manufacturers means many highly effective plant medicinals remain out of the hands of the people who need them the most. Educational programs too have been plagued with a lack of interest and funding.

In American universities, pharmacognosy programs (the study of biologically active compounds derived from living organisms) have been closing in recent years. There are only half a dozen left. Ethnobotany programs, the study of how cultures use plants, are also in trouble. "We have more people studying the surface of Venus than out in the field studying plants," says Dr. Paul Alan Cox, a professor of botany at Brigham Young University in Provo, Utah, who has been studying American Samoa since 1985 (Stix, p. 142).

In sharp contrast, research on plant extracts is booming in such industrialized nations as Germany, Japan and South Korea. (New Zealand, England and Sweden also have expanding programs.) A U.S. Department of Agriculture (USDA) report warns that the U.S., still the world leader in drug development, is in danger of falling out of the race if these other countries successfully tap the world's ecosystems for new remedies. We all lose the race when our world forests, oceans and rangelands are burned and developed before our scientists have had a chance to investigate their medicinal resources.

Fortunately, some good comes out of this research. Manufacturers of herbal remedies and supplements (when not stopped by government agents) use this research to create products available in your health food stores. The isolation of vitamin B17 and amygdalin came from such research. Once we know what the active ingredients are, we can look to local sources for our plant medicinals. The following list are foods determined to have anti-cancer properties. Best to purchase them in organic form through farmers' markets, in health food supermarkets, or grow, pick or sprout them yourself.

Seeds

Alfalfa
Sesame (unhulled)
Flaxseed
Chia (sprouted)

Vegetables

Wild Cabbage, Brussels sprouts
Brassica Oleoracea, Cauliflower
Broccoli, Turnip
Black mustard, White mustard

Radish, Kohlrabi
Shepherd's purse, Collard greens
Kale, Squash
Spinach, Sweet Potato
Watercress, Yams

Berries

Almost all edible wild berries contain vitamin B17 and in more abundance than cultivated berries.
Blackberry
Chokeberry, Cranberry
Elderberry, Gooseberry
Huckleberry, Loganberry
Mulberry, Raspberry
Strawberry

Sprouts

Vitamin C content is 10 to 30 times richer when these sources are sprouted.
Alfalfa, Bamboo
Fava, Garbanzo
Mung/Wheat berries

Legumes

Chickpeas
Fava, Kidney
Lentils (sprouted), Limas
Mung (sprouted), Navy
Peas, Scarlet runners

Grains

Barley, Buckwheat (Kasha)
Chia, Millet
Flax, Oats
Rice (brown), Rye
Vetch, Wheat berries

All kernels and fruit seeds are high in nitrilosides. When cooking or eating any of the fruits listed below, I try always to include the seed. Particularly delicious is the apricot kernel wrapped in a dried apricot, which detracts from the kernel's bitter taste.

Fruits

Apple, Apricot
Crabapple (wild)
Cherry (choke)
Currants, Nectarine
Peach, Pear
Plum, Prune
Papaya, Quince

Nuts

Bitter almonds
(Are grown mostly in China and are illegal in this country.
Ordinary sweet almonds have no substantial B17 content.)
Cashews
Macadamia

Miscellaneous

Sorghum, Molasses
Clover (white and red)
Wheat grass

CHAPTER 22:

Detoxifying with Vitamin C

"... Preventive pathology instead of curative pathology."
— *Buckminster Fuller,*
Futurist and Writer

Although this book accents nutrition, it also reveals other preventive methods — other ounces of prevention that add up to a ton of cure.

The following chapters examine the various major types of cancer, starting alphabetically, and consider what can be done to prevent the greatest scourge that mankind has ever known: cancer of the bladder, the breast, the cervix, the colon, the eye, the prostate and the skin.

Some of the information that follows appears in my book, *FOODS THAT HEAL.*

What the Scientists Say

It is widely accepted by scientists today that at least 50 percent of human cancers can be attributed to specific causes, including tobacco smoke, ionizing radiation, occupational exposures to toxic chemicals such as asbestos and benzene, heredity and viruses that alter the immune system.

The extent to which the remaining 50 percent of cancer is due to pesticides and industrial chemicals in our food, water and air is subject to debate, in large part due to politics. The National Cancer

Institute supports the theory that the high fat content of the American diet promotes cancer. And chlorinated tap water is associated with higher rates of breast cancer in virtually every study conducted, according to Dr. William Marcus, Ph.D., of the Environmental Protection Agency (Kugler, p. 169).

Michael A. Evans, Ph.D., associate professor at the University of Illinois College of Medicine at Chicago states that 70 to 90 percent of human cancer is a result of the environment, including cigarette smoke, synthetic chemicals, food additives, agricultural chemicals, and other factors such as sunlight and dietary fat. Dr. Evans believes many of the factors are not in and of themselves problematic, but probably act together or in combination with other environmental and genetic factors to create a carcinogenic effect (Kugler).

Some people experience spontaneous remission of their cancer, without any treatment whatsoever. Why does this happen? Why do some get cancer and others don't? The answer basically lies in the extent of their health and well-being. A poor digestive system will not only lower the immune system through malnourishment and malabsorption, but it will encourage the body's absorption of chemicals and toxins. Constipation not only creates pathways of least resistance, but the longer toxins remain in the bowel, the better the chance of chemical poisoning. Many chemical food additives are not problematic unless they are held in the body long enough to react with digestive bacteria.

Scientists do know, without a doubt, that cancer can be prevented through optimal dietary supplementation. There are more than 500 naturally-occurring carotenoids which are potent antioxidants and immune stimulants that can help prevent cancer (Hematology).

Ordinarily, cancer can be induced in 85 to 90 percent of experimental mice fed the cancer-causing chemical dimethylbenzanthracene (DMBA). That number can be reduced to five to fifteen percent with antioxidant nutrients, reports Dr. Richard Passwater in his book *The New Supernutrition*.

In another study, vitamin B12 and vitamin C together prevented the growth of transplanted mouse tumors and produced a 100 percent survival rate. However, neither vitamin alone at the same dosage had any effect on prevention of tumor growth (Poydock, p. 210).

Smoker's Preventative

A pair of Tulane University researchers scored a stunning victory over bladder cancer some decades ago. A victory, of course, that mainstream medicine ignored. However, ignoring it did not make it go away, particularly for cancer victims desperate for a successful solution.

Dr. Jorgen U. Schlegel, then head of the Urology Department of Tulane, New Orleans, and biologist George Pipkin, made the exciting breakthrough. They discovered that vitamin C (ascorbic acid) can destroy cancer-producing substances that precede bladder cancer in smokers (Schlegel, p. 155).

Of course, they blew the whistle on continued smoking by victims of bladder cancer. Statistics over the years have shown that bladder cancer is twice as prevalent in smokers as in non-smokers. (In more recent times, we learned that second hand smoke also can help to bring on cancer.)

Schlegel and Pipkin administered 1,500 mg. of vitamin C in three time-spaced doses of 500 mg. each.

The success rate was so phenomenal that Schlegel recommended such a regimen for "individuals who, due to age, cigarette smoking or other factors may be prone to bladder cancer formation."

Bowel Tolerance

Vitamin C enters the bloodstream, creating a buildup beyond the body's normal needs, so that it spills into the urine stored in the bladder. Before the bladder can discharge the vitamin C-saturated urine, the second 500 mg. dose of this vitamin enters the bloodstream.

Later, the third dose follows, keeping the ascorbic acid concentration in the urine so high bladder cancer in smokers often regresses, if patients continue taking 1,500 mg. of ascorbic acid or more each day, as demonstrated by a later study of Schlegel.

Let me explain the concept of bowel tolerance. Large amounts of vitamin C stimulate the bowel, causing diarrhea. It is your body's way of telling you you've taken more than it needs at that time. Although disconcerting, the effect is temporary. Simply reduce the dosage, working your way up to your desired dosage. The more vitamin C required to achieve bowel intolerance, the more toxins need to be washed out of the system. Diarrhea occurs because the bowel contains no more toxins for the vitamin C to absorb.

Because your body excretes any vitamin C it does not immediately use, purchase time-release supplements or take supplements at regular intervals. For 1,000 mg. total, take 250 mg. four times a day. Take vitamin C just after eating, when stomach acid is optimum for absorption. If this isn't possible, chewable tablets or a liquid vitamin formula can be used.

Foods high in vitamin C include rose hips, acerola cherries, parsley, green peppers, watercress, strawberries, broccoli, tomatoes, sprouted alfalfa seeds and spinach. All of these foods have more vitamin C than oranges.

CHAPTER 23:

Guarding Against Breast Cancer

Breast cancer is the most common type of cancer in women. The American Cancer Society estimates that in 1994 in the United States 182,000 women will be diagnosed with breast cancer and 46,000 will die of it. The number of deaths among women attributed to breast cancer have doubled in the last thirty years from 22,871 in 1959 to 42,837 in 1989 (*Cancer Facts & Figures 1993*, ACS). Gradually, women are finding out how it can be prevented and successfully cured with a minimum of stress to body and mind.

Some of the preventive methods for breast cancer also apply to guarding against other types of cancer. For instance, making sure your thyroid gland has enough iodine so it can function properly.

A survey by Dr. J.G.C. Spencer, of Frenahay Hospital in Bristol, England revealed higher than average cancer rates in goiter belts in 15 nations on four continents. Goiter belts are geographical areas where the soil has only about one-seventh the amount of iodine needed to assure efficient thyroid function, easily identified by the high incidence of goiter among its populace (Spencer, p. 393).

Lower than normal thyroid function seems to invite cancer, as shown by many animal experiments. Cancerous tissue from rats grafted onto other rats took hold readily in the animals whose thyroid glands had been removed, but hardly ever in those with normal thyroid function.

Studies of thousands of laboratory rats and human beings by Dr. Bernard Eskin, Director of Endocrinology, Department of Obstetrics and Gynecology, Medical College of Philadelphia, show that a lack of iodine, the thyroid gland's most essential nutrient, encourages breast cancer (Langer, p. 121).

Iodine-Poor Soils Undo Us

Dr. Eskin learned that the highest incidence of breast cancer, and deaths from it, are in the goiter belts of Austria, Poland, Switzerland and the United States.

The United States' goiter belt is in the northern area of the nation from the mountains of New England to Washington and includes the provinces of Canada following this path along the border. These states are: Maine, New Hampshire, Vermont, New York, Pennsylvania, Ohio, Michigan, Indiana, Illinois, Wisconsin, Minnesota, North Dakota, Montana, Idaho and Washington.

Breast cancer death rates in the United States are the highest in the Great Lakes area. The world's lowest death rates from cancer (as well as the lowest incidence of goiter) are in Japan and Iceland. The breast cancer death rate in Japan, where iodine is liberally supplied in seafood and seaweed eaten daily, is just one-fifth that of the United States. Kelp is the best source of iodine and available in any health food store. Just as important as getting enough iodine is getting too much. Either extreme can be deadly. Doctors recommend dietary sources and supplementation not exceed 1 mg a day. Like all essential minerals, iodine should be combined with other minerals for proper nutritional balance. Look for an easily absorbable, derived-from-nature liquid mineral blend. Liquid formulations provide the optimal absorption ratios.

Selenium, The Secret Weapon

Much evidence indicates that, like iodine, selenium is a prime breast cancer preventative. Patrick Quillin, Ph.D., explains how authorities mapped the soil selenium levels across the United States, then overlaid a map of cancer cases in each state (Quillin, p. 129).

An amazing correlation surprised the researchers. States with the lowest levels of soil selenium (supporting selenium deficient crops) correlated with the highest incidence of cancer cases.

South Dakota, with the highest amount of soil selenium, had the lowest number of breast cancer cases. And Ohio, with the lowest amount of soil selenium, had the highest incidence of cancer, 200 percent higher than that of South Dakota.

Cancer patients often have a lower-than-normal blood level of selenium, so critics of this study claim that cancer might have brought on the low selenium readings, states Quillin.

However, a second study involving 10,000 Americans shatters this objection. Blood samples were taken, then frozen and stored over the years. As individuals developed cancer, their blood samples were thawed out for analysis. Those with cancer turned out to be the ones who, at the start of the study, had the lowest blood selenium levels. Scientists conducting the study found that low blood selenium doubled the chance of developing cancer.

Special credit for discovering that selenium may be effective in protecting against breast cancer is given to Gerhard N. Schrauzer, Ph.D., of the University of California at San Diego.

An experiment by Schrauzer revealed when a trace amount of selenium was added to the drinking water of mice susceptible to breast cancer, their incidence of such cancer dropped from 82 percent to 10 percent (Langer, p. 14).

Still another Schrauzer study contributed to documentation that selenium can prevent breast cancer. In analyzing samples from blood banks in 17 nations, Schrauzer found selenium blood levels in the United States were only one-third as high as in Asian and Latin American nations and death rates from breast cancer were two to five times higher in the United States and in Europe than in Asia and Latin America.

Dr. Richard Passwater asserts that both selenium and vitamin E must be present in the body at ample levels in order to prevent cancer, and in his excellent book, *The New Supernutrition*, cites numerous studies to back up his contention. Vitamin E extravagant foods are wheat germ, safflower seeds, sunflower seeds, sesame oil, walnuts, corn oil, hazelnuts, soybean oil, almonds, olive oil and cabbage. Look for a quality source of vitamin E (d-alpha tocopherol). It should be taken with at least eight ounces of spring water, between meals.

Selenium Food Sources

Most diets, especially in the western states where soil selenium is plentiful, offer about 100 micrograms (mcg) daily. Most nutrition-oriented medical doctors set an upper limit on selenium intake at 200 mcg daily, inasmuch as this trace mineral is beneficial in moderate amounts and poisonous at high levels.

An incredibly rich source of selenium is Brazil nuts, as disclosed by researchers from the department of podology at Cornell University's Toxic Chemicals Laboratory and the Gannett Health Center.

Six Brazil nuts eaten daily can increase selenium blood levels by 100 to 350 percent.

"Selenium shows up in your blood immediately," states Donald J. Lusk, Ph.D., director of the lab. Lusk and associates found that Brazil nuts contain 2,500 times as much selenium as most other nuts.

The Cornell researchers identified other rich sources of selenium: organ meats (from animals grazed on selenium-rich fields), fish, whole grains and eggs. Still others are corn, cabbage, beans, peas, vegetable oils, onions, chicken, beets, barley, tomatoes, soybeans, saltwater and freshwater fish, brown rice, alfalfa, peanuts, meat and garlic.

A word about the absorption of minerals. It's important, whenever emphasizing supplementation, to understand the connection between digestion and assimilation. Doctors recommend pills be taken with meals because that is when stomach acid is at its strongest and best able to liquefy food. The small intestines cannot absorb nutrients if the food is not in solution (liquefied). Some people do not have adequate amounts of hydrochloric (stomach) acid and therefore cannot adequately break down food. These people should choose a liquid mineral formula derived from natural sources. A new patent-pending method, Solucell, adds even more efficiency by delivering nutrients directly to the cells. Look for supplemental formulas that use this innovative Solucell method.

Just as the addition of iodine and selenium to a diet deficient in these minerals can guard against breast cancer, so can the reduction of fat. One study shows women who reduce their fat intake from an average of 40-45 percent of total calories to 20 percent or less can reduce their chances of developing breast cancer.

Fat Out, Vegetables In

Overweight individuals are often vulnerable to breast cancer. Stanford University researchers found that women overweight in their college years are eventually more likely to develop breast cancer than normal weight persons (Harder, p. 367).

Among the strongest pieces of evidence in support of the fat/cancer connection is cancer incidence among immigrants. When European and Asian women migrate to the United States and begin eating American style, their breast cancer rates rise to approximately that of American women within one or two generations. Reduce fat intake, add whole grains and fiber, and you may slash the chances of breast cancer by 50 percent.

A study at the University of Toronto suggests lignans may prevent colon and breast cancer. Lignans inhibit tumor growth, and countries with diets high in lignans have low breast cancer rates. Stabilized flax tops the list with a hefty 800 parts per million of lignan compounds, 100 times more potent than any other grain. Buckwheat and wheat also contain lignans, as do vegetables, which contain small amounts of the compound (Mora, p. 101).

Included in our hopeful cornucopia, broccoli and its assorted kin stand out. The foods highest in the most potent cancer-fighters are the so-called cruciferous vegetables. They include broccoli, cabbage, cauliflower, Brussels sprouts, mustard, kale and collard greens.

University of Minnesota pathologist Lee Wattenberg has shown that mice exposed to a strong carcinogen then fed meals rich in broccoli or cabbage (the equivalent of eating three-fourths of a pound a day) are half as likely to develop cancer as mice who have never munched a broccoli floret or crunched a cabbage leaf. Even those mice that get the disease develop only a third as many tumors as the others (Jaret, p. 58). In areas of rural China, where cabbage is a staple, breast cancer is extremely rare.

It turns out broccoli and its cruciferous cousins are loaded with substances called indoles ("indole-3-carbinols" to food scientists), which appear able to block carcinogens before they do their dirty work. Most cancer-causing chemicals aren't innately harmful, says Wattenberg. They're simply useless. So various enzymes produced by the liver and other organs break them down to get rid of them. In the process, unfortunately, these harmless substances can turn dangerous. Some become unstable and damage the DNA of healthy cells. Others form deadly partnerships. The nitrates abundant in hot dogs and pickled foods, for instances, aren't a problem until they react in the digestive tract to samines, which can turn healthy cells into cancerous nitrosamines.

Broccoli's indoles may also trigger the enzymes that expose cancer cells to white blood cells. Indoles work to prevent breast cancer by triggering certain enzymes that dismantle the hormone estrogen, helping to protect against breast cancer. Any natural substance that lowers estrogen levels inherently lowers the breast cancer risk. This is because high estrogen levels promote estrogen-dependent breast cancers (Herbert, p. 472).

H. Leon Bradlow, who directs the Institute for Hormone Research in New York, says studies have shown capsules of purified indoles – about as much as you'd get in half a head of cabbage – speed up the breakdown of estrogen in humans.

Whole foods are best, but if their source or shelf life is uncertain, their nutrient content will be also. Sometimes your choices in produce are limited to the vegetable with the least number of brown spots. When your produce shelves are either rotten or raw, look for a supplement that includes freeze-dried whole foods, like sprouts, broccoli, green peppers, spinach and carrots, combining them with digestive herbals such as rosemary and licorice root, and immune-boosting garlic and green tea extract.

Non-Dietary Preventive Measures

Studies indicate women who breastfeed their first or second child for one to six months reduce their breast cancer risk by 10 to 25 percent. Those who nursed for seven or more months slashed their risk of breast cancer by 50 to 75 percent (Harder, p. 367). Exercise apparently plays an important role. A study by the University of Southern California Comprehensive Cancer Center revealed that two hours per week of dancing, aerobics, swimming, jogging or tennis may decrease the likelihood that adolescent girls will develop breast cancer later in life.

Even if you do everything right, prevention should still include breast self-exams. Experts suggest women check for lumps once a month to become familiar with the usual appearance and feel of the breasts. Familiarity makes it easier to notice any changes from one month to the next.

It is recommended women first examine their breasts visually, in the mirror, holding the arms up and down. Then in the shower or bath with soap gently moving the fingers in a circle, from the outside to the nipples. It is important to also examine the area surrounding the breasts, including the armpits, chest and neck. Self exam may not discourage the development of breast cancer, but measures taken following disclosure can keep it from being fatal.

Many women don't know how to do self-exams properly, says Jean Richardson, a University of Southern California assistant professor of preventive medicine, who tested 540 women's efficiency with a foam rubber breast model (Women).

Only one percent of the women found the five lumps present. Why such a small rate of success?

"Even when the women were told to press hard on the model, and try to find the lumps, almost half of them didn't find a single one," says Dr. Richardson.

Although the American Cancer Society claims the radiation cancer risk from periodic mammogram for lump detection is negligible, many women choose to be tested by nuclear magnetic resonance (NMR), a procedure that gives off no radiation and can show whether or not lumps are cancerous or benign, eliminating the need, expense and discomfort of a biopsy.

Something You Should Know

In a major breast cancer study, researchers have confirmed that lumpectomy, in which only the cancerous tumor is removed, is just as safe and effective as a mastectomy, in which surgeons remove the entire breast. The research, performed at the University of California, Irvine, looked at 5,892 Orange County women in 126 Southern California hospitals. Not only did they find that women who chose lumpectomies with radiation were just as likely to survive as those who had mastectomies, but their survival rate was affected by the kind of hospital they were in.

The Irvine study examined the medical records of a group of white women whose breast cancer was diagnosed between 1984 and 1990. Regardless of whether they had lumpectomies or mastectomies, patients in large hospitals – those with over 200 beds – were 26 percent less likely to die in the five years after surgery than those who received treatment in small hospitals. Patients in small health maintenance organization hospitals were the most likely to die from their cancer; 63 percent greater than small non-HMO hospitals and almost twice as likely to die than large non-HMO hospitals (JAMA, April 20, 1994).

CHAPTER 24:

Conquering Cervical Cancer

A generation ago, cervical cancer was a rarity. Now it is one of the most common. One of the reasons is the presence of diethylstilbestrol (DES), a synthetic hormone, currently given to meat-source animals, and, in the '50s, commonly prescribed to pregnant women to prevent miscarriage. Now experts agree the drug can be traced to a high incidence of vaginal and cervical cancer among the daughters of these women.

The first reported connection came in the spring of 1971 from gynecologist Dr. Arthur L. Herbst and associates at Harvard Medical School (*New England Journal of Medicine*, April 22, 1971). While researching an unusual incidence of seven cases of adenocarcinoma of the vagina, he found each had mothers who were administered DES in the '50s. Prior to these cases, the occurrence of this type of cancer was extremely rare.

According to an abstract submitted by Herbst to the 24th Annual Meeting of the Society of Gynecologic Oncologists, held February 7-10, 1993, in Palm Desert, California, (Herbst, p. 18): "It has been approximately 20 years since intrauterine Diethylstilbestrol (DES) exposure was associated with the subsequent development of CCA of the vagina and cervix in young females. At that time a registry was created to study these cancers. A recent NCI-sponsored multidisciplinary conference emphasized both renewed interest in research in this area, and the fact that these cancers are continuing to occur.

"As of June 1992, 589 cases had been reported to the registry and 60 percent of the investigated cases have a positive DES history. The oldest exposed patient in the U.S. was 42 years of age when diagnosed in 1991. This indicates these tumors are continuing to develop as the at-risk population ages. A recent informal G.O.G. survey indicates 15-18 cases (not all exposed) are being seen annually in the U.S. While the peak age is 15-28 years, it is not known if a secondary rise in the age incidence curve may occur for patients in their 40s and 50s. The cancers are rare with a risk of about 1 per 1000 among DES female offspring. Currently, 20 cancers have developed in DES-exposed females who were identified as having vaginal adenosis or cervical ectropion on initial examination and then developed clear cell adenocarcinoma. Risk factors in addition to DES exposure are a maternal history of miscarriage, the daughter's birth in the fall, and prematurity."

Unfortunately, we can't do a retake of the past, Hollywood-style, so we have to deal with what preventive measures can be taken. It is a sad fact that many pregnant women may still be ingesting synthetic estrogen unknowingly.

DES is used to increase the weight of cattle and chickens before being marketed. It is illegal to include it in animal or poultry feed, but the U.S. Department of Agriculture would need an army of agents to monitor the more than 50 million cattle and many times that many chickens to determine residues of DES in meat and chicken.

Implants of DES are permitted in cattle and chickens, and supposedly the residues vanish prior to marketing time. However, who knows how much DES a pregnant woman, any of us for that matter, is ingesting along with that juicy hamburger?

Does such a small amount of DES amount to anything? Researchers have shown this hormone is so potent just two parts per billion is poisonous to mice. Only an infinitesimal amount daily – .07 millionths of a gram – is needed to cause cancer in mice (Encyclopedia, p. 301).

Whenever the DES issue rears it hideous head, agricultural economists use the threadbare argument that meat and poultry would cost a fortune if it weren't for diethylstilbestrol. Are they saying cancer doesn't cost our medical system a fortune in treatments and hospitalization, not to mention the pain and anguish to cancer patients and loved ones?

The tempered "good news" is an estimated 25 percent of market cattle is raised without DES. Such wholesome meat – poultry as well – is sold by health food stores that have the appropriate refrigeration. And yes, it costs more. But isn't it worth the price?

Highest Risk Candidates

Various studies reveal cervical and vaginal cancer occur most in the following: lower economic groups, those with virus-caused genital infections, such as warts and possibly herpes – and in individuals who start practicing sex at an early age and have had numerous partners (Morgan, p. 60).

Prolific women are more prone to cervical cancer. Mothers of five or more children are twice as likely to get cervical cancer as those with one to three children. Some authorities claim wear and tear on the cervix during labor and delivery and pregnancy-related inflammation contribute to developing cervical cancer.

Studies at Emory University School of Medicine and at the Centers for Disease Control in Atlanta reveal cancers and other tumorous conditions of the cervix develop more readily in smokers than non-smokers. And the more smoking the woman does, the greater the hazard (Medical p. 4).

Women who use birth control pills run a higher risk of cervical dysplasia than non-users (Practical, p. 109). Dysplasia, an abnormal multiplication of non-malignant cells, is suspected of leading to cervical cancer. While doctors aren't positive this triggers it, they find these abnormal cells along with cervical cancer cells. It is estimated it takes from ten to fifteen years for cervical cancer to develop. Regular pap smears, therefore, can go a long way toward avoiding this type of cancer.

Preventive efforts should especially be taken if there is a family history of cervical cancer.

A Need for Folic Acid

Women on birth control pills often are deficient in folic acid, a nutrient vital to an unborn baby's development. A lack of this B vitamin is also common among women with cervical hyperplasia. Either the Pill depletes the existing supply of folic acid or the women may not be getting enough.

A University of Alabama research team headed by medical doctors Charles E. Butterworth and Kenneth Hatch, discovered ten milligrams a day of folic acid may arrest or possibly even reverse early dysplasia (Butterworth, p. 73).

Twenty-two of the women were placed on this regimen for three months. Twenty were given placebos. Eighteen of the twenty-two on folic acid found their condition arrested. The remaining four were rewarded with total reversal of their conditions.

Inasmuch as folic acid is essential to proper cell division, some researchers think that a deficiency of this vitamin might cause abnormal cell division.

Help From Beta Carotene and Vitamin C

Many conventional doctors don't take into account the numerous studies linking cervical cancer with vitamin and mineral deficiencies. Up to 67 percent of patients with cervical cancer have been found to be deficient in one or more nutrients (Orr, p. 632). As a group, they have a level of beta carotene only one-half of normal women (Dawson, p. 612).

A study by Dr. Sylvia Wassertheil-Smoller and associates at Albert Einstein College of Medicine disclosed healthy women ingest more beta carotene, a vitamin A precursor, and vitamin C than women with abnormal pap smears.

The conclusion of Wassertheil-Smoller is that women prone to cervical cancer might get protection from a daily intake of beta carotene and at least 90 mg. of vitamin C daily (Wassertheil-Smoller, p. 714).

Is it possible to get enough folic acid, beta carotene and vitamin C from natural foods to offer protection from cervical dysplasia and possible cancer? Inasmuch as folic acid appears in foods only in micrograms – thousandths of a gram – it is difficult but not impossible to obtain the 10 daily grams used in the Butterworth-Hatch study.

Richest sources of folic acid are torula yeast, brewer's yeast, alfalfa, endive, chickpeas, oats, lentils, beans, wheat germ, liver, split peas, whole wheat, barley, brown rice, asparagus, green peas, sunflower seeds, collard greens, spinach, hazelnuts, kale, peanuts and most fresh, raw vegetables.

Beta carotene and vitamin C are far easier to derive from foods.

Yellow and green leafy vegetables, like carrots, sweet potatoes, squash, cantaloupe, spinach and broccoli are rich in beta carotene.

Beta carotene foods that also include significant amounts of vitamin C are spinach, cantaloupe and broccoli.

CHAPTER 25:

Colon Cancer Can Be Avoided

A merica's dietary habits: over-eating, under-exercising and going heavy on junk foods, probably do the most to bring on colon cancer.

Although much has been made about being overweight as a contributor to cancers of every type, little has been mentioned about the hazard of a major cause of excess poundage: over-eating.

David Kritchevsky, associate director of the Wistar Institute of Philadelphia, the nation's first institute established for biological research, conducted a most revealing animal study.

Kritchevsky and associates fed a group of rats five times as much fats as the control group, but 25 percent fewer calories. In spite of their super high fat diet, the rats on the lower calorie diet developed significantly fewer tumors.

Does this mean it's OK to eat all the fat we want? Of course not. Kritchevsky concludes from his study that ingesting more calories than we need and burning off too few with exercise is a contributor to colon cancer and all other types of cancer.

Limit Fat Intake

Other eminent cancer authorities believe excessive fat intake – 40 plus percent of the daily diet seems to be the national average – is one of the main causes of colon cancer.

Several research studies reveal individuals on a high fat diet double their chances of developing colon cancer. Fat promotes cancer by stimulating production of bile, a greenish liquid secreted by the liver to aid in the digestion of fats, found to contribute to tumors in animals.

One experiment revealed a 100 times increase of anaerobic bacteria – those that need no oxygen to exist – in patients who eat a great deal of fat. These bacteria are capable of changing bile acids in fecal matter into chemicals that can cause cancer and also converting bile into estrogen hormone, which triggers tumor growth (Kunin, p. 81).

A recent six-year study of Chinese individuals found those living in the U.S. who ate an average of only 100 calories of saturated fat more per day than participants living in China had colon cancer risks nearly double that of their counterparts. In women, increasing saturated fat intake has also been shown to increase risk for colon and breast cancer (Brohier, p. 1).

Fat is the dietary component most often linked to cancer. Diets of patients with colorectal cancer contain significantly more fat and sugars and far less fiber compared to diets of healthy individuals. Intake of dietary fat is also strongly associated with intestinal cancer. Frequent consumption of high fat foods among blacks, especially, is directly associated with the incidence of colon cancer (Lieberman, p. 10).

Fat intake is very high in Finland, where the incidence of coronary heart disease is one of the highest in the world. The incidence of colon cancer, however, is less than one third that of the United States. These lower colon cancer statistics have been attributed to consumption of a popular coarse, whole-grain rye bread. The bread increases fecal bulk to three times that found in most Western nations.

An experiment by Dr. Robert Bruce, director of the Toronto branch of the Ludwig Cancer Research Institute, disclosed waste matter in the large bowel contains potential cancer-causing substances. The longer it presses on the colon wall, the greater the threat of colon cancer (Pauling, p. 347).

Eat Basic Foods

If too little fiber is present in the large bowel, the waste matter becomes small and hard to move. Anything in the feces that the small intestine can't absorb into the body is stored here: man-made chemicals containing carcinogens, particulates from polluted air, even objects swallowed by children. Without adequate fiber to move the waste through, this undigested garbage sits, and the large intestine continues to absorb water and any chemicals contained in it. The longer it sits, the harder it will be to expel and the more likely the body is to be poisoned or damaged by it.

Too little water can also encourage slow waste movement. Without water, nothing moves, especially fiber.

We can blame civilization for colon cancer. Our early ancestors had few of the problems we experience today in as much as they ate a myriad of foods including nuts, seeds, roots and wild plants, mammals, rodents, bugs and reptiles. One can only wonder at the magnificence of the human body when we see that we are a highly-efficient processing plant capable of breaking down even the roughest of food, squeezing out every bit of nutrient, and eliminating the leftover waste.

With its grain mills and food processing, grains lost their roughage when reduced to flour, and seeds gave way to oil processed from them. Whole foods became conveniently chopped, pressed and formed, like some packaged sliced meats, and the fiber in fruits became soft, sweet and denatured in cans.

Great Britain's Dr. Denis Burkitt, world-famous for his expertise in fiber in relation to proper waste elimination, has found that a lot of refined carbohydrates, like white sugar and refined flour products, encourage the multiplication of cancer-causing bacteria in the colon and, consequently, chemical changes that can invite cancer (Null, p. 146).

Vegetables for Vitality

Most vegetables contain quality fiber, although not at bran level, and offer special protection against colon cancer, as underscored by a significant study made by Dr. Saxon Graham, chairman of Social and Preventive Medicine at The State University of New York at Buffalo, and co-workers (Carper, p. 57).

The Graham team compared the diets of 256 male colon cancer patients at Roswell Park Memorial Institute and 783 non-cancer patients of the same age. They focused mainly on how frequently they ate 19 vegetables, including the now well-known cruciferous cancer fighters: cabbage, broccoli, brussels sprouts, cauliflower and turnips, and other veggies such as beta carotene-rich carrots, yams, watercress, squash, peppers and tomatoes.

Colon cancer patients ate few vegetables regularly, compared with the others. Those who consumed the most vegetables ran the least risk of cancer. The more frequently they ate them, the less likely they were to develop colon cancer.

Consumption of tomatoes and strawberries are strongly associated with low cancer risk. A 20-year study found a negative correlation between eating green and yellow vegetables daily and the risk of various cancers. In other words, the higher the consumption of these vegetables, the lower the risk of colon cancer.

Seventh Day Adventists, mainly vegetarians who eat fresh vegetables, whole grains and legumes (beans and peas) develop little colon cancer or any other kind of malignancy.

Battle with Bacteria

Vegetarian fare is not the only cancer preventive. High quality yogurt, rich in lactobacillus acidophilus, body-friendly bacteria, is usually well-tolerated by even those sensitive to milk lactose. Acidophilus helps reduce enzymes in waste matter that lower the body's defense against cancer-causing agents.

Researchers Goldin and Gorbach have tested yogurt on fecal enzymes in human subjects and observed changes in them, indicating a lower risk of colon cancer (Bland, p. 302).

Numerous studies show a connection between cancer of the bowel and the amount of animal protein in the diet. One of the most highly publicized studies to suggest such a connection is the Nurses Health Study of 122,000 women. Researchers found that women in that study who ate beef, pork or lamb daily were 2-1/2 times more likely to develop colorectal cancer than those who ate red meat less than once a month.

Sunshine Vitamin Converts Carcinogens

Not all carcinogens are environmental. Some are created by our bodies. Thanks to our Creator, we have been given a valuable gift to fight with: sunshine and vitamin D.

According to Dr. Cedric Garland, director of the epidemiology program at the University of California, San Diego (UCSD) Cancer Center, normal body processes create fatty acids and free bile acids in the colon. These acids are suspected carcinogens or cancer-causing agents. However, we're given protection from this process because vitamin D (obtained from sunlight) appears to convert carcinogens into safe, insoluble calcium salts (McGuire, p. 18).

Vitamin D is a fat-soluble vitamin, and can be acquired either by ingestion or exposure to sunlight. It is known as the "sunshine" vitamin because the action of the sun's ultraviolet rays activates a form of cholesterol present in the skin, converting it to vitamin D. However, air pollution, clouds and window glass inhibit the sun's action on the skin.

UCSD epidemiologist Edward Gorham found the average intake of vitamin D in Japan is ten times that in the U.S. This is most likely due, he believes, to the popularity of fish that are rich in vitamin D. Anago, a type of eel favored by many Japanese, contains 5,000 international units of vitamin D per 100 grams. That's over ten times the U.S. RDA! But is there any evidence suggesting individuals with colon cancer have abnormally low vitamin D levels?

To look at this question, the UCSD team and researchers from the Johns Hopkins University Training Center compared serum 25-hydroxy vitamin D levels in individuals with colon cancer. They relied on frozen blood samples drawn from 25,620 Washington County, Maryland volunteers in 1974. Thirty-four of these individuals subsequently developed colon cancer. Their samples were thawed and compared in a blind fashion to 67 other samples that served as controls (McGuire, p. 18).

The results? Those with the highest blood levels of 25-hydroxy vitamin D had the least risk of developing colon cancer. Overall, risk of colon cancer decreased 75 percent to 80 percent for individuals with the highest vitamin D levels.

"Both epidemiologic and laboratory evidence suggests that vitamin D, whether from sunlight exposure or diet, is of major importance in reducing the risk of colon cancer," said Dr. Garland. Only natural vitamin D has been shown to have this beneficial effect. A warning here about the vitamin D in milk. An intake of dairy foods fortified with vitamin D, like milk, results in decreased magnesium absorption. This is because the so-called vitamin D added to milk is actually a hormone – and a synthetic one at that.

Beware of synthetic vitamin D because it can actually contribute to aging by depositing calcium in the soft tissue at the surface of the skin. Get your vitamin D from foods and sunlight instead. Foods containing high amounts of vitamin D are cod liver oil, salmon, sardines, herring, egg yolk, organ meats and bone meal.

The colon cancer bottom line? Eat less sugar, more fiber, more vegetables (preferably fresh and organic) and less fat. You can add lactobacillus acidophilus to your diet through yogurt or supplements. Add vitamin D supplements or get moderate amounts of unprotected sunshine (Garland suggests 10 to 15 minutes per day). Watch out for antibiotics, which not only lower your immune system, but kill off friendly intestinal bacteria. If you find yourself prescribed a lot of antibiotics, try an extract of goldenseal/echinacea instead. It's a great body-booster and is available in health food stores.

CHAPTER 26:

Lung Cancer Precautions

G iving up smoking and avoiding secondhand cigarette smoke are two of the best ways to prevent lung cancer.

I've been emphasizing the dangers of chemicals in relation to cancer. Here's something I bet you didn't realize: cigarettes contain more than just tobacco – a lot more. Recently, National Public Radio (NPR) got a list of 13 additives that tobacco companies *add* to their cigarettes. The chemicals are on a secret list of about 700 additives that tobacco companies report to the government each year. Federal law prohibits government officials from releasing information from the list.

As reported in an Associated Press article (April 9, 1994), these chemicals are so bad, FDA doesn't allow any of them to be used in food and five are designated as hazardous substances by the Environmental Protection Agency. Among them are ammonia, which irritates the skin, eyes and respiratory tract, and freon, a chlorofluorocarbon which contributes to damage of the earth's ozone layer. Add up even minute amounts in each cigarette and multiply that by the millions of people who smoke packs a day and we've got a major environmental problem here.

An independent toxicologist consulted by NPR said the two chemicals that most concern him are ethyl furoid and sclareol.

Ethyl furoid is a chemical in the family of "notorious liver toxins," said Dr. Barry Rumack, a professor at the University of Colorado. Little is known about this chemical except it causes liver damage when tested on animals, and that it was discussed as a possible chemical warfare agent in the 1930s.

Sclareol causes convulsions in laboratory rats, Rumack said. When used in combination with other chemicals, "it lowers the threshold at which a human being can convulse," he added.

I've always suspected it was more than just tobacco. People have been smoking tobacco for centuries, and only since it became commercialized has lung cancer become so epidemic. Now we know why.

The Danger from Air Pollution

Where we live can be just as much a factor of lung health as how we live. A shocking six out of every 10 people in the United States today live in areas which fails to meet air quality standards set to protect human health (Paul, p. 24). This situation exists despite two decades of efforts to control air pollution in this country. In 1970, the Environmental Protection Agency, recognizing the danger, enacted the Clean Air Act of 1970, establishing national standards for six pollutants: ozone, carbon monoxide, sulfur dioxide, nitrogen dioxide, lead and particulates.

An April 1993 report by the American Lung Association ("Breath in Danger II,") estimates that more than 31 million children and over 18 million elderly people in the U.S. are at risk for lung disease or respiratory irritation because they are exposed to unhealthful levels of air pollutants, adding that 55 percent of Americans live in areas that do not meet current health standards for air quality (estimated by many to be too low).

In 1959, when the American Cancer Society started keeping track, they recorded 29,335 men died from lung cancer. Thirty years later, the number was 89,052. The number of women who died of lung cancer increased most alarmingly from less than 5,000 in 1959 to a little over 48,000 in 1989. Since 1987, more women have died of lung cancer than breast cancer, which for over 40 years was the major cause of death in women. An estimated 56,000 women and 93,000 men were estimated to succumb to lung cancer in 1993 (*Cancer Facts & Figures, 1993*).

Lung cancer among males has gone up nearly 2,000 percent since 1914. Dr. Eugene Houdry, a petroleum chemistry expert, reported that this increase corresponds exactly with the increase of gasoline consumption. He also noted that lung cancer declined 35 percent during the war years 1941-1945 when gas consumption was rationed (Encyclopedia, p. 311).

Researchers led by Douglas Dockery of the Harvard School of Public Health in Boston, Massachusetts have found prolonged exposure to microscopic pollutants, especially high in cities where transportation is dependent upon gasoline-powered engines, increases mortality rates from lung cancer and heart disease.

The Dockery study tracked more than 8,000 adults over a 14- to 16-year period and measured air pollution levels in the six American cities where they lived. The researchers found those who breathed air with the highest concentration of fine particles such as smoke and soot had a 26 percent higher death rate than those who inhaled the least polluted air (*Cancer Researcher Weekly,* December 1993).

They found high levels of fossil fuel pollutants (gasoline is a fossil fuel) were associated with elevated rates of lung cancer and cardiopulmonary disorders such as heart attacks, emphysema and pneumonia.

While past studies have linked air pollution to higher death rates, the Dockery study went one step further by taking into account individual differences such as smoking, diabetes, obesity, education and occupational hazards. After controlling for these factors, they still saw an association between air pollution and increased mortality.

The most significant aspect of the study is that the particles the investigators measured are smaller than those currently used by the EPA to set air quality standards.

The EPA evaluates larger particulates. These "not only have a different chemical composition, but are effectively removed by your nose and upper airways before they get to your lungs," Dockery said.

"But the microscopic particles the study gauged are more toxic, as well as more likely to reach lung tissue."

The American Lung Association believes the current standards for two pollutants, ozone (smog) and sulfur dioxide, are too low and fail to protect the health of many Americans, said ALA President Lee B. Reichman, M.D. (Breath).

Invisible, Odorless, Deadly Radon

The American Cancer Society warns of two other risk factors: exposure to industrial chemicals and substances such as asbestos, and exposure to residential radon.

For the benefit of those who don't know what radon is and what it does to lungs, let me start from the beginning.

Radon is a radioactive gas that comes from traces of uranium in soil and rock. It seeps through bedrock and soil into homes and is especially damaging in tightly insulated dwellings.

Prevalent in greatest amounts in the nation's southwest, it is present throughout most of the United States, even the east, where it emanates from granite, shale and phosphates. Radon-created free radicals damage normal cells, making them vulnerable to cancer.

Trapped in well-insulated homes, radon concentration sometimes builds up to such a high level that the incidence of lung cancer increases. A recent National Academy of Sciences study indicates that perhaps 10 percent of the approximately 150,000 annual fatalities from lung cancer can be traced to over-exposure to radon.

Mine workers with often direct exposure to underground radon have been noted for developing lung cancer from as far back as the year 1556, states Richard Passwater, Ph.D., in his book *The New Super Nutrition* (Pocket Books).

An estimated 20 million American homes are polluted with radon, reports the Environmental Protection Agency (EPA). Local and state health agencies can tell you where to buy kits to test for radon levels in your home and workplace.

Individuals living in warm climates can protect themselves to some extent by keeping house windows wide open as much as possible to dissipate the radon. Another strong preventive measure is taking antioxidants, particularly beta carotene.

Fight Back with Antioxidants

Dr. Passwater states that a "combination of antioxidant nutrients" protects the lungs against cancer, whatever its source – radon, cigarette smoke or air pollution.

Several studies reveal that on a diet deficient in vitamin A – even without inordinate exposure to tobacco smoke, radon or concentrated city air pollution – lung tissues change their character and become more vulnerable to cancer.

Beta carotene is perhaps the greatest defender against lung cancer. Dr. Passwater points out it can destroy the dangerous, cell-damaging "singlet oxygen" found in tobacco smoke and polluted air. Low levels of beta carotene has also been directly associated with the development of human lung cancer (Nutrition).

High amounts of air pollutants tend to use up large quantities of vitamin A. Then the liver produces reinforcing vitamin A from beta carotene. So that vitamin A is not destroyed by oxidation enroute to the lungs, vitamin E and selenium let themselves be destroyed to assure safe delivery of vitamin A to the lungs. For optimum performance, take these nutrients together.

See Chapter 33, Free Radicals, for more on the benefits of antioxidants.

CHAPTER 27:

Prostate Cancer, An Unnecessary Evil

In 1993 an estimated 35,000 men died in America from prostate cancer, according to The American Cancer Society. It is the second leading cause of cancer deaths in men, behind lung cancer. The news doesn't get any better. Nearly 60 percent of men between the ages of 40 and 59 years of age have enlarged prostate glands. Because of the often subtle symptoms, many don't even know it. Researchers at John Hopkins University and at Roswell Park Memorial Institute found men with an enlarged prostate were four times more likely to develop cancer than those with normal prostates (Faelton, p. 427). For early identification, watch for the following symptoms:

* Weak or interrupted urinary stream
* The feeling you cannot empty your bladder completely
* A feeling of delay or hesitation when urinating
* A need to urinate often, especially at night
* Dribbling

Any or all of these symptoms can indicate an enlarged prostate (benign prostatic hypertrophy or BPH), or chronic inflammation (prostatitis).

If a cancerous tumor develops, it usually grows on the outer portion of the prostate and may not exhibit symptoms. By the time a tumor causes symptoms, it has grown so large it forces pressure on the urethra. An early-stage tumor can be detected during a regularly-scheduled rectal exam or by the use of ultrasound or x-ray.

The prostate, whose function is to secrete a milky white fluid to carry sperm cells out of the penis, surrounds part of the urethra, the tube that carries urine from the bladder.

With advancing age, the prostate enlarges or inflames, a condition called prostatitis.

Because enlargement is common to any prostate problem, difficulty urinating is the first symptom. As the prostate enlarges, it squeezes the urethra, causing urine to back up into the bladder, making it feel full most of the time; and partially blocking the urethra, making it difficult to urinate. As the urethra narrows, you have to push harder to urinate. This can cause the bladder walls to thicken and stretch out of shape, becoming less efficient (when not overdistended, the bladder's capacity is one pint). If urine stays in the bladder, infections and even bladder cancer (from carcinogens in the urine) can develop. The kidneys may fail if they can't drain into the bladder because it's full.

Surgery is the usual course of action for prostate problems. The *New York Times* (June 23, 1992) reported that each year 400,000 American men spend at least $3 billion on prostate surgery. Unfortunately, many men have to repeat the procedure within five years.

Possible complications include infection, blood clots, excessive bleeding, loss of bladder control, impotence and sterility. During surgery, a muscle that is involved in ejaculation may be cut. If this happens, semen may move backward into the bladder, instead of traveling out of the body (Krames Communications, 1991).

Conventional therapy inadequacies make prevention the most solid bet. Pre-cancerous prostate problems, fortunately, can be managed with diet.

Think Zinc

Nutrition-minded physicians often prescribe zinc for prostate disorders since the prostate gland is a major storehouse of the mineral. It just so happens one of the major symptoms of a zinc deficiency is an enlarged prostate. Andrew Weil, M.D., recommends 60 mg of zinc picolinate daily. When symptoms subside, reduce that amount in half and continue taking it (Murray, p. 26). A super high level of zinc is found in the prostate gland and semen of men with no prostate problems.

Upon examining 755 enlarged prostate patients, Irving M. Bush, M.D. and associates at Cook County Hospital in Chicago, found most of them had a low amount of zinc in prostate tissue and semen. Nineteen of these patients were given a 34 mg. zinc pill daily for 60 days, then put on a maintenance program of 11 to 23 mg. daily. Every one of them reported less pain. An examination revealed that the prostate of fourteen patients diminished in size. Semen levels showed increased zinc.

Two hundred patients with infectious prostatitis were given 11 to 34 mg. of zinc daily for 16 weeks, and 140 experienced relief from symptoms and had higher amounts of zinc in their semen (Faelton, p. 429).

Only about 10 to 20 percent of the zinc we ingest from foods is properly absorbed. Large amounts of calcium, phytic acid (from grains, nuts and legumes), and cadmium (from pollution and cigarette smoke) can deplete zinc stores in blood and tissues.

For a prostate-healthy diet, emphasize the following foods high in zinc: oysters, shellfish, fish, whole grains, oatmeal, eggs, legumes, and nuts. Pumpkin seeds and sesame seeds are particularly zinc-rich.

Two nutrients must be considered along with zinc: vitamin B6 and copper. Too much copper will deplete zinc stores; they must be equal for optimum usage. Include 2-4 mg. of copper with any zinc supplement and eat these foods that contain copper: seafood, nuts, legumes, molasses and raisins.

Because zinc and vitamin B6 are intricately involved in hormone metabolism, a deficiency of one or both of these nutrients can be a contributing factor in prostate problems. Vitamin B6 also enhances zinc absorption. Foods high in vitamin B6 include brewer's yeast, brown rice, whole wheat, royal jelly, soybeans, rye, lentils, sunflower seeds, hazelnuts, alfalfa, salmon, wheat germ, tuna, bran, walnuts, peas and beans.

The EFAs Solution

There's a folk remedy used for an enlarged prostate which can be explained nutritionally. Pumpkin seeds contain both zinc and essential fatty acids. Dr. Jonathan Wright, of Tahoma Clinic in Kent, Washington, recommends his patients eat lots of foods high in essential fatty acids (EFAs), substances that can't be made by the body. EFAs are most highly concentrated in seeds: safflower, evening primrose, sesame, borage and flaxseed.

Dr. Wright first learned of this treatment through a study done by James P. Hart and William L. Cooper, two medical doctors. They fed daily EFAs to 19 men with BPH and every one experienced a reduction in prostate size (Hart, p. 2).

Based on this study, Dr. Wright has his prostate patients take a 400 mg capsule of EFAs three times a day (Wright, p. 281). This equals two handfuls of pumpkin or sunflower seeds. Flaxseed and borage oil are the most beneficial oils to ensure adequate and quality EFAs in the diet. Remember, purchase natural, unadulterated oils from health food stores. They must be raw as much as possible, and eaten fresh. If rancid, they could cause harm.

Amino Acids – the Newest Discovery

Recently, two doctors accidentally discovered three amino acids important to prostate health. The physicians were treating a group of allergic patients with a mixture of three amino acids – glycine, alanine and glutamic acid. One of the patients volunteered the information that his urinary symptoms had disappeared while on the amino acid mixture. This led to a trial of the same compounds on non-allergic patients with urinary symptoms. Patients with enlarged prostates experienced prompt and rather spectacular relief. The combination of glycine, alanine and glutamic acid has been shown in several studies to relieve many of the symptoms of BPH (Feinblatt).

Prostate Protocol

(From *Life Extenders and Memory Boosters*, Hans Kugler, Ph.D., *et al*, Health Quest Publications, Reno, NV.)

Amino Acids

Alanine: 200 mg/day
Glutamic Acid: 200 mg/day
Glycine: 200 mg/day

Vitamins

Beta Carotene: 25,000 IU/day
Vitamin B6 (pyridoxine): 100 mg/day
Vitamin E: 400 IU/day

Oils

EPA/DHA
Flaxseed or Borage: 1-2 tsp./day

Minerals

Zinc Picolinate: 50 mg/day

Herbs/Plants

Bee Pollen Extract: two tablespoons/day
Equisetum arvense (horsetail): 250 mg/day
Hydrangea arborescens: 250 mg/day

Panax ginseng: 25-50 mg ginsenosides/day
Serena repens (saw palmetto): 160 mg twice daily

Other Sources

Pygeum Africanum (bark of pygeum tree)
Pumpkin seeds
Raw prostate
Note: Health food stores carry a variety of formulas for "maximum prostate nutrition."

Pass the Vegetables, Please

A link has been established between the intake of dietary fat and prostate cancer. Some studies have shown vegetarians, who have a low dietary fat intake have a lower incidence of cancer of the prostate than men with high fat intake. The same studies show a vegetarian diet lowers circulating testosterone levels and a non-vegetarian diet raises them. Prostate cancer grows on testosterone and slows when testosterone is lowered. A study of Japanese men conducted in 1977 noted that the marked increase in mortality from prostate cancer paralleled the increase in fat intake in the Japanese diet since 1950 (Life Extenders, p. 169).

Eliminating most of the fat in men's diets would greatly reduce the number of prostatic maladies, according to Dr. Carl P. Schaffner, Ph.D., professor of microbial chemistry at Rutgers University.

Dr. Schaffner discovered that by reducing cholesterol levels in aged dogs, he was also able to reduce the size of the animals' enlarged prostates.

Another study, reported to the American Urological Association, corroborates the possibly harmful effects of high cholesterol levels on prostate disease. Dr. Cammille Mallouh, M.D., Chief of Urology at Metropolitan Hospital in New York, examined 100 prostates from men of all ages and found an 80 percent increase in cholesterol content of enlarged prostates. Cholesterol has been shown to accumulate in an enlarged or cancerous human prostate (*Cancer Research*, December 1979).

Cancer of the prostate may be associated with our typical "civilized" Western diet. Peter Hill, Ph.D., of New York City's American Health Foundation, noted that rural black South Africans who typically eat a low-fat, whole-food diet had healthy prostates. He conducted a test to see if their diet was to blame. Dr. Hill and his associates put a group of volunteers on a typical Western diet of lots of meats and fats. At the same time, a group of North American volunteers, blacks and whites, were put on a low-fat diet. Dr. Hill and his colleagues then tested the subjects for diet-induced hormonal changes associated with prostatic cancer.

After three weeks, Dr. Hill found that the South Africans eating the Western diet excreted notably more hormones, while the reverse occurred with the North American subjects. The metabolic profile of the North Americans now resembled the low-risk group. Dr. Hill stated, "This study is a preliminary indication that a low-fat diet is one of the factors which can lower the risk of prostatic cancer. By reducing total calorie intake, and substituting fruit and vegetable calories for animal calories, a high-risk prostatic cancer group has switched to a low-risk one" (Herbert, p. 472).

The American Cancer Society and the American Urological Association recommend that beginning at age 50, all men have a PSA test every year along with a digital rectal exam. A rectal exam to men is like the breast exam to women. It's considered the best way to detect an early-stage tumor.

The PSA test measures levels of prostate-specific antigen, a protein that seeps out of the prostate if a tumor is present or the gland is enlarged.

CHAPTER 28:

Sun (Skin) Cancer

While it is true you don't expose the average 20 square feet of your skin to the sun, there is a lot you do expose on a hot summer day, if you don't wear sunscreen and cover up. It is this exposure, all experts warn, that increases your likelihood of getting skin cancer. For our purposes here, my use of "skin cancer," will refer to all skin cancers collectively.

Since World War II, there has been in increase in skin cancer, due to the increasing popularity of suntanning and outdoor recreation. While most cancers respond promptly to treatment and are not life-threatening, malignant melanoma is one of America's fastest-growing cancers, estimated to have struck 32,000 people in 1993, killing 9,100. Almost 75 percent of all skin cancer-related deaths will be from malignant melanoma. Since 1973, the incidence of melanoma has increased a frightening four percent a year, according to the American Cancer Society. An additional 10,000 invasive non-melanoma skin cancers was estimated to have occurred in 1993, mostly sarcomas, including Kaposi's sarcoma, with 2,300 deaths from these types (*Cancer Facts & Figures*, 1993).

The Early Warning Signs

Fortunately, there are warning signs to watch out for. If you sport moles, know where and how large they are. On a piece of paper map out the locations and sizes of your moles. It may sound silly, but if a new one appears or a mole starts growing, changing color (especially black) or shape, starts scaling, peeling or bleeding, at least you'll be aware of it. Typically, a mole that becomes malignant enlarges considerably.

Authorities blame this epidemic of skin cancer on two factors: the thinning ozone that permits more of the sun's ultraviolet rays to penetrate to earth, and sun-worshippers who brown themselves to a "well-done" condition.

Once considered an ailment of the middle-aged and older, the result of a lifetime working and playing unprotected in the sun, melanoma now appears in young people.

"There is no such thing as a safe tan," says Darrel Rigel, M.D., clinical associate professor of dermatology at New York University, Manhattan. "Why does the body tan? Because the body is being injured by ultraviolet [UV] radiation that hits it. This causes the body to make melanin, a natural sunscreen. To get tan, you must get injured first" (Greeley, p. 30).

Melanin is the dark pigment skin cells make to block out damaging rays in response to injury from UV radiation.

UV radiation comes in two wavelengths: UVA and UVB. Both cause skin damage. According to Arthur Sober, M.D., associate professor of dermatology at Harvard University Medical School, the damage is potentially serious whether it is caused by direct sunlight or tanning devices, or by light reflected off snow or water, or passing through clouds. "On a cloudy day, a person feels cooler, but is still getting a good amount of UV exposure," he says.

Janusz Beer, Ph.D., D.Sc., senior scientist in the radiation biology branch of FDA's Center for Devices and Radiological Health, explains that in natural light, and depending on the time of day, most UV radiation comes from UVA. Both UVA and UVB can cause damage but most of the damage to DNA (genetic material) in skin cells comes from UVB. This can lead to cell and tissue damage and possibly to skin cancer. In addition, he says, scientists know that UVB impairs the body's immune system, which normally defends against disease.

Both UVA and UVB are present year-round, but UVB is more intense in the summer, at higher altitudes, and near the equator, according to the American Academy of Dermatology.

UVA speeds up skin aging by causing changes in the skin's collagen, the protein in the skin's connective tissue. "Just look at pictures of people who work outside, like farmers and fishermen. They all have wrinkly faces," says Beer. "The more exposure, the more wrinkles."

Sunburns and blisters are the most obvious, and painful, result of short-term sun damage. Long-term damage, such as wrinkling, can be disfiguring and, in the case of skin cancer, life-threatening.

Barbara Gilchrest, M.D., chairman of the department of dermatology, Boston University School of Medicine, says to think of skin damage symptoms as occurring on two tracks that can cross each other at any point. One track has freckling and wrinkling and the other has skin cancer (Greeley, p. 30).

Cosmetic changes – wrinkling, coarseness, and irregular pigmentation – are on one track. The more sinister changes, such as actinic keratosis – scaly, rough, and red, tan, brownish, or grayish spots on the skin that can lead to cancerous tumors – occur on the other. These changes occur as a person is exposed to UV light, even in infancy, she says. The age when you first can see these changes depends on your complexion, how much and how often you're exposed to the sun, and other factors.

According to data presented by NYU's Dr. Rigel to the American Cancer Society, there are six risk factors associated with malignant melanoma:

* three or more blistering sunburns during adolescence;
* blond or red hair;
* marked freckling of the upper back;
* actinic keratosis;
* other family members with melanoma; and
* three or more years of outdoor summer jobs as a teenager.

Protecting Yourself

Regardless of your skin color, if you're going to be out in the sun, even for a short time, apply a sunscreen to all skin that will be exposed. Apply the sunscreen generously before going into the sun and reapply it often. Formulated as a solution, lotion, or cream, sunscreens are rated by a sun protection factor (SPF). An SPF of 6, for example, means that you can stay in the sun six times longer before burning than if you were wearing no sunscreen. The American Academy of Dermatology suggests that everyone use a product with at least an SPF 15.

UV radiation from the sun can also damage your eyes, particularly if you are often out in the sun at midday. You should wear sunglasses when on the beach, on the snow, and all the time when outdoors in the tropics or subtropics, or in high altitudes.

When buying sunglasses, look at the label to help you make the best selection. Most sunglass manufacturers label sunglasses according to standards established by the American National Standards Institute in New York. There are three categories:

1) cosmetic use glasses block at least 70 percent UVB, 60 percent UVA; 2) general use glasses block at least 95 percent UVB, 60 percent UVA; and 3) special purpose glasses for intense sunlight block at least 99 percent UVB, 98 percent UVA. Polarized glasses cut down on sun glare but do not necessarily block UV.

The rays from tanning lamps and beds used in "tanning parlors" are no safer than natural sunlight. Some manufacturers and parlor owners tell their clientele their devices use UVA rays, the so-called "tanning rays," but not UVB, or "burning rays."

"We now know that UVA rays are high intensity and do damage," explains Sydney Hurwitz, M.D., clinical professor of pediatrics and dermatology at Yale University School of Medicine. Many parlors use UVB rays in combination with UVA, which gives people more color. But once they get the color, it only lasts for a few days so they often go back for repeated treatments, which is not healthy for the skin (Greeley, p. 30).

Lorraine H. Kligman, Ph.D., of the University of Pennsylvania Medical School, says research shows people who use tanning devices often show signs of suppressed immunity.

Also, faulty timing devices may allow people to get more UV exposure than expected. People who don't wear goggles may suffer eye damage from the long wavelengths that penetrate eyelids, she adds. Closing your eyes does not help.

Madhu Pathak, Ph.D., research professor in dermatology, Harvard Medical School, believes there are various ways in which people can shield themselves (Kintish, p. 48).

Antioxidant Protection

Dr. Pathak recommends using cosmetics and moisturizers that contain antioxidants, such as vitamins E and C and beta carotene, to counteract the skin oxidation caused by sunlight that damages cell membranes, DNA and skin proteins.

"An antioxidant-enriched formulation will retard or minimize these damaging reactions both on the short term and long-term," said Dr. Pathak. "The potency of cosmetics and moisturizers is limited and they won't work like sunscreens, but they might help minimize the damaging reactions, especially if used in conjunction with sunscreens."

Selenium is a power-packed antioxidant helpful for any disorder that involves damage or breakdown on the cellular level. Because "low plasma selenium levels have been linked to increased risk of non-melanoma skin cancer in human patients," E. Delver and B.C. Pence of Texas Technical University Health Sciences Center, Lubbock, Texas decided to see if increased selenium reduces the potential of skin cancer (Delver, p. 17).

Using hairless mice exposed to high doses of ultraviolet rays, the researchers supplemented the diets of three mice groups varying amounts of selenium. Those fed the highest amount of selenium had the least number of tumors. Tests showed the mice produced high levels of glutathione, an enzyme essential for detoxification. Selenium helps the body produce glutathione.

In an abstract presented to the Experimental Biology '93 FASEB Conference, the researchers concluded, "selenium has potential as a chemo-preventive agent for human skin cancer."

When scientists surveyed the vitamin-taking habits of 131 people with skin cancer and 200 similar people without, they found that vitamin supplementation of any type was associated with a 60 percent reduction in skin cancer risk. More specifically, getting more than 100 international units (I.U.) of vitamin E (tocopherol) a day was linked to a 70 percent drop in risk; with more than 5,000 I.U. of vitamin A daily linked to a 90 percent reduction, according to a study presented at the American Society of Preventive Oncology. It's not the first time these antioxidants have been mentioned as possible skin-savers, but it is the first time average amounts of supplements have been linked to such a significant drop in risk (*Prevention*, February 1994).

When it comes to cancer, take no chances. If you are at high risk, check with a qualified physician well-versed in nutritional therapy. In the meantime, there are issues to keep in mind regarding taking vitamins E and A.

Several substances interfere with, or even cause a depletion of vitamin E. When iron and vitamin E are taken together, they cancel out each other. Dr. Wilfred Shute in *Vitamin E for Ailing and Healthy Hearts*, (p. 75) suggests it be taken in one dose and all iron taken 8 to 12 hours later for proper absorption. The best time to take vitamin E is before mealtime or bedtime. Chlorine in drinking water, ferric chloride, rancid oil or fat and inorganic iron compounds destroy vitamin E in the body. Large amounts of vegetable oil (polyunsaturated fats) in the diet increases the need for vitamin E. For optimal benefit, apply vitamin E to the skin as well as taking it internally.

Factors interfering with absorption of vitamin A and beta carotene include strenuous physical activity within four hours of consumption, intake of mineral oil, excessive consumption of alcohol and iron, and the use of cortisone and other drugs.

Antioxidant Foods

Selenium-rich foods include tuna, herring, brewer's yeast, wheat germ and bran, whole grains and sesame seeds. Selenium works closely with vitamin E in some of its metabolic actions and in the promotion of healthy cells.

Vitamin E-extravagant foods are wheat germ (and its oil), safflower seeds, sunflower seeds, sesame oil, walnuts, corn oil, hazelnuts, soybean oil, almonds, olive oil and cabbage.

Beta carotene boosters are carrots, beet greens, spinach, broccoli and most other green leafy vegetables. Beta carotene is not toxic in large doses, but if you eat too much, your skin may turn orange or yellow. Beta carotene is converted into vitamin A in the body.

Foods rich in vitamin A include cod liver oil (the best source), dandelion greens, carrots, yams, kale, parsley, turnip greens, collard greens, chard, watercress, red peppers, squash, egg yolk, cantaloupe, persimmons, apricots, broccoli, crab, swordfish, whitefish, Romaine lettuce, mangoes, pumpkin, peaches and cheese. Look to raw, fresh fruits and vegetables that are orange or yellow.

Foods high in vitamin C include rose hips, cherries, parsley, green peppers, watercress, strawberries and spinach. All of these foods have more vitamin C than oranges.

CHAPTER 29:

Cancer Authorities Tell All

"The real leader has no need to lead; he is content to point the way."
– Henry Miller

There are many eminent, well-qualified physician/researchers out there who know what works best to prevent cancer. They are highly knowledgeable about the way the body works and the way cancer insidiously takes advantage of the body's weaknesses. Who better then to tell you what you can do to prevent and minimize cancer?

Seeds, beans and soybeans are the favorite anti-cancer foods of Dr. Walter Troll, New York University Medical Center. He recommends peas and beans (legumes) as being particularly good for reducing the chances of developing breast cancer.

Robert Good, M.D., Ph.D., longevity authority and long-time president and director of the New York City-based Memorial Sloan-Kettering Cancer Center, has for many years followed a low-calorie, low-fat diet to prevent cancer, and he suggests this for others.

Dr. Sidney Mirvish, of the University of Nebraska Medical Center, states vegetable protein may buffer the stomach against cancer by preventing the formation of certain carcinogens.

The Pauling Protocol

Renowned worldwide for his research of vitamin C (ascorbic acid) to assure sound health, Dr. Linus Pauling, two-time Nobel Laureate, set an example by taking 18,000 milligrams daily to protect himself against cancer and other diseases.

A study Dr. Pauling conducted with Dr. Ewan Cameron, then associated with the Vale of Leven Hospital, Loch Lomondside, Scotland, indicates that a 10,000 milligram daily intake of vitamin C can significantly prolong life with advanced cancer and, in some cases, even halt or reverse the progress of the disease.

The study was conducted with patients who had tried conventional therapy first, which failed them. Survival times for the vitamin C-takers was between 114 and 435 days longer than for comparable placebo groups. At the end of the experiment, eight percent of those on vitamin C were still alive, compared with none of the controls.

A similar study conducted at Fukuoka Torikai Hospital in Japan produced almost the same result. Then, two controlled studies were done at the Mayo Clinic that supposedly refuted these studies.

However, the Mayo Clinic researchers failed to follow the exact protocols of the favorable studies, so the results were different. Pauling cried "foul" because the Mayo patients had been so heavily dosed with toxic chemicals their immune systems were too damaged to respond to the vitamin C treatment.

Over and above taking 18 grams of vitamin C daily, what did Pauling do to prevent cancer?

"I cut down on sugar (sucrose) and fructose," he had told me at the Second World Congress on vitamin C. "Dr. Yudkin and other authorities warn about the harmful effects of sugar, especially relative to heart disease. However, I believe that these effects carry over to cancer as well.

"My daily vitamin intake averages about 25 times the RDAs: 800 I.U. of vitamin E, and a super vitamin B complex tablet with 50 mg of the major components.

"As for minerals, I usually take a standard vitamin and mineral tablet daily, too. Sometimes I take extra selenium, but not every day."

Dr. Pauling believed vitamin C is especially effective in preventing bowel cancer, since it most directly effects the bowel (see the principle of bowel tolerance in Chapter 21).

He believed large doses of vitamin C inhibit cancer by increasing the synthesis of collagen (a fibrous protein found in connective tissue).

Experts agree on Vitamin C

At the first World Congress on Vitamin C some years ago, Dr. Albert Szent-Gyorgy, who first isolated ascorbic acid from vegetable sources, told me, "I take a minimum of 1,000 milligrams of vitamin C daily to prevent cancer and to assure my good health."

Other prominent biochemists and medical authorities say that simple eating measures can prevent and possibly even reverse cancer.

Dr. Edward J. Calabrese, University of Massachusetts, Amherst, says yes when offered a steaming, seductive piece of pepperoni pizza, even though the sausage contains sodium nitrite which, with other chemicals, can become a carcinogen in the stomach.

Knowing sodium nitrite joins amines in the stomach, forming a cancer-causing agent called dimethyl nitrosamine, Calabrese follows his pizza binge by eating a whole orange. He believes the vitamin C prevents nitrites and amines from forming nitrosamines.

Calabrese knows organically grown vegetables and fruits are not always available and supermarket produce often carries carcinogenic pesticide residues, so he gets protection from an orange, some other vitamin C-rich food or a vitamin C capsule.

Tree and garden-fresh fruits and vegetables, rich in beta carotene (a vitamin A precursor) and vitamin C, with a little vitamin E, tend to cancel out cancer-causing oxidizing agents, asserts Calabrese. Their fiber also efficiently and quickly helps to move food through the intestines so that ever-present carcinogens have too little contact time to work on them.

Best bet vitamin C supplements or foods, starting with the highest content, are: rose hips (a health food store item), acerola cherries, guavas, black currants, parsley, green peppers, watercress, chives, strawberries, persimmons, spinach, oranges, cabbage, grapefruit, papaya, elderberries and kumquats, dandelion greens and lemons, cantaloupe, green onions, limes, mangoes, loganberries, tangerines and tomatoes.

The Davis Safeguard

An eminent student of cancer preventives and therapies, Jay M. Davis, M.D., Ph.D., Eureka, California, has made it part of his practice to thoroughly research chemical substances that protect against cancer, examining studies recorded in responsible medical publications such as *Lancet* and the *New England Journal of Medicine.*

"I was trained as both a physician and a researcher," he writes in his book, *Until A Cure Comes...* (Millet Press, 1840 Myrtle Avenue, Eureka, CA 95501). "During my years of Ph.D. training, a major task was learning how to evaluate research – to examine a scientific experiment and see if its conclusions are sound..."

On the basis of his research and medical practice experience, Dr. Davis takes the following daily for cancer prevention: selenium, 300 mcgs; vitamin E, 400 I.U.; beta-carotene, 15-30 mg; vitamin A, 10,000 I.U.; and vitamin C, 500 mg.

Sometimes Dr. Davis wonders if he may be overdoing it with supplements over and above a balanced diet. Then he hears of some friend, colleague, or patient who has been diagnosed with cancer.

"It always comes as a kick in the stomach, and convinces me of the correctness of my decision. Mind you, I have no guarantees I will not get the disease. But, as I've told my friends, I'll never die of cancer. After all my preaching about prevention, I'd die of embarrassment."

Prevention, Czechoslovakian Style

Emil Ginter, Ph.D., head of the department of biochemistry, Institute of Preventive and Clinical Medicine, Bratislava,

Czechoslovakia, has his own program for preventing cancer, emphasizing vitamin C and pectin in relation to cholesterol metabolism.

His regimen was derived from his extensive research in the synergism between vitamin C, vitamin E and bioflavonoids aimed at lowering the extremely high mortality rate from cardiac disease and cancer in his native country.

Being a highly "civilized" society like ours, the cancer problem is just as acute there. Czechoslovakia's highly industrialized society includes old industries that pollute inordinately and streets are jammed with cars with no anti-pollution devices.

Adding to their cancer hazard is the Czechoslovakian diet that features mostly animal fat and refined sugar and salt.

"Fresh, raw fruits and vegetables are available only in summer and autumn, not year around as in the United States, says Dr. Ginter. "Little citrus fruit is imported, so the consumption of natural vitamin C is low.

"Unfortunately, we don't have access to vitamin C and bioflavonoid preparations in our country, so we have to depend on getting these nutrients from natural sources, which is the best way," he states.

"One of the major anti-cancer preparations I take, when available, is 200 mcg. of selenium daily. I am working to manufacture this and other anti-cancer nutrients so desperately needed in Czechoslovakia.

"There's one thing we have in my country that is superior to what you have (in the U.S.): heavy whole grain breads, which I eat in large amounts daily to nourish myself well and to prevent bowel cancer."

The Packer Anti-Cancer Pattern

Like Dr. Ginter, Lester Packer, Ph.D., a world-renowned researcher in biochemistry at the University of California at Berkeley, emphasizes antioxidants in his cancer-prevention program. Well-known for his experiments using vitamin E to encourage cells to multiply far beyond the usual 55 replications, Dr. Packer is presently working at reversing the damage caused by free radicals.

"Most cancers are avoidable if you control the environment against food pollution, smoking and alcohol. Ninety-seven percent of head and neck cancers are caused by smoking and alcohol.

"My cancer prevention program is simple: vitamin C, 750 mg daily; vitamin E, to 800 I.U.; beta carotene, 23 mg every other day; Coenzyme Q-10, 100 mg daily; and thioctic acid, 30 mg. Thioctic acid is available in Germany. Friends bring it to me from there."

Suggestions From Dr. Abram Hoffer

Abram Hoffer, M.D., the Canadian physician famous for his biochemical treatment for schizophrenia (mainly niacin and vitamin C) with Sir Humphrey Osmond, hesitates to offer a cancer prevention program, but he is willing to relate what he recommends to his patients.

"No program will guarantee you won't get cancer, but this one will greatly improve your chances of preventing it," he told me. "I start by recommending a junk-free diet that eliminates food additives, sugar and sodium."

"My second rule is to ease back on fat, particularly dairy products, from 40 percent of the diet to about 20 percent. The third rule is to increase the consumption of fresh and raw vegetables.

"I think everybody should take vitamin C. For a person in reasonably good heath, I recommend anywhere from three to six grams daily (3,000-6,000 mg). I take 10 to 12 grams. It doesn't guarantee you won't get cancer. I have had patients taking three grams daily, and they still developed cancer.

"I also recommend a good vitamin B-complex, supplying 50 to 100 mg of the major B components, to which you might want to add for special indications. For instance, if there's an indication you lack vitamin B6, you would want to add more of that. If you are smoking a lot, you might want to add folic acid.

"We should all take vitamin E. I take 800 I.U. daily. Also cod liver oil is helpful, particularly in winter or in climates where there's not much sunshine, because of its vitamins A and D.

"You should also get plenty of calcium and magnesium. That doesn't necessarily mean you have to take mineral supplements, because a good diet not too high in protein will provide enough of these minerals. A high protein diet increases the need for calcium. Even though natives of Third World countries ingest little calcium, they seldom develop osteoporosis because protein is in such short supply.

"A daily intake of 500 mg of calcium is enough for the average person, with 1,500 mg a day for pregnant or lactating women. This should be balanced out with magnesium – not on a two-to-one ratio, but on a one-to-one ratio.

"On a junk-free diet, people will get enough beta carotene and potassium in fresh raw fruits and vegetables and in whole grain cereals and bread. However, if they can't stay away from the junk, it will be necessary to supplement with potassium. For my cancer patients, I recommend extra beta carotene.

"Selenium is critically important for cancer prevention. The average diet probably provides 100 mcg. I recommend 200 mcg a day for my patients."

Girth Control and More

Charles Thomas, Ph.D., president of Pantox, a San Diego-based company that measures the concentration of antioxidants in human blood for doctors, is well-qualified to make anti-cancer recommendations. He bases his program on extensive experience as a biochemist and eleven years as a professor of biological chemistry at Harvard University Medical School and, prior to that, 10 years as a professor of biophysics at John Hopkins University.

"My major way of preventing cancer is practicing girth control – eating less. In our society that means eating less fat, the simplest way of cutting down on calories.

"My wife and I don't eat butter or cheese. We use the skimmest skim milk on our whole grain cereal in the morning, but we enjoy a steak once in a while and eggs occasionally. I enjoy dry, crisp bacon. That's one thing I find difficult to eliminate. We don't use other dairy products or spreads such as mayonnaise.

"We take two grams of vitamin C daily and a nutritional formula that has 40 different nutrients including a gram of vitamin C, half a gram of magnesium, twice that amount of calcium, 200 mcg of selenium, and among others, 300 mcg of chromium in two different forms.

"We don't use salt in our house, but we do eat lots of fresh fruit and vegetables. In Pantox, we're always analyzing new things, not necessarily just antioxidants. We've found most people are short of folate, (especially) the elderly, alcoholics and children. Fresh fruits and vegetables are the major source of folate (folic acid)."

"I emphasize folate, because people who are deficient in this B vitamin break down their DNA faster than those who are replete in it. Folic acid is an important part of the synthesis of one of the nucleotidase that goes into DNA.

"A deficiency would probably make you more vulnerable to cancer, in that it causes a DNA repair reaction. Nothing in life is perfect. Mistakes can be made, and those mistakes are mutations," says Dr. Thomas.

"One third of all the cancers are colon and rectal cancers, caused mainly by the high fat content in the diet. When fats go into the lower colon, they are soaps. Soaps kill cells by disrupting the cell membranes. The epithelium, the surface layer of the colon, is then subject to much cell-killing, which eventually stimulates cell proliferation."

The Rimland Experience

Bernard Rimland, Ph.D., of San Diego, is known worldwide for his nutritional therapies for psychological and emotional disorders. He waged a successful battle against the cancer that threatened his teenage daughter, and offers his family's daily anti-cancer formula.

"Each of us take 10 to 12 grams of vitamin C in water or juice; 200 micrograms of selenium; 400 to 800 I.U. of vitamin E; and 25,000 to 50,000 I.U. of vitamin A. Of course, we eat a lot of fresh vegetables, adding about 1,000 mg of calcium, which is very important to prevent colon cancer," he told me at the Second World Congress on vitamin C.

"I started studying cancer intensively some 17 years ago when my teenage daughter was found to have what was then considered to be a terminal type of cancer: Hodgkins disease, stage 4B.

"Her liver and kidneys were deeply invaded, as radio assay revealed. Doctors had never seen anyone with kidneys so impaired. They gave her six to eight months to live. My in-depth reading of medical literature showed me there was a tremendous amount of knowledge about this disease that wasn't being utilized.

"So I immediately started her on 40 grams of vitamin C a day, orally. I also gave her a gram of niacinamide, 50 mg of the other B vitamins, 800 I.U. of vitamin E and 75,000 I.U. of vitamin A, as well as calcium, magnesium and other minerals in normal amounts.

"Although the oncologists were giving her chemotherapy – those horrible chemicals – and she lost all of her hair, they assured me their efforts wouldn't help a case this far gone. (Despite their contentions), she began to improve at a spectacular rate," Dr. Rimland says.

"Seeing her great improvement – as the oncologists did, too – I kept photocopying copies of medical literature about the efficacy of vitamin C and folded reports into thirds to fit into my jacket pocket to take to the oncologists. They paid no attention to them. I would return to the doctor's office two or three weeks later, and the reports were still on the desk, not even unfolded.

"Meanwhile, the (other) kids – in my daughter's words – most of them with leukemia – were dying like flies. I remembered Irwin Stone's writing which noted that the symptoms of leukemia are identical with those of scurvy.

"Stone used to say, 'If you run a vitamin C blood test, someone with leukemia would have almost zero vitamin C. If you gave that person a lot of vitamin C, the blood level would still measure zero. So you have to give them massive amounts to get the blood level anywhere near normal.

"And, if you did, the symptoms of leukemia would go away. Stone published case histories of people who recovered and did very well, just as my daughter did. She's perfectly normal today.

"The super-nutritional program saved her life and probably could have saved the lives of many of the little kids in her ward. However, there's no way of convincing the oncologists of this. It has to be their way or no way," concludes Dr. Rimland.

CHAPTER 30:

Fruits and Vegetables, Acknowledged Cancer Fighters

"Your foods shall be your remedies, and your remedies shall be your foods."

– Hippocrates

Looking at cancer statistics, researchers have had to acknowledge a link between cancer and diet. How else can they explain communities and cultures with a low incidence of cancer, whose only commonality was what they ate? Over the decades numerous researchers have produced study after study showing a relationship between vegetables and fruits, and cancer prevention and survival.

No one had a clue how cruciferous vegetables worked against cancer until a prominent researcher, Ernest Bueding and associates at John Hopkins University, accidentally came up with a partial answer.

Bueding's team of investigators, searching for a treatment for schistosomiasis, a parasitic disorder afflicting hundreds of millions worldwide, tested dithiolthiones, chemicals plentiful in broccoli, brussels sprouts, cauliflower and cabbage, against the worm responsible for it.

It surprised them that dithiolthiones depressed the level of glutathione in the worms. This had frightening implications because in human beings glutathione helps keep metabolism normal and is a detoxifier, a free radical fighter.

In subsequent tests on mammals, the Bueding team discovered that the effect of dithiolthiones in humans was just the opposite; they increased available glutathione.

Antioxidants

Antioxidants, vitamins C, E and beta carotene, in vegetables and fruits protect cells from damage by free radicals, which nutrition writer Patrick Quillin, Ph.D., calls "Great white sharks in the biochemical sea of life." These cell saboteurs have long been suspected of triggering various cancers.

Evidence unearthed by Gladys Block, Ph.D., University of California nutrition researcher, reveals vegetable and fruit antioxidants are staunch defenders against numerous types of cancer.

Dr. Block conducted an in-depth analysis of 99 studies to see whether there is actually a connection between diet and cancer. Eighty-nine of the studies disclosed vegetables and fruit, indeed, are a first line of defense against many types of cancer.

Thirty-three of the studies show vitamin C and related nutrients in cantaloupes, citrus fruits and green leafy vegetables protect us against cancers of the cervix, the esophagus and stomach.

Other research reveals vitamin E in corn, green leafy vegetables and soybeans guards us against cancers of the breast, pancreas and stomach.

A Japanese researcher, T. Harayama, conducted a 10-year study of 265,118 subjects who answered questions about their dietary intake. Harayama discovered that people who ate liberal amounts of vegetables containing beta carotene (carrots, sweet potatoes, yams, cantaloupe, apricots, spinach, squash and leafy green vegetables) had a lower risk of lung, stomach and prostate cancer.

In a study reported in the *American Journal of Clinical Nutrition,* biochemist G.A. Colditz took dietary information on 1,271 Massachusetts residents 66 years of age and older for more than five years, calculating the amount of beta carotene ingested. Assessing the volunteers' health at the end of this period, he found those who ate vegetables with the highest beta carotene content had 70 percent fewer cancers than those who consumed the least.

Numerous other studies bear out the fact that people who eat the most vegetables containing the largest amounts of beta carotene seem best protected from all types of cancer.

One authority, Dr. Marilyn S. Menkes, of John Hopkins School of Hygiene and Public Health, found that few people with high levels of beta carotene in the blood develop cancer. The opposite is true for individuals with low blood levels. Asked how many carrots a person would have to eat daily to get enough beta carotene to cancer-proof him or herself, Dr. Menkes responded, "One carrot." That's low cost insurance.

While we're on Bugs Bunny's favorite subject, there is a new carrot developed by a University of Wisconsin research geneticist, Phillip Simon, Ph.D., that out-carrots them all. Called Beta III, this one is tops of the carrot kingdom, deep orange in color and containing two to four times more beta carotene than more common carrots.

Frederick Khachik, Ph.D., a research chemist at USDA's Human Nutrition Center in Beltsville, Maryland, lauds the new carotene-rich carrot and beta carotene, saying that beta carotene not only prevents cancer by quenching free radicals, which contribute to turning normal cells into cancerous ones, but also slows down the aging process and revs up the immune system.

For those who don't care for raw carrots, beta carotene is also found in peaches, cantaloupes, apricots, nectarines, squash, green peppers and green peas.

Folic Acid

Now biochemists know it's more than just beta carotene and vitamins C and E in vegetables and fruits that help to prevent cancer. Folic acid, one of the B vitamins, is a powerful nutrient, and often deficient in those who need it the most.

Some studies indicate folic acid may help to turn off cancer genes. So says researcher Edward Giovannucci, Harvard Medical School.

However, alcohol blocks absorption of folic acid, so alcohol may be a cancer promoter. In the presence of alcohol, cancer genes synthesize a protein that may cause cells to proliferate, says Giovannucci.

The Harvard research team discovered a high intake of folic acid, gotten from fresh vegetables and fruit and vitamin supplements, lowered the risk of tumor development. Volunteers who had two alcoholic drinks daily turned out to have an 85 percent higher risk of developing tumors than non-drinkers.

Other research shows folic acid directs the growth of new cells in the body. A shortage or lack of this nutrient may contribute to improper or abnormal cell formation.

It is a well-established fact few individuals eat enough fresh fruits and vegetables to obtain sufficient folic acid. Furthermore, use of birth control pills increases the requirement for this nutrient.

Quercetin

One of the newer superstar anti-cancer nutrients in health food stores is quercetin. Dr. Terence Leighton, a biochemistry professor at the University of California, Berkeley, a world authority on this subject, has unrestrained enthusiasm for it:

"Quercetin is one of the strongest anti-cancer agents known," he says.

Various lab studies reveal that quercetin unleashes a one-two punch against cancer. Leighton says it blocks cell changes that invite cancer and, if a tumor has already started, stops the spread of malignant cells.

Richest sources of quercetin are onions, broccoli, zucchini, grapes, green algae, and eucalyptus leaves.

Red and yellow onions contain an incredible amount of quercetin – 10 percent or more of their dry weight. Not so white onions or, for that matter, garlic, the onion's odoriferous cousin.

Niacin

Several years ago 200 diet and cancer researchers from 21 countries gathered in Fort Worth, Texas, to share research on the relationship of cancer and niacin, which is found mainly in chicken, eggs, fish, meat, nuts and whole grains.

"There's no question that niacin is one of the building blocks of the body to make it resistant to enemies," Dr. Nathan Berger, professor of oncology at Case Western Reserve University in Cleveland, told the conference.

Various publications presented there convinced researchers that niacin-deficient cells develop cancer 10 times more readily than normal cells, although participants could not explain the reason why.

Phytochemicals

Adding to what we know about cancer and nutrients, scientists have isolated and identified the many healing chemicals contained in fruits and vegetables. They are collectively called phytochemicals ("phyto" is derived from the Greek word for plant).

Phytochemicals are neither vitamins nor minerals, yet they are equally potent and vital to the healthy functioning of our bodies. They are isolated from plants and are known technically as anthocyanosides, limonoids, glucarates, phenolic acids, flavonoids, coumarins, polyacetylenes and carotenoids. One example of the multiple capabilities of phytochemicals is echinacea, an herbal most often found in extract form, containing substances that destroy infection germs directly, and bolster the immune system by magnifying the white blood cell count.

Many of mainstream medicine's pharmaceuticals are derived or synthesized from phytochemicals, including aspirin from willow bark and an anti-cancer medication from the Pacific yew tree.

Some naturally-occurring phytochemicals throw a biochemical wrench into one or more of the mechanisms leading to a tumor. "At almost every one of the steps along the pathway leading to cancer," says epidemiologist John Potter of the University of Minnesota, "there are one or more compounds in vegetables or fruits that slow or reverse the process" ("Beyond Vitamins," *Newsweek,* April 25, 1994).

The cruciferous (family crucifera) vegetables: broccoli, cauliflower, Brussels sprouts, turnips, kale, turnip greens and bok choy are the most highly-regarded anti-cancer foods. Researchers have isolated sulforaphane as responsible for their cancer preventive properties.

"The results are quite dramatic," says Dr. Paul Talalay of Johns Hopkins Medical Institutions. In his initial studies he found that among lab animals exposed to carcinogens and given sulforaphane, few developed tumors.

Two years ago Talalay added sulforaphane to human cells growing in a lab dish and reported that it boosted synthesis of anti-cancer enzymes. In the April 1994 *Proceedings of the National Academy of Sciences,* his team reported conclusively that the compound protects living animals against cancer.

Phytochemicals in the whole tomato have also been identified in a first line of cancer defense. Scientists at Cornell University reported that two of tomatoes' estimated 10,000 phytochemicals, p-coumaric acid and chlorogenic acid, stop the formation of cancer-causing substances.

During digestion, the body routinely makes carcinogenic compounds, called nitrosamines, out of nitric oxide and amines, by-products of certain foods we eat (including those containing man-made chemicals). Tomato acids take away the nitrosamines before they can do any damage. Cornell's Joseph Hotchkiss gave volunteers tomato juice and found less nitrosamines in their bodies, emphasizing use of the whole tomato.

Cabbage and turnips contain phenethyl isothocyanate (PEITC), a cousin of the broccoli phytochemical. Reports Gary Stoner of Ohio State University, PEITC inhibits lung cancer caused by chemicals in mice and rats. Ellagic acid in strawberries, grapes and raspberries also neutralizes carcinogens before they can invade DNA.

In 1993, German researchers announced they had isolated a chemical in soybeans that prevents tumors from growing. Called genistein, it might be why Japanese men who relocate to the West and adopt a soy-poor diet for even a few years have a greatly elevated risk of prostate cancer.

Onion and garlic contain allylic sulfide, which creates a family of enzymes that detoxifies carcinogens. Capsaicin in hot peppers keeps toxic molecules from attaching to DNA, which can initiate cancer; so does a phytochemical in turmeric and cumin. And almost every fruit and vegetable, from berries to yams to citrus and cucumbers, contain flavonoids. In a cellular version of musical chairs, these compounds race to sites on the cell where cancer-causing hormones, including estrogen, attach themselves. When the music stops, the flavonoids keep the hormones from sitting down on the cell's surface.

Make fruits and vegetables part of your daily diet and you'll be on the road to a cancer-free lifetime.

CHAPTER 31:

Garlic and Green Tea, Guerrilla Warfare

"That which we call a rose by any other name would smell as sweet."

— *William Shakespeare*

After all the talk about dangerous chemicals we eat and drink and the importance of cleansing the body to remove toxins, the only thing left is to find that one special food that absolutely cleans and purifies the body. Here it is: *garlic* is one of the best natural antioxidants and systemic detoxifiers. To recount the studies here would take up the whole book. All you need to know is it has been proven over and over again to work effectively.

If garlic were a pharmaceutical, you would see advertisements in all the magazines, and the lucky company with the patent would earn hundreds of millions of dollars a year. Everyone would learn of garlic's vast power and flock to their doctors for a prescription. Fortunately for those of us in the know, garlic is available easily and inexpensively.

Unfortunately, because it's not patentable, few cancer patients are aware of the many benefits they can derive from raw garlic and, especially, my favorite, Kyolic® aged garlic extract. If garlic were an over-the-counter medicine, Kyolic® would be touted as maximum-strength.

Garlic may be news to you, but it is old news to our ancestors.

Garlic's History

Egyptian slaves stopped work on the great pyramid of Cheops until the pharaoh restored their daily ration of garlic. They believed it was the key to their health, strength and endurance. No doubt their gardens were laden with breath-restoring peppermint also.

Babylonian cuneiform writings from 3,000 B.C. reveal garlic was used as a cure for many ailments. The Talmud recommends it as an aphrodisiac for married people on the Sabbath evening.

The venturesome Vikings, who supposedly discovered America before Columbus, and the ancient Phoenicians, stowed a liberal supply of garlic aboard to keep themselves healthy during long voyages.

The Chinese, Romans and Greeks used garlic to cure stomach and intestinal ailments, lung infections, worms, skin rashes, ulcers and to stay young. Egyptians, Greeks and Indians saluted garlic with festivals for thousands of years. At the present time, Gilroy, a small Northern California city which declares itself the Garlic Capital of the world, attracts hundreds of thousands to its annual garlic festival held each summer.

Modern Day Studies

Garlic's most lofty purpose is in preventing cancer. Dr. Herbert Pierson, former program manager of the National Cancer Institute (NCI), says researchers agree cancer's future is in prevention, and garlic plays a starring role.

Pierson whole-heartedly supports the NCI-backed research on garlic and other food products as "more cost-effective than looking for new drugs." The vast number of drugs that fail government scrutiny and the delays in new drug approval have forced science and the government to see food as the preventive medicine of the future.

One reason garlic may protect against cancer is its ability to help the body inactivate, metabolize and eliminate cancer-causing substances (carcinogens) without damage. Garlic is also believed to enhance the body's immune system.

Biologist Dr. Michael Wargovic and colleagues at the Univei Texas, M.D. Anderson Cancer Center, report a series of studie ing the cancer prevention power of garlic. They discovered that a water-soluble organosulfur compound, S-allyl cysteine (SAC), in Kyolic® aged garlic extract, significantly blocks the development of colon cancer in mice.

Additionally, they found S-allyl cysteine enhances the body's production of glutathione S-transferase, a powerful enzyme that detoxifies many carcinogens. Because S-allyl cysteine is considered safe and causes fewer side effects than diallyl sulfide in raw garlic, Dr. Hiromichi Sumiyoshi, a prominent researcher, considers it a "prime candidate" for further cancer-prevention study.

Kyolic® aged garlic extract has numerous patents pending due to its ability to protect the liver from tumor growth.

Dr. Sidney Belman, New York University Medical Center, demonstrated that applying garlic oil directly to the skin of mice prevented skin cancer induced by DMBA, a potent carcinogen used in most studies of cancer.

Several epidemiological studies have linked the large amounts of garlic, onions and scallions eaten in Italy and China with their low stomach cancer rate.

Many cured meats, such as bacon, ham and sausage, contain nitrates and/or nitrites, chemical preservatives that link with amino acids and become nitrosamines, potent carcinogens.

Nitrosamines are a by-product of our "civilized" daily living. They are caused by chemicals in air pollution, cigarette smoke and processed foods. Nitrosamines are found anywhere you have chemical pollution, known or unknown.

Jinzhou Liu, a Chinese biochemist at Penn State University, has discovered that Kyolic® odorless aged garlic extract is much more effective than vitamin C in preventing nitrosamines from being formed – in lab experiments with animals and people.

Researchers at UCLA began using aged garlic extract to treat malignant melanoma (skin cancer), discovering that Kyolic® suppresses the growth of cancer cells. Dr. S.B. Hoon claims Kyolic® may be the perfect means for preventing melanoma.

Troubled by the rapid rise of bladder cancer each year —more than 50,000 cases — West Virginia researchers led by Dr. Donald Lamm tried the aged garlic extract.

"The reduction of tumor growth with Kyolic® aged garlic suggests it may prove to be an extremely effective form of immunotherapy" he states.

Still another study by J. Liu and J. Milner, Division of Nutritional Science, University of Illinois at Urbana and Penn State University, tested the effectiveness of this garlic product with and without selenium on breast cancer.

In a study using laboratory mice, Kyolic® aged garlic extract was added to their basic diet, resulting in a 66 percent reduction of carcinogenic breast tissue binding. When a trace amount of selenium was added, there was a 99 percent reduction in this binding.

Dr. Milner found the studies most impressive. In a follow-up experiment, raw garlic was found to be almost as effective as the Kyolic®. However, the side effects to those on raw garlic were too toxic to give credence to the experiment.

A study by Dr. Benjamin Lau of Loma Linda University, published in the *Journal of Urology*, showed that the aged garlic extract completely stopped the growth of cancer in mice, while treatment with a live vaccine only reduced cancer growth by about 55 percent.

Why is garlic such a worthy opponent to cancer?

Garlic has large amounts of the amino acid cysteine, an incredibly powerful antioxidant/free-radical destroyer/detoxifier. Remember, antioxidants snuff out free radicals that attach to cell membranes and DNA and reprogram normal cells to become cancerous.

It also contains glutathione, a term familiar to you by now, which is an enzyme that helps rid the body of toxins and heavy metals. Heavy metals such as cadmium, lead and mercury are often present in industrial waste and contribute heavily to our cancer epidemic. Kyolic® increases glutaghinone in the liver, helping the body rid itself of chemicals, pesticides and other toxins.

Aflatoxin Remedy

Research by Loma Linda University scientists suggest Kyolic® may help solve an acute worldwide health problem: aflatoxin, a deadly poison produced by molds found on peanuts, cottonseed, corn, beans, rice, grains and sweet potatoes.

Aflatoxin has multiplied the incidence of liver damage and liver cancer to astronomical levels in Africa and Asia, and other parts of the world where agricultural technology is primitive and food inspection is almost non-existent. Liver damage or cancer may be caused by aflatoxin but often cannot be traced to it. Aflatoxin in expectant mothers can result in their babies being born mentally retarded.

Even with our advances in screening, the United States is not exempt from this deadly threat.

In his excellent book, *Healing Nutrients* (Contemporary Books), Patrick Quillin, Ph.D., discusses a part of rural Georgia which has two times as much mental retardation as the rest of the nation. He suggests the area's food source may be tainted with aflatoxin.

Kyolic® was found in studies to be particularly effective in preventing mutation of healthy cells and their attacks by aflatoxin's cancer-causing compounds.

Maximum Strength

One of the reasons for my bouncy good health and young looks is I have taken deodorized Kyolic® every day for more than a decade. Raw, odoriferous garlic would have destroyed my social and business life.

During a speaking tour of Japan, I visited the factory and laboratories of Wakunaga Pharmaceutical Co., Ltd., manufacturer of Kyolic®, to see for myself how they manage to enhance the incredible power of raw garlic.

First of all, Kyolic® garlic is grown in special organically rich mineral soil. If you've been paying attention, you'll remember that any food, be it animal, vegetable or mineral, requires a nutritionally rich source to grow from. A nutrient-rich garlic can't possibly be grown in mineral-poor soil. Commercially grown garlic is treated with formaldehyde, sprayed with two herbicides, and fertilized with artificial and incomplete nitrate fertilizers.

I was amazed at the size of the facilities and the beauty and spaciousness of the Wakunaga property. The grounds are landscaped with flowers and shrubs which have been planned to display an array of colors as the seasons change.

Wakunaga focuses on producing quality, natural pharmaceuticals from extracts of natural herbs. I saw for myself how they maintain strict quality control throughout the entire production process, from cultivation of raw materials to finished products.

Wakunaga's unique aging process – more than 18 months – produces a garlic that is safer, more valuable and more effective than raw garlic. The company employs over 25 Ph.D.'s and has more than 500 employees. Some 125 garlic researchers worldwide conduct scientific studies on Kyolic® as well.

Kyolic® is included in my personal anti-cancer regimen as one of my most important nutritional supplements. I also use a liquid mineral solution with B12, biotin and silica; a B vitamin supplement made from organic seed sprouts; a special vitamin C formula that includes green tea extract; 400 IU vitamin E; and antioxidants.

I avidly follow international garlic studies, and am convinced the science of garlic is truly the science of Kyolic®. More than 100 published studies of Kyolic® cover a vast range of subjects from AIDS to cancer, to cholesterol and allergies. The company has 14 international patents and patents pending on Kyolic®, which is perhaps the only garlic that promotes friendly flora in our intestinal tract – so vital to our health and well-being.

In summarizing the major studies – some of which you have read about here – Dr. Herbert Pierson reports "excessive amounts of raw garlic can be toxic, but when aged" it "enters the body's cells and stimulates immune response."

Dr. Tariq Abdullah, Panama City, Florida, conducted studies showing that raw garlic and Kyolic® enhances natural killer cell activity to fight cancer. He says, "No other substance, either natural or synthetic, can match garlic's proven therapeutic versatility and effectiveness. Garlic is the best example of the philosophy, "Let your medicine be your food, and your food your medicine."

Garlic has been the medical arsenal mainstay of past civilizations. A good thing gets passed around, which is why history teems with civilizations utilizing garlic's healing power. Before the advent of antibiotics, garlic was the last word in battling infections. Knowing what we do about conventional pharmaceuticals, doesn't it make sense to depend on Kyolic® for our health needs instead?

Green Tea in the Limelight

At an annual meeting of the American Association of Cancer Research, April 10-13, 1994 in San Francisco, conventional researchers made the startling announcement that enough evidence has been found to proclaim that green tea (Camellia sinensis) does indeed appear to protect against cancer (Green). For many researchers following green tea and its epidemiological evidence, this is nothing new. Asian populations consume great quantities of green tea, and, not coincidentally, have one of the lowest cancer rates in the world. Even the Japanese, who have one of the highest populations of smokers, experience fewer cases of cancer than the Americans.

Green tea is extremely rich in flavonoids, which are potent antioxidants. It also contains polyphenols, which are strong free radical scavengers. The caffeinated version can be used as a coffee substitute because it contains the caffeine but not the roasted hydrocarbons which are known to be potent carcinogens (Posniak, p. 127).

Conventional Medicine Concurs

In 1993, the National Cancer Institute prepared a review of hundreds of studies on tea and cancer. Their conclusion? "On the basis of many epidemiologic observations and numerous laboratory studies, we believe that tea consumption is likely to have beneficial effects in reducing cancer risk." Let me summarize some of the more impressive studies that elevate green tea to medicinal status.

Lung Cancer

One of the NCI researchers, Zhi-Yan Wang, of the College of Pharmacy, Rutgers University, found mice that were given decaffeinated green tea as their sole source of drinking water, then exposed to the chemical carcinogen NNK, had fewer lung tumors than those who did not receive the tea. The effect occurred both if the tea was administered prior to and during the time of exposure to NNK or if tea consumption did not begin until afterward.

Similarly, Santosh K. Katiyar, of the Department of Dermatology, Case Western Reserve, reported that green tea polyphenols protected against chemically induced forestomach and lung tumors in mice. Katiyar found the result held for two different carcinogens: diethylnitrosamine and benzo(a)pyrene.

Breast Cancer

In an in-vitro study, Nitin T. Telang, of the Strang-Cornell Cancer Research Laboratory, Cornell University Medical College, found epigallocatechin gallate (EGCC), a major component of green tea polyphenols, effectively suppressed c-myconogene-induced mammary cell transformations (the beginnings of breast cancer) in tissue-cultured mouse cells. Telang suggested the results may be due to the compound's ability to reduce estrogens (Green).

Stomach Cancer

A recent study in Shizuoka Prefecture, Japan indicated that the cancer death rate, especially from stomach cancer, was lower than the national average and that inhabitants of towns having lower incidence rates tended to drink green tea more frequently than did inhabitants in other areas (Oguni, p. 332).

A case-control study in Kyushu, Japan showed that individuals consuming green tea more frequently or in larger quantities tended to have a lower risk of gastric cancer (Kono, p. 1067).

Skin Cancer

Scientists from Rutgers University, the American Health Foundation and the Cancer Centre of Tokyo reported a series of studies on green tea at a 1991 meeting of the American Chemical Society in New York. Japanese scientists called tea extract "a practical cancer chemo-preventive agent to be implemented in everyday life" (Charles, p. 17).

One leading tea researcher in the U.S., Allan Conney of Rutgers University, exposed groups of mice to various cancer-inducing treatments while giving them green tea to drink instead of water. Whatever the carcinogen, the tea-drinking mice developed fewer cancers than a control group of mice. Skin cancers resulting from exposure to ultraviolet radiation were reduced by between 39 and 87 per cent compared to controls, and the incidence of stomach cancers and lung cancers was about 50 percent lower among tea drinkers (*ibid*).

CHAPTER 32:

The Healing Power of the Mind

"The mind has great influence over the body, and maladies often have their origin there."

— *Jean Baptiste Poquelin Moliere,*
17th Century French Playwright

Innocent as they seem, statistics can be killers, particularly when issued by orthodox physicians about a cancer patient's survival prospects.

"Nine out of ten people with your kind of cancer die," is a typical ominous prediction.

This is exactly the type of statement that annihilates hope, shatters morale and almost assures the patient will die. Never assume anything, I always say.

Using reverse English on such a prediction works wonders for Bernie Siegel, M.D., cancer surgeon and author of best-sellers, including *Love, Medicine and Miracles.* He tells patients, "One out of ten survives this kind of cancer – you could be the one!"

Dr. Siegel's super-charged positivism contributes to his phenomenal number of cancer patient healings, the envy of many oncologists.

Some years ago, *Reader's Digest* ran a thought-provoking article, "Avoid the Habit of Dying." A quote from Mark Twain neatly sums up its theme:

"Man is the only animal that lives by vital statistics and dies before he has to."

People calculate how long they will live by the longevity of their parents and, by accepting this limitation for their lives, create a self-fulfilling prophecy for death at a certain age.

By predicting how long a cancer patient or disease sufferer has to live, arrogant orthodox oncologists try to play God. Two factors seem to escape them: their poor qualifications for the job, and the fact that the position is already admirably filled.

Belief Can Cure or Sicken

Despite a mountain of studies showing the mind has a powerful influence over the body, much of medical orthodoxy clings to the dinosaur concept that the body and mind are separate, disclaiming or at least discounting the evidence that stress and positive thinking influence the body.

As a species, we are incredibly suggestible.

During an athletic event in a small stadium in the Southern California city of Highland Park, six people found themselves feeling sick. They crowded into the tiny first aid office complaining of dizziness and nausea.

The nurse questioned them and found they had one thing in common: they all had a soft drink from the stadium's single vending machine.

Quickly, she phoned an emergency doctor who rushed to the scene and after talking to the nurse, announced over the public address system no one should use the beverage vending machine or finish his or her drink taken from it. He told the crowd six people who had drunk a soft drink from it were being treated for dizziness and nausea.

Within five minutes, 200 more people crowded the corridor outside the room. All of them were dizzy and felt like vomiting. The nurse phoned for ambulances.

The ambulances, packed with people, tires screeching, raced to the seven nearest hospitals.

Meanwhile, an expert examined the vending machine, its pipes, water source and soft drink syrup. He found nothing amiss and reported this to the doctor, who announced via the public address system that it was all right to use the vending machine. Then he phoned the hospitals to inform stadium patients that a careful examination had revealed that there was nothing wrong with the beverages from the vending machine after all.

Within 10 minutes, all the "victims' " symptoms disappeared, and they were released.

Psychoneuroimmunology: The Science of Belief

When patients' illnesses were found to have no physical cause, they were dismissed as psychosomatic. But when physicians realized how many could also cure themselves of illnesses that had physical causes, researchers began to investigate the ways the mind communicates to the body. The psychosomatic syndrome has been conventionally legitimatized through the field of psychoneuroimmunology, pioneered over 25 years ago in an effort to understand the influence of emotional states on human health and resistance to disease. The goal has been to define the pathways and mechanisms of communication between the nervous system, the endocrine system, and the immune system. Research in this rapidly growing field actually started with Claudius Galen, an eminent physician and medical writer of the second century, A.D., who found melancholy women were the most likely to develop cancer.

Eighteen centuries later, researchers are corroborating Galen's observation. In one study, people who showed depression at the start of the investigation were twice as prone as non-depressed individuals to contract cancer, even when use of alcohol and tobacco, occupational hazards and heredity had been considered.

Melancholy and depression are not the only emotional characteristics that apparently invite cancer.

Nothing to Live For

Repressed emotions seem to contribute to cancer, a s.
L. Graves, John W. Schaffer and colleagues at John
University School of Medicine disclosed.

Based on psychological data gathered between 1948 and 1964 on
almost 1,000 Johns Hopkins male medical students, Graves revealed
people who live or stay alone are 16 times more prone to develop cancer than others.

In a landmark study, women with breast cancer who participated in
a support group lived twice as long as women who didn't.

No one knows how social ties influence good health, but theories
abound. Some researchers theorize having social support encourages
people to take better care of themselves. But some studies also suggest that people who participate in support groups or have someone
whom they trust and confide in are physiologically affected by an
increased immune response. In fact, a recent study suggests that as
your social network expands, so does the number of certain
disease-fighting cells, known as monocytes and lymphocytes.
Researchers at the University of Arizona and Canyon Ranch, in
Tucson, Arizona, measured the number of these killer cells in a group
of 110 elderly people when they enrolled in an 11-day health promotion program. Researchers also assessed their levels of social support
and perceived stress. After three months, patients who reported an
increase in social support saw their monocytes increase.

The importance of a positive emotional life for cancer prevention
or management is illustrated in a study by Janice Kiecolt-Glaser, Ohio
State University, and immunologist Ron Glasser.

There were startling differences in DNA repair in the white blood
cells of psychiatric patients when compared with people not suffering
from emotional illness. Blood drawn from volunteers taken from both
groups was exposed to X-rays, causing DNA damage.

Measurements were then taken on the speed and efficiency with
which certain white blood cells were able to repair the DNA damage.
The blood from psychiatric patients showed less ability to repair
DNA.

The researchers concluded: emotional stress may be "directly associated with an increased risk of cancer and infectious disease."

Loneliness, or "social isolation," was linked to cancer mortality in a 17-year study of 7,000 individuals by epidemiologists Peggy Reynolds and George Kaplan. For the purpose of this study, loneliness was defined as either having little or no contact with close friends and/or relatives, or feeling alone and isolated even when with friends and relatives.

Women who felt socially isolated were three times as likely to die from cancer as women who were socially fulfilled.

Based on his contact with thousands of cancer patients over the years, Dr. Bernie Siegel believes that repressed emotions and feelings of helplessness make a person a higher cancer risk and shortens his or her life.

One of Siegel's favorite expressions is that instead of turning fighters into victims, doctors should be turning victims into fighters. He claims that "nice" people have to quit being doormats, get up and express, rather than repress, their emotions if they want to prevent or beat cancer.

Positive-cancer patients live longer than others, indicates a study of 40 malignant melanoma patients by Lydia Temoshok, M.D., of the University of California in San Francisco.

All the patients studied had this type of cancer to approximately the same degree with almost an equal chance of cure. The emotional profiles of the patients who died revealed twice the level of anger-hostility, depression-dejection, fatigue-inertia, tension-anxiety, confusion and distress as the survivors.

The Missing Link

The late Norman Cousins valued positivism and credited laughter for extending his life appreciably after a grave illness. He told me, "There's one thing that patients who have lived far beyond the time doctors predicted for them have in common. Although they didn't deny the seriousness of their diagnosed illness, they did deny the doctor's verdict that went along with it."

There's a growing body of evidence to suggest that the brain talks directly to the immune system. For one thing, it's been discovered there are nerve fibers in the thymus, the immune system's master gland, as well as in the spleen, the lymph nodes, and the bone marrow – all vital parts of the immune system. And it has been found immune system cells have receptors for neuropeptides, chemicals that are produced within the brain itself.

Sometimes this electrochemical link between brain and body can be mobilized to produce astonishing, seemingly miraculous results. A middle-aged woman is diagnosed with terminal lung cancer and given only a few months to live. "I can't die," she says, "I have four children to raise." Ten years later, her cancer in remission, she watches her youngest child graduate from college. A man with a terrible secret – he knows that his father has committed murder – suddenly develops throat cancer. The night before surgery to remove the tumor, he breaks down and tearfully reveals his father's crime. Within four hours he's able to eat for the first time in a week, and the surgery is canceled. Four days later, the tumor has entirely disappeared.

Obviously, many things that happen to us are unavoidable. But how we react to them is avoidable. Taking control is the key to survival, and having something to live for is the key concept. Whatever it takes, be it changing your diet, spending hours buried in medical books, or seeking out an alternative medical practitioner, or feeling in control of the situation can be the telling factor in your chances for survival.

Never underestimate the power of the mind and the stress of emotions. Doctors find that arthritis often develops in middle-aged women after the last child has left home. Patty Hearst suffered a lung collapse after she was found guilty of bank robbery. President Richard Nixon developed phlebitis when pressured to resign. Hubert Humphrey and Robert Taft both came down with cancer following unsuccessful bids for the United States presidency. When faced with stressful situations, seek out stress relievers and hope builders.

Something to Live For

For inspiration, let me finish out this chapter with a couple of documented case histories. The first comes from the September 6, 1985 issue of the *Journal of the American Medical Association* (JAMA).

Jane A. McAdams' mother had cancer and was expected to die within several weeks. To lift her spirits, Jane bought her the most luxurious and expensive robe she could find. However, as Jane watched her mother unwrap the gift, she showed not a flicker of pleasure and for a long time said nothing.

When she finally spoke, her mother said, "Would you mind returning it? I really don't want it." Picking up the newspaper on her bed, she pointed to an ad for an expensive summer purse. "This is what I really want."

Jane couldn't believe what she was hearing. It was still winter, and her mother wanted an expensive summer purse that she couldn't possibly use for five or six months. Why, she might not even be alive in the spring, not to mention summer!

Then, as if a lightning bolt had struck her, Jane realized the significance of the request: she needed her daughter's faith to beat the odds.

That same day – in the heart of winter – Jane bought and delivered the summer purse to her mother. It must have been what her mother needed because she wore out the original purse and a half dozen purses that followed. Her mother was alive and well at eighty-three and happy to receive another summer purse birthday gift.

Little things are big things in the minds of the sick who need hope – a word of encouragement, future plans, an optimistic attitude or a confession of love.

Love can work miracles. Bill Robertson and Catherine McLeod, both in their fifties, were undergoing chemotherapy for leukemia in Scotland's Edinburgh Western General Hospital. Each had been given only a few weeks to live. Then, as they talked, recalled pleasant memories, they found something beautiful was happening to them. They fell in love.

Life was again worth living. They felt new surges of optimism running through them — enough to tell themselves and each other they were getting better. In their excitement, they began making plans.

The power of their love and faith gave them purpose, hope and a determination to live. Each subsequent laboratory test showed a definite improvement in their conditions. Within months, they were pronounced free of cancer.

Now they are happily married and five years later are still well, invalidating the predictions of doctors who tried to play God.

CHAPTER 33:

Cancer Causes and Promoters

"Men are like plants, the goodness and flavor of the fruit proceeds from the peculiar soil and exposition in which they grow."
— *Michel Gillaume Jean de Crevecoeur,*
18th Century agriculturist and essayist

Insidious enemies of good health invade us everywhere we turn. From the vegetables grown in toxic soil to the fish caught in waste-laden waters, to the items in our households we use to clean our homes and make ourselves beautiful. Even the ground we walk on is coated with carcinogenic automobile oil and antifreeze. The water is polluted with chemicals designed to kill bacteria but which have unknown long-term side effects, and the air is polluted with everything that evaporates or is spewed from exhaust systems.

These frightening disclosures made one patient wryly tell his alternative doctor, "I'd be better off if I stopped eating, drinking and breathing."

Fortunately we have the power to minimize the exposure and maximize our bodies' potential to overcome the effects. The first step is to consider what we eat.

Cancer in Food

One way to detour around an army of possible carcinogens is to avoid processed foods and their additives. Approximately 5,000 food additives are permitted in America's food supply by the FDA. Avoid them as though your life depended on it, which it does. Included among these are: antibiotics given to meat-producing animals, anti-foaming agents, foaming agents, bleaches, chemical sterilizing agents, coating materials, colorings, emulsifiers, flavorings, humectants (smoke agents), modifiers, organic solvents, preservatives, sweeteners, synthetic dyes and thickeners.

This is not to say all synthetic additives cause cancer. The problem is one food product may contain many and it's impossible to predict their interactions with each other. Some reactions to natural body chemicals may create carcinogens.

Food additives are regulated by the Food and Drug Administration (FDA), and are typically tested on animals. The Delaney Clause of the Food, Drug and Cosmetic Act mandates any additive found to induce cancer cannot be deemed safe. It does not, however, specify how cancerous, and this is the loophole not only FDA but Congressional representatives are using to get out of it. As of this writing, Congressman Henry Waxman (D-Calif) is replacing the Delaney Clause with a "negligible risk" standard, meaning it will be legal for processors to include carcinogenic additives in food. Certain food dyes (Red No. 3, used in candy and baked goods; Yellow No. 5, used in pet food, beverages and baked goods, and Yellow No. 6, used in beverages, candy and desserts) have been found in studies to be carcinogenic, yet continue to be sold on our supermarket shelves with the excuse they pose a "negligible risk."

The more additives listed on a food product label, the more reasons for avoiding it. At an annual meeting of the International Union Against Cancer in Rome, Dr. W.C. Hueper, of the National Cancer Institute, stated there are 20 groups of possible cancer-causing additives as well as 17 groups of suspect food contaminants. He concluded by stating many chemicals introduced into foodstuffs "possess carcinogenic properties."

The *New York Times* printed the frightening story, and the FDA was so inundated with angry phone calls, telegrams and letters that it publicly branded Dr. Hueper an "alarmist," saying the nation is well protected against harm from food additives. No more was heard on this issue from Dr. Hueper.

Worldwide, a clear association consistently appears between the highest rates of breast, colon and prostate cancers and nations that have the fattiest diets. But the link between cancer and meat eaters goes even deeper. *All* fried and broiled foods contain mutagens, chemicals that can damage cellular reproductive material. But fried and broiled meats have far more mutagens than similarly prepared plant foods. One study indicates some 20 percent of American meat eaters may have toxic mutagens in their digestive tracts. These mutagens can be absorbed into the bloodstream where they attack cells. The same study indicates vegetarians are unlikely to have mutagens in their digestive tracts (Wynder, p. 11).

More evidence abounds to warn us away from meat altogether. Commercial meat is laden with carcinogens in the form of nitrates. It would be far simpler if it were just smoked meats, but nitrates are used to color and preserve meats, as well as being shellacked onto our croplands every year in fertilizers. Fully eight billion pounds of beef and pork, mostly in the form of hot dogs, luncheon meats and canned hams are impregnated with nitrates (Encyclopedia, p. 324).

A recent study has some saying "I told you so!" For years hot dogs have been suspected of playing no role in childhood nutrition. Then we learned of the preservatives contained in them. Now it's official. A headline in the *Los Angeles Times*, June 3, 1994 proclaimed "Hot Dogs Linked to Cancer." John Peters, a University of Southern California epidemiologist, reported in the scientific journal *Cancer Causes and Control* that children who eat more than 12 hot dogs a month have nine times the normal risk of developing childhood leukemia. Two other reports in the journal suggest children born to mothers who eat at least one hot dog a week during pregnancy have double the normal risk of developing brain tumors, as do children whose fathers ate hot dogs before conception. Researchers point to these reports as explaining why the incidence of childhood leukemia and brain tumors has increased over the last two decades.

The food processors will tell you the truth, it's not their added nitrates that hurt you. What they don't tell you is that nitrates turn to nitrites in the human stomach. In a process called nitrosation, nitrites combine with substances called secondary amines to form nitrosamines, which have been proven to cause cancer.

If someone told you holding your head over a fire and breathing the smoke was safe would you believe him? Of course not. Yet, when you eat smoked food, you are essentially doing the same thing. When meat is exposed to smoke to preserve it, millions of tiny carbon particles are trapped in it. If you inhale the smoke, you increase your chances of getting lung cancer. By eating it, you increase your chances of getting stomach cancer. Dr. Charles C. Stock, biochemist in charge of experimental cancer chemotherapy at the Sloan Kettering Institute, delivered a report to the Montreal Medico-chirurgical Society in Montreal, Canada showing the incidence of stomach cancer is extremely high in regions where meat and fish is smoked (Encyclopedia, p. 323). Other researchers, especially in areas of high smoked meat and fish consumption, have borne out this connection.

Not surprising to most is the fact that industrial and agricultural pollution of the earth's rivers, lakes and oceans has lead to widespread environmental contamination. Many of the most popular seafood dishes today are contaminated with pesticides and industrial chemicals that have been shown to cause cancer and birth defects. Industrial chemicals such as PCBs (polychlorinated biphenyls) and methyl mercury tend to accumulate in significant amounts in some fish and crustaceans. It's hard to believe the U.S. government used to allow the dumping of hazardous mercury into our coastal oceans, but it did. And we're still seeing the results in our food chain.

Studies in Michigan indicate that PCB exposure during pregnancy causes a delay in infant brain development, resulting in slower neuromuscular development, as well as causing decreased head circumference, birth weight and gestation. Such birth defects were reported among infants whose mothers ate only two or three Great Lakes fish a month over several years (Fein, p. 315).

By rule, it is safest to avoid all freshwater fish, including farm-raised catfish, as well as swordfish and shark. Deep water fish such as red snapper, grouper, halibut and flounder are generally safe.

Cancer in Drinking Water

The water we drink – like the food we eat – is loaded with carcinogens: chlorine, fluoride, arsenic and pesticides.

Chlorine a carcinogen? Who says? After all, we've lived with chlorinated water since the birth of the 20th century, and it has wiped out typhoid fever and cholera plagues.

A clue to chlorine's cancer contribution came originally from statistics showing New Orleans had the nation's highest rate of bladder cancer – 15 percent higher than the national average. Its water comes from the Mississippi River which ends its long downhill trip to the Gulf of Mexico at New Orleans.

A study by the Environmental Defense Fund found "there is a significant relationship between the incidence of certain types of cancer" in New Orleans and the drinking water.

Until these findings, Dr. Jorgen U. Schlegel, head of the Urology Department of Tulane University, New Orleans, had thought tobacco smoking was the cause.

The Environmental Protection Agency (EPA), in announcing 66 possible carcinogens in New Orleans water, theorized it was not the chlorine alone that caused bladder cancer but its blending with industrial and agricultural wastes. Then the EPA announced 79 other U.S. cities, including New York City, Boston, Los Angeles, Seattle, Evansville, Indiana, Cincinnati, and Duluth, Minnesota had carcinogens in their water supplies.

Nobel-Prize winning Dr. Joshua Lederber, of Stanford University, then announced chlorine had never been properly checked for safety. He said chlorine's incredible ability to annihilate bacteria comes from undermining the microbes' DNA, the nucleic acid that contains the genetic instructions for cells.

Inasmuch as DNA is a basic unit for cell replication and the continuity of life, the fact that chlorine damages it is frightening!

Almost a generation ago, University of Tokyo researchers discovered chlorinated water can cause red blood cells to clump. The National Cancer Research Institute in Tokyo referred to chlorine as a "co-carcinogen."

Dr. K.P. Cantor and colleagues at the National Institutes of Health believe that at least 12 percent of bladder cancers are attributable to drinking chlorinated tap water.

An equally insidious and harmful Trojan Horse that attacks us from the inside is fluoride in municipal water supplies.

For years consumer groups, led by the National Health Federation, Monrovia, California, urged the EPA to investigate the dangers of fluoride added to drinking water.

Fluoride has been added to drinking water for decades now, based on the assumption fluoride fights tooth decay among children. Fluoride is a waste product of synthetic fertilizer processing and aluminum smelting. As municipalities were sold on the belief that fluoride strengthens teeth, these industries were able to get rid of a toxic waste and bolster their bottom line.

The EPA ignored pleas to investigate the possible dangers of long term fluoride ingestion. Finally, the continued efforts of two scientific gadflies, Dr. John Lee and Dr. Dean Burke, senior biochemist with the National Cancer Institute, stung Congress into having fluoridated water impartially investigated.

Several years ago, the contention of consumer groups and Drs. Lee and Burke that fluoride could be cancer-causing was borne out. The government-sponsored animal research showed that fluoride contributes to bone cancer.

Despite these findings, and the fact that seniors on fluoridated water sustain more falls and shattered hips than seniors on non-fluoridated water, the EPA made no efforts to ban fluoridation.

In fact, several years ago, the EPA compounded the assault on our health by increasing the maximum allowable level of fluoride in municipal water from 1.4 to 2.4 parts per million (ppm) to four ppm.

One of the hush-hush scandals in Washington is the battle between an EPA union representing scientists and attorneys, and EPA policy makers.

Local 2050 at the National Federation of Federal Employees, led by Robert Carton, Ph.D., an EPA staff toxicologist, claims the EPA is whitewashing the dangers of fluoridation, and its fluoridation review is "scandalous" and "borders on scientific fraud," and the EPA is "politicizing science," manipulating scientific conclusions to meet predetermined political goals.

In May 1990, William L. Marcus was a senior toxicologist in the EPA's Office of Drinking Water. He was the only board-certified toxicologist. He wrote a memo warning there is strong evidence that adding fluorides to our drinking water increases the cancer death rate. Marcus declared there could be in excess of 10,000 avoidable fluoride-related cancer deaths per year. Marcus was sternly ordered by his supervisor to stop writing anything to anyone about it. He responded that to stop would violate his oath of office. He was fired.

In April 1994, Labor Secretary Robert Reich ordered the EPA to reinstate Marcus, compensate him for legal costs and pay him damages. Reich determined the reason the EPA fired Marcus was retaliation for Marcus' criticism of fluoride. According to the National Whistleblower Center, "The Department of Labor found EPA guilty of falsifying employment records, discrimination, and retaliation against an employee whistleblower (Miller, p. 585).

Scientific evidence now reveals that, over and above contributing to bone cancer, fluoride mottles teeth, weakens bones, muscles and tendons, causes premature facial wrinkling and speeds up the aging process.

Numerous comparative studies show no dental advantages in communities with fluoridated water – only grave disadvantages. Conservative publications such as the *Journal of the American Medical Association* and the *New England Journal of Medicine and Epidemiology* have printed articles indicating that even as little as one ppm of fluoride in water actually weakens bones and aggravates fractures two to three times more than water without fluoride.

Remember too, the EPA authorizes communities to use up to four times that amount. After all, industry has to get rid of its waste product – at a fat profit!

Even if you don't live in one of the U.S. communities that fluoridates water, you may still be exposed to hidden and unwanted fluoride in water used to make beer, soft drinks, canned goods, reconstituted fruit juices, dry cereals or spaghetti. It is also in some children's vitamin drops and tablets, and in mouthwashes and dental solutions applied to children's teeth.

Like fluoride, arsenic, a deadly poisonous chemical element, is not a new cancer threat. It has been in the earth's crust since the beginning of time. However, in water it is a far more serious health hazard then previously thought.

So says Joseph P. Brown, a toxicologist with the California Environmental Protection Agency in Berkeley. Brown states that a new risk assessment of arsenic danger by his agency indicates "it ranks right up there with radon and second-hand tobacco smoke."

This means drinking water at the present U.S. EPA allowable level of 50 parts per billion (ppb) for a lifetime creates a one in 100 risk of cancer.

Brown cities Taiwan as "almost a laboratory for studying the epidemiology of arsenic."

The super-high mortality rate in Taiwan and incredible number of bladder, kidney, liver, lung and prostate cancers there are related to the 83,656 wells serving the population with water contaminated by 150 to 800 parts per billion (ppb) of arsenic.

In order to reduce the cancer risk from arsenic to about one in a million, Brown recommends that California's Department of Health Services lower its 50 ppb standard to two parts per trillion – not a bad anti-cancer standard for the nation!

And while considering carcinogens in your drinking water, particularly if you're in a rural area, don't forget lawn and garden fertilizers that add nitrates to your well.

Ingested nitrates, when they join amino acids in your stomach, form carcinogens. Vitamin C taken several times a day prevents the nitrates from hooking up with amino acids.

For your own health's sake, please check to find out whether or not your community water supply is fluoridated and whether its arsenic level is higher than two parts per trillion. If the answer is yes in either case, you might wish to buy bottled spring water.

Cancer in the Air

How's your community air? Not so good if you live in 182 major cities, where the EPA rates the air unhealthy. Unfortunately, most of the U.S. population lives in or near industrial haze. For those who don't, there are other threats to clean air.

How many times have you found yourself quickly rolling up your car windows and shutting off your outside vents, as a diesel-belching bus, truck or car pulled in front of you? The smell is inescapable, the black soot unquestionably polluting; yet, experts have said for years diesel is not a health risk – until now. Assessing for the first time the health effects of everything that comes out of a diesel pipe, the California Environmental Protection Agency (Cal-EPA) concluded high exposure to diesel fumes can increase the risk of lung cancer by 20 to 70 percent (*Cal/EPA Report*, June 1994). Aside from its chemical composition, it contains 30 to 100 times the exhaust particulates of auto engines; and you're inhaling it as you drive down the road.

Use your vehicle's air conditioning system to keep out invisible and odorless carbon monoxide, as well as the black soot that belches from diesel exhausts on buses, trucks and cars.

Even small town America can't escape the toxic effluent from autos, service stations, body paint shops, dry cleaners, industrial plants, power grass mowers, smelly leaf blowers, tobacco smoke and, of course, pesticides.

Numerous studies show that smog contributes to lung cancer and that the best weapon against it – other than avoidance – is at least 400 I.U. of natural vitamin E daily.

Although not as widespread as smog, radon gas probably kills more people annually than smog – between 20,000 and 30,000 according to a National Cancer Institute estimate.

Radon is a radioactive gas formed through the natural breakdown of uranium-238. It seeps through bedrock and soil into about 10 percent of U.S. homes and is especially damaging in tightly insulated dwellings. It attaches itself electrostatically to surfaces throughout the house, especially to dust and tobacco smoke. When you breathe, these particulates lodge in your nose, mouth, throat and lungs and release their radioactivity.

Prevalent in greatest amounts in the nation's southwest, it is present throughout most of the United States – even the east, where it emanates from granite, shale and phosphates, as well as in and around uranium mines or dumps. Radon-created free radicals damage normal cells, making them vulnerable to cancer.

How can you tell if your home is radon polluted? You can't without a radon test kit or without help from pros with the proper equipment. Radon test kits are available in catalogs and stores.

On its own, tobacco smoke can be a killer without help from radon – particularly by causing emphysema and lung cancer. As many newspaper and magazine articles have shown, second-hand smoke can harm, sicken and even kill those who share the smoker's home.

Heavy Metal Exposure

One of the most powerful toxic metals in cigarette smoke is cadmium, a prime carcinogen. Cadmium also enters your life through soft water, which has a high acid content and erodes cadmium, copper and lead from water pipes.

Can anything be done to nullify or cancel the negative effects of cadmium? An animal experiment shows that with a high intake of calcium, less cadmium is absorbed. It was just the opposite in animals on a low calcium diet.

Lead is another heavy metal that can cause cancer. Lead poisoning affects the nervous system and blocks the body's absorption of iron and copper, which is necessary to produce hemoglobin, the red substance that carries oxygen to our trillions of cells.

Although leaded gasoline is a thing of the past, its memory lingers on – in the soil, vegetation and water. We also get lead from old water pipes, earthenware dishes and mugs whose lead glaze was fixed at too low a temperature, in toothpaste tubes, from food and beverage can sealants and from fruit on trees sprayed with lead and arsenic (lead-arsenate).

Lead can be taken out of the body, as an experiment by researchers at the Brain Bio Center (Princeton, New Jersey) demonstrated.

Electric battery factories are notorious for lead-polluted air. In this study, twenty-two factory employees with lead poisoning were given 2,000 milligrams of vitamin C and 60 mg. of zinc each day. Within 24 weeks, their blood levels of lead plummeted by 26 percent.

Lead can also be removed by a qualified physician practiced in chelation therapy. In 1948 the U.S. Navy began using EDTA (ethylenediaminetetraacetic acid) to safely and successfully treat lead poisoning. At the same time, EDTA was being used to remove calcium from pipes and boilers. EDTA is approved by the FDA for heavy metal toxicity.

Electromagnetic Fields

If the entry of lead into the human system is a subtle process, the entry of electromagnetic radiation is even more so. It comes to us from many sources.

Many household items give off radiation: electric clocks, computers, computer monitors, electric blankets, ceramics with uranium glazing, radium dial clocks and watches, leaking ionizing smoke detectors, heated water beds, hair dryers, toasters, refrigerators, electric drills, light dimmers, microwave ovens, TV sets, beepers and pagers.

Major outside sources are radio and TV transmission stations, microwave towers, electric power lines, transformers and power stations. Hand-held radar detectors also give off radiation.

Highway patrolmen who hold their radar detectors close to their bodies have more cases of testicle and penis cancer. Telephone and electric power linemen are subject to higher rates of leukemia.

A 20-year study published in the May 1994 *American Journal of Epidemiology* involved 220,000 Canadian and French utility workers. It found that utility workers with heightened exposure to magnetic fields had three times the risk of acute myeloid leukemia than those with less exposure.

Epidemiological studies have typically found residents living close to power lines have a higher incidence of cancer and leukemia. Even electric blankets have been suspected to play a role in cancer.

Many authorities feel that X-rays are abused and may cause cancer. The University of Southern California Dental School advises fewer mouth X-rays. Several studies find that orange juice may help to neutralize the effects of anti-cancer radiation.

A study published in the *Journal of the American Medical Association* disclosed that the cancer risk of long-term exposure to low level radiation may be as much as 10 times greater than previously believed.

A 40-year study of 8,318 employees of the Oak Ridge National Laboratory found their deaths to leukemia and cancer were 10 times higher than that of the Japanese survivors of the atomic blasts in Hiroshima and Nagasaki.

These findings were matched by biologist Colin Hill at Argonne National Laboratory in Illinois. Dr. Hill directed a single small dose of neutron radiation at mouse embryo cells.

Then he beamed one-twentieth the amount of radiation 20 times at another set of mouse embryo cells. Both sets of cells developed cancer, but there were nine times the malignancies in the ones who got the 20 jolts of radiation. The same results were obtained in small animal experiments.

The New York State School of Public Health measured electromagnetic radiation in homes close to power sources. Even when all power was shut off, researchers found the electromagnetic fields were still powerful in homes of child cancer victims.

Authorities believe 10 to 15 percent of cancer in children is probably linked to low frequency electromagnetic field exposure.

Another study, by the New York State Department of Health, revealed children living near power lines have more brain tumors, as well as leukemia.

Controllable factors

In some instances we invite environmental enemies into our body, even though we know they harm or even may kill us. These preventable factors include birth control pills, alcohol and, of course, cigarettes, which University of Southern California researchers have discovered are major risk factors for liver cancer.

Women who use birth control pills for more than five years have 5.5 times a greater risk of developing liver cancer than women who have never used the Pill. Cigarette smokers have 2.1 times the risk of non-smokers, and heavy drinkers have a 4.3 better chance of developing cancer than teetotalers or light drinkers.

These findings by Mimi Yu, Ph.D., a professor of preventive medicine at the USC School of Medicine, and associates, were reported in the *Journal of the National Cancer Institute.*

"Our findings for oral contraceptives and cigarette smoking are probably the best data to date," says Dr. Yu. "The association with alcohol consumption has already been studied extensively. So has infection with viral hepatitis, the leading risk factor for liver cancer."

Although this research shows birth control pills are a high risk factor, presumably due to their estrogen content, no significant association was found for Premarin or other forms of estrogen replacement therapy.

Liver cancer is a rapidly-fatal disease that's common among Asian populations but relatively rare in non-Asians. The major cause of this degenerative disease is infection with hepatitis B virus, an ailment prevalent in Asian populations.

Yu and fellow USC researchers conducted a study with non-Asians to limit the confounding role of hepatitis infection. Blood samples of all subjects were taken to make certain that they were free of hepatitis infection.

The study sample consisted of 74 cases of liver cancer occurring in white and black residents of Los Angeles country, aged 18 to 74, and 162 healthy controls of comparable age, sex and race.

Results of the study showed that use of birth control pills increased the risk of liver cancer threefold and use for five or more years increased the risk 5.5 times.

These findings are indeed alarming. However, the risks may be even greater, because the research included women who were too old to need birth control when oral contraceptives became available. When the statistics were limited to women ages 64 and younger – women in their reproductive years when birth control pills were introduced (the 1960s) – the risk for more than five years of use jumped to almost 30 times that of women who had never used birth control pills.

Several other studies implicate birth control pills too, and tests with animals show that estrogen contained in birth control pills promote liver cancer.

"Increased risk of liver cancer is a factor women may want to take into account when they consider oral contraceptives – especially for long term use," says Dr. Yu. "For example, if a woman smokes cigarettes and has been infected with hepatitis B or C, she may not want to push her luck by taking birth control pills."

The data on alcohol consumption implicated only heavy drinkers. Moderate drinkers showed no increased risk. The greatest risk (4.7 fold) was for men who drank more than nine cans of beer, nine glasses of wine or nine shots of spirits daily. Men slightly below that had a 2.6 fold increased risk.

The female subjects drank relatively little and thus provided an opportunity to demonstrate the independent effect of cigarette smoking, inasmuch as drinking and smoking often go hand in hand. The data for both non-smoking women and men clearly indicate that cigarette smoking alone is a definite risk factor for liver cancer, states Yu.

A careful analysis shows that among non-Asians, 54 percent of the liver cases in women can be attributed to cigarettes and birth control pills, and 56 percent of these cases in men can be attributed to alcohol and/or cigarettes.

The identification of cancer-causing substances does not end here. As free-thinking scientists become more creative in the search for the cause of cancer, more and more of what is around us, and what we do, eat and ingest will be under scrutiny. In fact, during the final edit of this book I found some research that associates cancer with conventional medicine.

The study, published in the May 18, 1994 *Journal of the National Cancer Institute*, has Canadian researchers concluding three common allergy drugs promote cancer growth in laboratory mice, even in low doses.

Researchers at the Manitoba Institute of Cell Biology in Winnipeg reported cancer tumors grew faster and larger in mice injected with loratadine, astemizole and hydroxyzine, three antihistamines. The antihistamines didn't cause the cancers, which were injected into the mice, but did make them bigger, the researchers said. Look to my book *Foods That Heal* for alternative solutions to dangerous medicines.

A synthetic hormone prescribed to women who have had breast cancer has been found in studies to cause other kinds of cancer, according to an article in *Science News* (April 16, 1994). Tamoxifen, manufactured by Zeneca Pharmaceuticals, Wilmington, Delaware, is given to women to prevent re-occurrences of their breast cancer malignancies.

Breast cancer patients randomly assigned to receive Tamoxifen in a nine-year Swedish study developed almost six times as many endometrial cancers as did participants taking a placebo, or inactive substance. The Swedish study also found an increased risk of gastrointestinal cancers in Tamoxifen users.

A U.S. study reported eleven times more endometrial cancers in breast cancer patients assigned at random to receive Tamoxifen. Some data even suggests Tamoxifen-induced uterine cancers may be unusually deadly.

Studies done by the pharmaceutical company itself showed adverse reproductive changes and cancer in animals whose mothers received Tamoxifen. Because the changes resemble those seen in the offspring of animals and women taking diethylstilbestrol (DES), FDA and Zeneca asked doctors to "stress that women should not become pregnant while taking (this drug)."

In an ongoing breast cancer prevention trial, NCI is giving Tamoxifen to 8,000 healthy subjects, who "will be at risk for the adverse outcomes," said Dutzu Rosner, a surgical oncologist from the State University of New York at Buffalo. Indeed, she says, "I'm questioning the philosophy of chemoprevention in healthy women using a toxic agent."

By now, most of us are familiar with the long-term dangers of inhaling asbestos. We've read about schools being closed while hazardous materials specialists carefully remove asbestos ceilings. Sources of asbestos abound. It wears off automobile brake linings and clutch facings, and is contained in such household items as ironing board covers and pot holders. Asbestos, once inhaled, continues to react in the lungs for a lifetime. It is associated with lung cancer.

Talcum powder has been shown to be as potentially deadly as asbestos. Asbestos and talcum are naturally occurring minerals, and are chemically and geologically related. They are often found in the same geological sites. In fact, a well-known brand of talcum powder in England was withdrawn from market after it was discovered to be laced with asbestos. They are also similar in the effect they have on the human body. It is known that older talc workers die of lung cancer at a rate four times higher than would be expected. Talc workers are also subject to talcosis, a disease that scars the lungs (Encyclopedia, p. 267).

Researchers have found particles of talc in approximately 75 percent of ovarian tumors and 50 percent of cervical tumors examined (Griffiths). How does talc find its way into ovaries and cervixes? Doctors used to apply talcum to preserve their rubber gloves during surgery. For the same reason, it is common for women to dust talc on their diaphragms to keep them dry and extend their shelf life. Any product that contains talc can be a potential killer, including some feminine hygiene sprays.

Dr. Langer, a mineralogist with the New York Mount Sinai Hospital believes it may be asbestos particles hidden within the talcum that causes these cases of cancer. He and his associates did a study on one of the ovarian slides used by Dr. Griffiths. Mount Sinai found asbestos fibers along with the talc.

After discovering talcum gave them skin lesions, doctors started using natural cornstarch instead. Cornstarch is an excellent non-toxic alternative to talcum.

CHAPTER 34:

Free Radicals, Nature's Decaying Process

"Without knowledge, life is no more than the shadow of death."
— Jean Baptiste Poquelin Moliere,
17th Century French Playwright

Obviously, the person who claimed "the best things in life are free," didn't know about free radicals. They're free all right. However, they're anything but the best things in life. Just in case the only free radical you ever heard of was Abby Hoffman, let me explain how they work.

Free radicals are molecules that lack one of their customary electrons. Since the natural order here is pairs, the molecule, now called a free radical, will steal an electron from another compound, rendering that compound unstable and setting up a chain reaction that damages vital cell structures. By one estimate, each cell sustains more than 10,000 of these hits a day, and not all the damage is repaired.

This electron-stripping is referred to as oxidation. Oxidation is what rusts metal and makes oils rancid, so imagine what it does to your body! Free radicals also cause cells to cross-link with each other, destroying collagen in the skin, causing sagging and wrinkles.

There are many, many factors that contribute to the formation of free radicals in our bodies: sunlight, X-rays, radiation of many kinds, ozone, smog, tobacco smoke, sugar, food additives and preservatives, nitrates in cured meats, charcoal-broiled meats, alcohol, many anti-cancer drugs, fats, polluted water and air, insecticides and herbicides, excessive intake of iron, heavy metals such as lead, cadmium and asbestos, vigorous exercise, infections, and every kind of stress – emotional, mental and physical.

Natural free radicals are nature's contribution to death and decay – nature's population controller, if you will. If the only free radicals we had to deal with came from sunlight, breathing and exercise, we would live long, age well and die of old age, not heart disease and cancer.

Civilized Free Radicals

All free radicals are not created equal. Man-made free radicals (a product of our "highly advanced" civilization) speed up the natural decay process, and cause early sickness and death. Those caused by radiation – ionizing (nuclear power plants and X-rays) and non-ionizing – are the worst. Biologist Dr. George Wald, Nobel Prize winner, pulls no punches in saying there's no safe dose of radiation. A few authorities warn against having X-rays, except in extreme situations.

Dr. Ernest Sternglass, Professor Emeritus of Radiological Physics, University of Pittsburgh Medical School, believes internally-deposited radioactivity is far more toxic than ordinary chemical toxins.

This is because each and every electron given off by a radioactive nucleus has several million volts of energy, enough to disrupt millions of organic molecules in living cells.

"Thus, radioactive isotopes that concentrate in specific organs (such as iodine 131 in the thyroid) are millions of times more damaging than ordinary chemical toxins such as lead or DDT," contends Lita Lee, Ph.D., in her book *Radiation Protection Manual*.

"Internally deposited radioactivity causes great cellular damage, including toxin production, enzyme deactivation/destruction, cell membrane damage, altered cell metabolism, mutations and abnormal cell division (inhibited, retarded or cancerous)."

Lita Lee also writes radiation isn't like smoke that dissipates. It hangs around for longer than we'll be around – for as much as 400 years in the cases of cesium 137 and strontium 90.

Radiation has entered our food chain through U.S. government experimental atomic bomb blasts in the West and the World War II atomic bombings of Japan. It also entered our food chain through radioactive accidents at Three Mile Island and Chernobyl.

How Free Radicals Cause Cancer

Once free radicals cause cross-linkage, the cell cannot reproduce properly. Free radical interference causes the RNA-DNA to change and give the wrong orders. A slightly different new cell then emerges, because mutation has taken place. Such mutations may, in time, lead to the development of cancer.

The development of cancer is not a one step process. Earl Stadtman, Ph.D., chief of the biochemistry laboratory in Bethesda, Maryland, says free radicals promote changes in DNA. The first step is when the cells change to a pre-cancer mutation in a process called oncogenesis. The next step is the formation of cancer cells.

Changes in DNA brought about by free radical assault don't have to be major to cause cancer. Dr. Theodore Krontiris and two Tufts University colleagues in collaboration with three Yale University School of Medicine collaborators, found a tiny piece of damaged DNA amid human genes may be the cause of one in every 11 cases of breast, bladder and colon cancer – 50,000 cases annually.

These researchers zeroed in on a fragment of DNA called "minisatellite DNA," distributed widely among human genes and seemingly without a function. A small alteration in one of them, seated against the growth-controlling RAS oncogeny is now being linked to cancer.

Not only did the biochemists study 796 cancer patients and 652 people without cancer, they also statistically analyzed 28 other studies. The results support their conclusions.

Krontiris says in time their discovery will help to "find people who are at very high risk" of cancer.

New concepts are often slow in converting the scientific community to their validity and value. So it was with the free radical theory of aging proposed by Denham Harman, M.D., some 34 years ago. At that time, he announced free radicals are the saboteurs causing cellular damage leading to degenerative diseases and premature death.

Few biochemists went along with Dr. Harman because no one had the tools to identify free radicals and prove they really exist in living organisms. However, in 1969, two scientists discovered superoxide dismutase (SOD), a natural body enzyme that forms hydrogen peroxide as it neutralizes free radicals, and were able to prove that Harman was indeed right. There is no way for SOD to form hydrogen peroxide without combining with superoxide, which is another name for a free radical.

Are we helpless against the attacks of free radicals? Not by any means. Now that we know their major causes, we can avoid some and quench others by means of certain enzymes present in cells and by substances called antioxidants in foods and supplements.

Researchers Pursue the Cancer Answer

Researchers at the University of Southern California's Institute for Toxicology (Los Angeles), one of the world's few labs operating exclusively to study free radicals, tell us there are two kinds of cell enzymes that oppose free radicals: defensive and repair.

These scientists are probing to discover how natural defenses operate to prevent or compensate for free radical damage – and to enhance these defenses.

One of their methods is to condition cells by exposing them to low levels of oxidative stress. The response is similar to the body's practice of creating specific antibodies when exposed to low levels of a disease. Cells respond by producing defensive enzymes "immunizing" them against greater exposures.

Findings by these researchers raise hopes it might someday be possible to "inoculate" the body against the damaging effects of oxidation (free radicals).

In a series of experiments, bacteria were exposed to hydrogen peroxide, a common oxidant. First, a lethal concentration was established that would destroy 98 percent of bacteria in a sample.

Then bacteria samples were pre-exposed to a low concentration of hydrogen peroxide, followed by exposure to a lethal concentration. Pre-exposed cells were much better able to cope with a lethal concentration and survive.

The degree of protection varied according to the degree of pre-exposure and to the amount of time before lethal concentrations were given. At best, only 10 percent of the cells died.

Researchers discovered that exposing cells to low levels of hydrogen peroxide brought about a typical form of resistance, the synthesis of 40 enzymes. Some of these enzymes can normally be found in cells, but, under this circumstance, were produced in greater-than-usual amounts. However, some of these 40 enzymes are not usually seen in such cells, says Kelvin J.A. Davies, Ph.D., a USC associate professor of toxicology and biochemistry.

The enzymes appear to be the keys to the adaptive response. Experiments showed that when the secretion of these enzymes was blocked, even pre-exposed cells were no longer able to withstand lethal concentrations of hydrogen peroxide.

About 25 percent of the protective enzymes were secreted within 20 minutes of pre-exposure, the USC researchers found, and the remaining enzymes were produced in a second wave, peaking 30 to 50 minutes after pre-exposure.

Many of the first-wave enzymes are antioxidants, which prevent damage from ever occurring by snuffing out free radicals. These enzymes exist normally in cells but are generated in greater amounts during stress from oxidation.

The second wave of enzymes repair damage from free radicals. They dismantle damaged proteins, fats and even DNA into their constituent parts, remove the destroyed parts and fill in the missing pieces, reassembling the damaged molecule.

"A great deal of work is being done with antioxidants, and it's been thought that the early enzymes are the ones that count," says Dr. Davies. "However, our research suggests that the later enzymes may be even more important." This evidence comes from bacteria mutants that Davies and his research team have constructed. These mutants lack the genetic element that regulates the first wave enzymes.

When the mutants are exposed to the stress of oxidation, the early (defensive) enzymes appear in even greater numbers and successfully protect the cells from lethal concentrations of hydrogen peroxide. "The ideal situation is to have both defensive and repair enzymes, but our findings show the repair enzymes alone can do the job of protecting cells," says Davies.

Results of these studies and similar findings from Davies' studies have spawned more research to single out each of the enzymes and learn its relative importance. Of particular interest to the USC researchers are the repair enzymes – especially those that repair DNA.

"If a DNA molecule is damaged and not repaired, the result will be a continuing mutation," Davies says. "So all damaged DNA needs to be repaired, or it can lead to aberrations like cancer."

The major target of USC scientists is to identify the regulators, or genetic switches that turn on the genes encoding for repair enzymes. "If those regulators can be isolated, it might be possible to use genetic therapy to introduce specific regulators into the cells of persons at high risk, say for heart attacks or stroke," says Davies.

"Then, when cells are subjected to oxidative stress, the regulators would turn on the repair enzymes. The body's own protective mechanisms would be marshalled to protect against heart attack or stroke."

Davies' team has discovered a regulator called hoxR in bacteria that turns on repair enzymes. Investigators at other universities, notably Bruce Demple, at the Harvard School of Public Health, and Bruce Ames, at the University of California at Berkeley, have discovered regulators that turn on defensive enzymes.

At this writing, no regulators in human cells have been found.

However, Davies says when they are, recent advances in genetic therapy would make it possible to use the regulators to prevent a host of diseases, including cancer. While we hope for the best in the future, it may be a long, and for some, deadly wait. I suggest that while you wait you utilize the rich natural sources given you in this book to both obtain more enzymes in your food and stimulate your body to produce them.

Antioxidants to the Rescue

While our individual cells are capable of fighting destructive free radicals, they need certain raw materials to form protective enzymes. Standard nutritional requirements maintain minimum health requirements. However maximum health is required to battle the ravages of our "civilized" world. Large amounts of antioxidants are required: vitamins A, C, E, beta carotene, selenium, zinc, copper, manganese, superoxide dismutase (SOD) and glutathione peroxidase (GP).

Each has a special cell protective or regenerating function. Vitamins A, C and E team up to protect blood vessels and other body tissues from free radical damage. Vitamin E fights to protect cell walls from attack by free radicals. Jeffrey Bland, Ph.D., exposed red blood cells to destructive ultraviolet light, some with vitamin E added. Those without vitamin E aged faster than those with this essential antioxidant. Further, the unprotected red blood cells bulged like an over-inflated bicycle tire, while those with vitamin E resisted the reaction far longer, demonstrating that vitamin E's antioxidant action actually extends cell life and therefore, human life.

Scientists at the Institute of Human Nutrition in Poland examined healthy subjects from 60 to 100 years old, discovering volunteers with the highest amount of vitamin E in their blood serum showed fewer fat peroxides and thus, fewer free radicals.

Then they divided the subjects into three groups taking daily amounts of nutrients, some taking 200 International Units of vitamin E, some taking 400 milligrams of vitamin C, and the last group taking the same amounts of both. Although all groups showed a drop in peroxide levels, an indication of fewer free radicals, those taking both vitamin C and E showed the greatest decline.

Strenuous exercise not only causes exhaustion but also an increase of free radicals. However, a generous intake of vitamin E can decrease free radicals and, consequently, the damage done by them.

Researchers led by Satoshi Sumida, of the Osaka Gaukuin University of Japan, tested 21 healthy college-age males. First the volunteers rode exercise bikes until exhausted.

Next the volunteers were given 300 milligrams of vitamin E each day for four weeks. Then the exercisers were retested. This time their blood cells showed far fewer signs of free radical damage, compared with their first test.

How does vitamin E perform its protective work? A 1988 *Mayo Clinic Proceedings* article, "Free Radicals in Medicine," states that vitamin E converts free radicals to less reactive forms by donating a hydrogen ion to the independent radical.

Japanese researchers not only created a means for testing antioxidant effectiveness but also how two prominent antioxidants, vitamins E and C, work together to protect us from free radicals.

To do this, the researchers dissolved a fatty substance in solvents and other solutions to create free radicals. Next they kept the mixture at body heat and measured the amount of oxygen it used. Then they added vitamin E to the mixture, observing that oxidation was suppressed until all the vitamin E was utilized.

When vitamin C was added to the mixture, it was found to be a little less effective than vitamin E as an antioxidant. However, it was discovered that vitamin C extends the life of vitamin E so it can suppress free radical damage longer. The researchers concluded vitamin E and C work best when taken or eaten together.

Antioxidant Food Sources

Best food sources of vitamin C are rose hips, acerola cherries, guavas, black currants, green peppers, strawberries, spinach, oranges, cabbage, grapefruit, papaya, elderberries, lemons, cantaloupe, limes and mangoes.

Vitamin E extravagant foods are fresh wheat germ, safflower seeds, sunflower seeds, sesame oil, walnuts, corn oil, hazelnuts, soybean oil, almonds, olive oil and cabbage.

Beta carotene, a vitamin A precursor, like most members of the family of carotenoids and vitamin A are powerful antioxidants and immune system boosters.

Beta carotene revs up the immune system by increasing the number of natural killer cells, increasing T-lymphocyte cells' production of interferon, and improving the ability of monocytes to fight off cancer.

Beta carotene boosters are carrots, sweet potatoes, spinach, most green leafy vegetables and orange or yellow vegetables.

Foods rich in vitamin A include cod liver oil, dandelion greens, carrots, yams, kale, parsley, turnip greens, collard greens, chard, watercress, red peppers, squash, egg yolk, cantaloupe, persimmons, apricots, broccoli, crab, swordfish, whitefish, Romaine lettuce, mangoes, pumpkin, peaches and cheese.

The trace mineral selenium is a noted cancer preventive, mainly through its ability to quench free radicals, as shown by 55 studies reviewed by Cornell University and University of California researchers.

Selenium and vitamin E work best together. A Finnish study of 51 cancer victims revealed that low blood levels of selenium increased the danger of cancer. Further, low levels of both selenium and vitamin E increased the risk even more.

Selenium and vitamin E are important members of the key antioxidant system glutathione peroxidase acid and glycine. Glutathione peroxidase also works with vitamins E and B2 to snuff out free radicals.

Glutathione peroxidase, like superoxide dismutase (SOD), renders free radicals harmless. SOD is not a biochemical loner. It unites with catalase (CAT) then transforms free radicals into hydrogen peroxide, which CAT then converts to water.

If this is getting pretty complicated and you want an easy way to make sure you're getting your essential antioxidants, look for a good, easily absorbable, derived-from-nature liquid mineral blend. Minerals in solution provide the optimal absorption ratios.

It is clear the key to the cure for cancer will be less in what it does than what it is. Enzymes, free radicals and toxic pollutants are part of the puzzle of cancer that, once fully understood and freely explored, will allow physicians to prescribe effective, viable and affordable preventives and treatments, freeing us from our modern-day plague.

CHAPTER 35:

Alternative Therapies, Your Freedom to Choose

"Freedom to differ is not limited to things that do not matter. That would be a mere shadow of freedom. The test of its substance is the right to differ on things that touch the heart of the existing order."
— *Justice Robert Jackson*

In this age of elastic statistics, can we believe the National Cancer Institute (NCI) when it says we are gaining on cancer?

An article by John Bailar and Elaine Smith in the *New England Journal of Medicine* revealed that despite statistics issued by the NCI to the contrary, the mortality rate from cancer is mounting. The sad truth is cancer is the number two killer of Americans today. Without the acceptance of a low fat diet and exercise to combat cardiovascular disease, soon it will be the number one killer. Among children ages 1-14, cancer causes more deaths in the U.S. than any other disease, according to the American Cancer Society.

A subsequent in-depth report by the General Accounting Office (GAO) backed findings by Bailar and Smith. The NCI had indeed used elastic statistics to make its research efforts look better.

Can we therefore trust an agency that protects its vested interests by dubious statistics to give us a fair evaluation of alternative cancer therapies?

That is essentially what the writers of a book, *Unconventional Cancer Treatments,* published by the U.S. Congress, Office of Technology Assessment, did. Despite strenuous efforts to be fair and unbiased, the authors almost invariably used the NCI as the final authority regarding the effectiveness of unorthodox cancer therapy.

The point I want to make here is: you have choices and options that are being denied to you. Mainstream medicine denies or rebukes valid information about alternative therapies that may work for you, instead choosing to promote and restrict your choices to therapies that not only have a poor track record but have too many unknowns to be comfortable with.

Without recommending any one therapy, let me show you what else is being done in the treatment of cancer. These therapies are offered through licensed medical practitioners, academically-trained researchers and other qualified professionals. Let's take a closer, less biased look at some of the more popular unorthodox therapies named after their founders or after a product used in connection with them.

The Gerson Treatment

One of the best known unconventional cancer therapies that can be done at home is the Gerson treatment, founded by Max Gerson, a German-born medical doctor who practiced in Germany, Austria and France before emigrating to New York in 1946.

Gerson's therapy consists of a low-sodium, high-potassium, no-fat, high fresh vegetable-fresh fruit diet, with various vitamin-mineral supplements and coffee enemas, all of which can be done in your own home. The details are outlined in his 1958 book, *A Cancer Therapy: Results of Fifty Cases*.

The treatment is based on detoxification, not just from internally generated toxins but also from environmental poisons like those outlined in Chapter 32. Gerson's rationale was that to treat cancer one must restore the body's innate healing mechanism by replenishing and detoxifying it. The body is restored through an intensive nutrition program flooding the body and its body cells with easily assimilated nutrients needed for improving metabolism healing.

The therapy includes 13 glasses of various fresh raw juices prepared hourly from organically grown fruits and vegetables, and three full vegetarian meals, freshly prepared from organically grown vegetables, fruits and whole grains.

In testimony before a subcommittee on foreign relations in 1946, Dr. Gerson estimated that 30 percent of "hopeless" cancer cases can be treated with his regimen to produce a favorable response. In one of his last published papers, he estimated about 50 percent positive results.

I personally know of people who have used this therapy. Ten years ago an acquaintance, Mrs. Sanger, and her husband left their fine home in Wisconsin, traveling to California so she could pursue treatment for her liver cancer under the care of a physician open-minded to the therapy. She and her husband moved into a small trailer, hiring someone to help her prepare her raw juices and meals. When last I saw her, she had beaten her conventional doctors' predictions by three years, and wasn't giving up until she was proclaimed cancer-free.

Presently, the National Institutes of Health, Office of Alternative Medicine, is conducting evaluations of nutritional treatments for cancer. The Gerson Therapy is among them.

Gerson died in 1959.

Burzynski Antineoplastons

Stanislaw R. Burzynski, M.D., Ph.D., holds what is probably the most promising and accepted alternative treatment, yet certain "authorities" would stop him. The story you are about to hear is just one of the many travesties of medical justice in the uphill battle to provide health-giving, effective alternative cancer treatments.

Burzynski, born in Poland, received his M.D. in 1967 and his Ph.D. in biochemistry a year later, both from the Medical Academy of Lublin. As a medical student in the late 1960s, his research led him to a revolutionary discovery.

He discovered cancer patients lack a certain group of peptides in their blood. He named these peptides "antineoplastons." He theorized that antineoplastons are part of a biochemical defense system (parallel to and separate from the immune system), and returning them to the human body would reverse the cancer process.

In 1970, Burzynski moved to the United States and until 1977, served as research associate and assistant professor at Baylor College of Medicine in Houston. While at Baylor he continued testing his theory. In 1973 he obtained a license to practice medicine in Texas, leaving Baylor in 1977 to found his own research institute and begin treating cancer patients with antineoplastons. He contacted officials at the Texas Department of Health and was told he would not be violating Texas Food, Drug & Cosmetic laws.

In the mid-1970s, he received funding from NCI to do research on how to efficiently extract antineoplastons from urine and test human cells.

This work proved successful and promising, but the NCI rejected Burzynski's 1976 application for follow-up experiments, finally granting supplemental funding to allow him to conclude initial work by July 1977.

In 1983, the FDA obtained an injunction against Dr. Burzynski, keeping him from shipping his medicines out of state. However, a federal judge granted him permission to manufacture and administer his treatments to patients in Texas.

From 1983 to 1989 Burzynski applied to the FDA for permission to determine the safety and efficacy of antineoplastons in human studies. In March 1989 FDA said it would permit a study of oral antineoplastons on a small number of women with advanced refractory breast cancer to be conducted at a U.S. medical center. As of April 11, 1994, nine antineoplaston clinical trials have been approved by the FDA, with five currently in progress. The study of antineoplaston is being conducted at the National Cancer Institute, Sloan-Kettering Memorial Cancer Center and the Mayo Clinic (Burzynski). The goal of these trials is FDA approval of antineoplaston as a cancer therapy drug available for use by all physicians.

Burzynski hypothesizes that antineoplastons may act by interfering with the action of certain enzyme complexes (methylation complex isozymes) that allow malignant cells to gain a growth advantage over normal cells. He also suggests that antineoplastons may interact directly with DNA.

Reports from the Burzynski Research Institute state that Burzynski has had the greatest success in treating cancers of the bladder, breast, brain, bone, prostate, non-Hodgkins lymphoma (the cancer that ended the life of Jacqueline Kennedy Onassis). A majority of his cancer patients "show positive responses to treatment" (*Unconventional Cancer Treatments*).

Burzynski feels that measuring naturally circulating antineoplastons in blood and urine "may help identify individuals who are more susceptible to the development of cancer or to diagnose the cancer at early stages."

In a press release, Burzynski stated by administering antineoplaston in oral form, as opposed to intravenously, "Some prostate cancer patients, even those who failed to respond to conventional therapy, have experienced a complete remission of their cancer in as little as five months."

Unconventional Cancer Treatments claims Burzynski's studies are outside mainstream science. Since when have major scientific discoveries conformed to mainstream science of the period? In 1867, when Dr. Lister first advocated antiseptic surgery, the other doctors laughed at him.

Unrecognized by status quo scientists in the United States, Burzynski has published papers in peer-reviewed medical journals around the world. His research publications have been presented at the prestigious International Congress of Chemotherapy. Further, in a recent meeting of this congress, fourteen papers on antineoplastons were presented – certainly a record for what the American medical monopoly considers "quackery."

Since his first discovery, other researchers have investigated the antineoplaston theory. Researchers at Kurume University in Japan found antineoplastons had an anti-tumor effect on mice, and National Cancer Institute researchers are looking at antineoplastons.

Several years ago, NCI medical experts and scientists visited Burzynski's facility to observe his work. They reviewed the records of patients with deadly brain cancers who had experienced either a complete or partial remission. One NCI physician remarked that, in twenty years, he had never seen comparable results.

Frank Wiewel, an advisor to the recently-established Office of Alternative Medicine (OAM) of the National Institutes of Health, visited the Burzynski Research Institute. He remarked, "Frankly, I was astounded by what I saw. Many people's tumors disappeared under this unique treatment. I was also impressed by Dr. Burzynski's honesty."

Despite the clinical trials underway and testimony by experts, the American Medical Association issued an article in its *Clinical Alert* warning doctors and patients away from Burzynski's therapy. This is the same AMA whose authorized therapies are contributing to cancer mortality rates.

Also, despite acceptance on a federal level, efforts are being made by the State of Texas to revoke Burzynski's medical license and close down his practice. In 1988, a Texas Department of Health official instigated proceedings that resulted in a Texas State Board of Examiners attempt to revoke his medical license. Officials charged Burzynski with violating the Texas Food Drug & Cosmetic Act (TFD-CA) by using non-FDA approved medicine on his patients, and violating the Texas Medical Practice Act (TMPA – unprofessional conduct based on the TFDCA allegation). The hearing was set for September 1988 but didn't actually get heard until May 1993 (Jaffe, p. 635).

By the time the hearing took place, officials had added another charge: violating the false advertising provision of the TFDCA which holds no one may claim a non-FDA approved drug affects a disease, whether or not the representation is true or false.

Burzynski defended himself by pointing out Section 5.09 of the TMPA provides a physician may administer any drug to meet the immediate needs of the patient. He argued the provision supersedes and overrides the general TFDCA provision which has never been and should not be applied to a practicing physician. During testimony on his behalf, a neuro-radiologist from NCI testified that Burzynski's treatment was the best he'd ever seen for brain cancer, and a dozen of his patients testified they'd die without Burzynski's continued treatment. Many of his patients presented the judge with letters from their doctors.

The Texas State Board of Medical Examiners hired the Texas Attorney General's Office to pursue the matter. In March 1994, the Texas administrative law judge accepted Dr. Burzynski's position and held that under the TMPA, he is permitted to use his own medication on his patients. Due to the wording of the Texas advertising statute in the TFDCA law ("whether or not representation is true or false"), the judge suggested Burzynski be issued a cease and desist order. However, he concluded that the statute was "dangerously close" to being unconstitutional.

The Texas State Board of Medical Examiners continues to pursue efforts to revoke Burzynski's medical license.

The Burzynski Research Institute is based in Stafford, Texas. Dr. Burzynski and associates treat patients at his outpatient clinic in Houston.

Macrobiotic Diet

Simply stated, the principle of the macrobiotic diet is to emphasize eating "live" food. Anything that grows if put in the ground is live food. Live food nourishes and heals the body. That's what macrobiotic promoters will tell you.

Originating in Japan, macrobiotics has a prominent leader, Michio Kushi, president of the Kushi Institute in Boston. Kushi states that macrobiotics is neither a treatment nor a therapy, but a common sense approach to daily living. It is intended for individuals to take charge of their health and to develop a natural, balanced way of living. The prime mover of macrobiotics is George Ohsawa who, several decades ago, is said to have cured himself of a serious illness by quitting the modern refined diet, then sweeping Japan, in favor of a simple diet of brown rice, miso soup, sea vegetables and other traditional foods.

Kushi maintains cancer is the body's healthy attempt to deal with toxins ingested and accumulated through many years of eating today's unnatural diet and living in a polluted environment.

A macrobiotic diet eliminates milk, cheese, meat, eggs and other oily, greasy foods, as well as foods and beverages with a cooling or freezing effect: ice cream, soft drinks and orange juice.

Accumulated toxins, Kushi says, show themselves as allergies, earaches, coughing and chest congestion, a bulging belly, swelling and weakness of the legs, dry skin, hardening of the breasts, prostate problems, vaginal discharge or ovarian cysts – potentially cancerous conditions. In his book, *The Cancer Prevention Diet*, he writes:

"As long as improper nourishment is taken in, the body will continue to isolate abnormal excess and toxins in specific areas, resulting in a continual growth of cancer. When a particular location can no longer absorb toxic excess, the body must search for another place to localize it, and so the cancer spreads."

These are the foods recommended by the macrobiotic plan to prevent or manage cancer: complex carbohydrates, not simple sugars; high fiber foods, rather than refined junk foods; unsaturated fats, not saturated; sea salt, not refined salt; natural vitamins and minerals found in food; natural, organically grown food, rather than that which is chemically fertilized; whole, unrefined foods; vegetable protein, rather than animal; and foods cooked by gas and wood-burning stoves, rather than by microwave ovens or electric stoves.

White fish is permitted one to three times weekly, if necessary. Non-aromatic and non-stimulating teas – bancha twig tea, stem tea, roasted brown rice tea, or cereal grain coffee are permitted – along with plain, non-iced water.

Two major criticisms of the macrobiotic diet is it lacks vitamins B12 and vitamin D. Kushi responds that occasional fish supply the vitamin B12 and the fish liver oil and daily exposure to sunlight fill the need for vitamin D.

A medical doctor, V. Newbold presented six case histories of patients with advanced cancer who followed a macrobiotic diet, in addition to using orthodox treatment. They are well described medically, with reference to appropriate diagnostic tests, with biopsy-proved backup in five of the six cases and follow up scans and tests.

Several physicians on the advisory panel of the Office of Technology Assessment (OTA) reviewed the cases. Three mainstream reviewers did not find these cases convincing. One reviewer felt the orthodox cancer treatment could have been the cause of recovery.

Two alternative physicians believed five out of the six cases, except the cancer unproved by biopsy, showed positive effects from the macrobiotic diet. The remaining unorthodox physician found two cases legitimate, two highly suggestive, one suggestive and one not convincing.

Chaparral

A popular herb in health food stores, chaparral has a long history as a folk medicine used for curing leukemia and cancers of the kidney, liver, lung and stomach. American Indians in the Southwest used it for arthritis, bowel cramps, bronchitis, colds, tuberculosis and venereal diseases.

Leaflets and twigs of the larrea divericata coville (creosote bush of the Southwest United States) are made into chaparral tea by steeping seven or eight grams of dried leaves and stems – a gram is 127th of an ounce – in a quart of hot water.

One of its main ingredients, nordihydroguaiaretic acid (NDGA), an antioxidant, has been found to have anti-tumor activity in certain kinds of cancers in animals. As summarized by two studies, NDGA has been reported to inhibit the development and promotion of certain carcinogen-induced tumors in rodents.

Fifty-nine patients with "advanced incurable malignancy" were treated at the University of Utah with either chaparral tea or NDGA.

Some patients drank two or three glasses of chaparral tea daily, while others received oral doses of NDGA (250 to 3,000 mg) daily.

Only 45 stayed with the treatment for the required four weeks. Tumor remissions, regressions of 25 percent or more, were reported in four patients. It was noted that 27 patients had "subjective improvement."

Although the authors of this study did not conclude chaparral tea or NDGA are effective anticancer agents, regressions of some tumors in advanced cancer cases suggest these agents are worth investigating.

The Hoxey Treatment

So far as acceptance is concerned, the Hoxey Treatment has had more ups and down than a busy elevator. It is based on an herbal formula bequeathed to Harry Hoxey (1901-1974) first, via his great grandfather (John Hoxey) second, via his grandfather and, third, from his father. Supposedly, John Hoxey discovered it in 1840 on his southern Illinois farm, when one of his horses with a cancerous growth was put in a special pasture with grasses and flowering wild plants and was healed.

Concluding the wild plants contributed to the horse's recovery, he combined them with old folk remedies for cancer and used the formula to treat other horses. Harry's father, a veterinarian, was the first Hoxey to use the formula for human cancers.

Harry's father commanded him to use the herbal concoction to treat cancer patients "if need be, in defiance of the high priests of medicine."

Despite the manifestation of cancer in certain localized areas, Hoxey believed that it was a systemic disease characterized by a chemical imbalance.

The first Hoxey clinic was launched in the early 1920s. In less than 30 years, the Hoxey Outpatient Clinic in Dallas became one of the world's largest privately-owned cancer centers. It had branches in seventeen states and a clinic load of 10,000 patients under treatment or observation.

However, Hoxey's boastful claims and confrontational style antagonized the American Medical Association (AMA) and the FDA. Before the end of the 1950s, the FDA closed the Dallas clinic.

It was inevitable that Hoxey would have to move south of the border. Since 1963, Hoxey's clinic in Tijuana, Mexico has been operated by Mildred Nelson, Hoxey's loyal and lifetime chief nurse, using the same formula.

In Harry Hoxey's book, *You Don't Have to Die*, he lists the products in his internal treatments for all cancers. They are: potassium iodine in concert with some or all of the following, depending upon the individual case, licorice, red clover, burdock root, stillingia root, berberis root, pokeroot, cascara, Aromatic USP 14 (an artificial flavor), prickly ash bark, and buckthorn bark.

Hoxey also had external preparations to apply topically to tumors. Burdock, buckthorn, cascara, barberry, some licorice components, one of pokeroot's components and one of stillingia's constituents have exhibited anti-tumor activity.

Hoxey and Nelson claimed a cure rate as high as 80 percent. Investigating groups throughout the clinic's history have challenged these statistics and have indicated that the therapy has little value.

The NCI announced no assessment of the Hoxey treatment could be made. However, they failed to verify his case records, which he opened to them. Their failure to cooperate, he felt, was deliberate, resulting from a widespread conspiracy against him by the AMA.

Neither the U.S. Public Health Service nor the Surgeon General, even with pressure from individual senators, investigated Hoxey's claims. Hoxey's point of view was represented in a report to the Senate Interstate and Foreign Commerce Committee by Benedict Fitzgerald, an attorney who examined records of Hoxey's litigation with the AMA and various branches of the federal government. Here's a direct summation of the situation from Congress' Unconventional Cancer Treatments: "After reading about the circumstances of these attempted case reviews, Fitzgerald wrote the NCI 'took sides and sought in every way to hinder, suppress, and restrict (the Hoxey Cancer Clinic) in their treatment of cancer.' "

"To date, no independent, comprehensive assessment has been made to resolve the many allegations and issues raised by Hoxey's tumultuous career."

Pau D'Arco

Available in health food stores in powder form, capsules or tea bags, Pau D'Arco, also called taheebo, lapacho, ipes, ipe roxo and trumpet bush, a product of South America, is a popular folk remedy for cancer, leukemia, Hodgkin's disease and among other ailments, malaria.

Derived from the inner bark of a purple flowered tree native to Argentina and Brazil, Pau D'Arco is considered a strengthener and cleansing agent with antimicrobial ability.

One of Pau D'Arco's principal ingredients, lapachol, has been extensively tested on animals and found to have anti-tumor properties in two types of cancer. However, in high daily oral doses – 1,500 mg or more – it was found in some cases, to cause nausea, vomiting and prolongation of blood clotting time.

The latter objection is usually overcome by taking vitamin K, noted for its aid in blood clotting. In one study, nine patients who had received orthodox cancer treatment were administered 20 to 30 mg/kg/day of lapachol for 20 to 60 days or longer.

The result was one total and two partial tumor regressions. A reduction of pain was noted in all patients. However, some of the patients had nausea, dizziness and diarrhea.

An unpublished study involving crude extracts of Pau D'Arco in mouse cells in culture (Lewis Lung Carcinoma) stimulated the activity of macrophages derived from mice that kill cancer cells. Used with mice, Pau D'Arco reduced the occurrence of lung metastases after surgery for removal of primary tumors.

The Gonzalez Nutritional Protocol

This regimen is a blend of therapeutic theories borrowed from William Donald Kelley, D.D.S., Melvin Page, M.D., John Beard,

M.D. and some from Gonzalez himself. A medical doctor in New York City, Nicholas Gonzalez felt the Kelley anti-cancer program had merit, so he borrowed it and made his own modifications to it.

Basic to the plan is Kelley's contention that human beings fall into three genetically-based categories: sympathetic dominants, parasympathic dominants and balanced types.

"Sympathetic dominants have evolved in tropical and subtropical ecosystems on plant-based diets," contends Kelley in his book *Unconventional Cancer.* He believes parasympathetic dominants evolved in colder regions on meat-based diets, and balanced types evolved in intermediate regions on mixed diets. While modern migrations have extensively mixed the three types, Kelley believes historically people belong to one of the three categories.

Starting from this base, Dr. Gonzalez tailors an individualized diet determined by an experimental blood test. The content ranges from entirely vegetarian to entirely meat with 90 variations in between.

Starting with the research and clinical findings of a turn-of-the-century physician, Dr. John Beard, who found that pancreatic enzymes – proteases, lipases and amylases – stop malignant cell growth, Gonzalez discovered pancreatic enzymes are the body's guardians against cancer.

Not only does Gonzalez emphasize pancreatic enzymes in his therapy, he administers hydrochloric acid for improved digestion, concentrations of beef organs in pill form, and vitamins and minerals – 150 pills daily in all.

Coffee enemas, colonic irrigations, cleansing the kidneys, lungs and skin are part of the purging and cleansing plan inherited from Kelley. Alcohol, cigarettes, soft drinks, white flour products and white rice, as well as fluoridated and chlorinated water are all no-nos.

Several people I know have reported cancer healings through the Gonzalez protocol.

Hydrazine Sulfate

Much of the credit for discovering hydrazine sulfate's use in cancer control goes to Joseph Gold, M.D., director of the Syracuse (New

York) Cancer Research Center and Rowan Chlebowski, M.D., Ph.D., and associates, University of California, Los Angeles (UCLA).

Dr. Gold theorized cachexia (condition of low weight, tissue loss and weakness) results from the breakdown of sugar in tumor cells and the production of new sugar in the liver and kidney.

Following trial and error, Dr. Gold chose to experiment with hydrazine sulfate. He found that in animal experiments hydrazine sulfate blocked the growth of tumors in rats and increased the effectiveness of certain chemotherapeutic drugs.

Gold noted a number of tumor regressions and subjective improvement in advanced cancer patients being given hydrazine sulfate by their doctors. However, there were some side effects: numbness in the extremities and transient nausea.

Dr. Chlebowski and his colleagues performed experiments with hydrazine sulfate and found it corrects abnormal glucose tolerance and decreases increased glucose production in cancer patients with cachexia.

In human trials, Chlebowski gave hydrazine sulfate to 65 patients with non-operable, non-small cell lung cancer. Half of the group received chemotherapy and a placebo.

Patients taking hydrazine sulfate had a better appetite, ate more and showed higher blood albumin levels than those in the chemotherapy group. Studies show higher albumin is predictive of a better two-year survival rate among patients having this type of cancer, with a poor survival time among individuals with low blood albumen.

Patients in fairly good condition taking hydrazine sulfate lived longer than those in a similar condition taking a placebo – 328 days, compared with 208 days. Forty-two percent of those on hydrazine sulfate were still alive a year later, compared with just 18 percent on the placebo.

To their credit, the NCI found the evidence convincing enough to sponsor additional study of hydrazine sulfate on human volunteers.

Vitamin C

Dr. Linus Pauling, two-time Nobel Laureate, was subjected to scathing criticism when he advocated vitamin C to extend the life and well-being of cancer victims.

Pauling's now famous collaboration with Dr. Ewan Cameron, a Scottish surgeon at the Vale of Leven Hospital, Loch Lomondside, Scotland, produced a study showing patients given one to two grams (1,000-2,000 mg.) of vitamin C daily, eventually working up to 10 or more grams according to bowel tolerance, outlived those who did not take the supplement (Cameron, p. 4538).

Not only did they live longer, patients reported greater well-being, improved appetite, increased mental alertness and decreased need for pain-killers. In their 1979 book, *Cancer and Vitamin C,* Cameron and Pauling wrote:

"Giving vitamin C in large doses to patients with advanced cancer produces subjective benefits in almost every patient by about the fifth day. The patient will claim to feel better, stronger and more mentally alert.

"Distressing symptoms such as bone pain from skeletal metastases diminish and may even disappear completely... The patient becomes more lively and shows more interest and also eats more food, indicating that he has a better appetite and is no longer feeling nauseated and miserable."

Three tests of vitamin C's worthiness to be used in advanced cancer patients were performed at the Mayo Clinic. Two were completed and the third abandoned because in early stages, said the researchers, it showed no promise.

Cameron and Pauling objected, saying the Mayo studies did not follow the original procedure, did not test the premise properly and, therefore, could not be considered a refutation.

Gladys Block, Ph.D., while with the National Cancer Institute, surveyed 46 studies on vitamin C and found that 33 showed statistically significant protection against cancer in eleven typical cancer sites (Block, p. 270).

"The strength and consistency of the results reported here for several sites suggests that there may be a real and important effect of ascorbic acid in cancer prevention," wrote Dr. Block.

Researchers at Albert Einstein College of Medicine discovered a striking revelation about vitamin C. They found women with vitamin C intake of less than 30 mg. daily (half the RDA, or half an orange) had a ten times greater risk of developing cervical dysplasia (a cancer precursor) than women with a higher intake of vitamin C.

Shark Cartilage

In the effort to discover a cancer cure, one ingredient has risen out of the waters: shark cartilage. Even conventional researchers have admitted there's something here worth investigating. A book written by Dr. William Lane, Ph.D., *Sharks Don't Get Cancer*, started the ball rolling.

In an interview with Mike Wallace on the TV news program, *60 Minutes* (February 28, 1993), biochemist Dr. Lane pointed out sharks have existed for more than 400 million years and rarely develop cancer, no matter how polluted the water in which they live. The fact that they are made up of mostly cartilage protects them from cancer, maintains Bill Lane.

Shark cartilage stops the development of new blood vessels, he contends. Like healthy cells, cancer cells in a tumor have to be fed. Within less than 14 days, they develop a system of arteries. Shark cartilage blocks this tumor-survival effort, causing it to starve to death.

Dr. Lane couldn't afford to run clinical trials in this country, so he took his research to Cuba, where a group of Cuban military doctors agreed to run trials on 29 cancer patients. Initially skeptical, the doctor in charge, Lieutenant Colonel Jose Menendez, agreed to be interviewed by *60 Minutes*, testifying that during the 16-week trial, the majority of patients treated with shark cartilage saw a reduction in the size of their tumors.

60 Minutes recruited the assistance of Dr. Charles Simone, a veteran orthodox oncologist who spent five years doing research at NCI.

He was given the opportunity to review the Cuban trial results and venture an opinion. He responded, "At this point, early in the stage of the history of shark cartilage, I think we have to say that there are intriguing data, enough to pursue in a more formal way. You know, in the last fifty years, we have not made any significant progress in the treatment of cancer in adults, so we need to look at other issues, like shark cartilage."

60 Minutes also sought the opinion of Dr. Eli Gladstein, University of Texas Southwestern Medical Center who reluctantly ventured, "there's some cases that had lumps of tumor get smaller. That's what we look for in this business."

The U.S. is behind the times when it comes to shark cartilage. Researchers around the world have been experimenting with shark cartilage and getting good results.

In 1988, Dr. Ghanem Atassi of the Institut Jules Bordet in Brussels, Belgium conducted an experiment in which 40 mice received grafts of human melanoma. Half the animals received no medication, while the other half received daily doses of shark cartilage. In 21 days the tumors in the untreated mice had doubled in size while tumors on the other mice decreased in size.

In Costa Rica, Dr. Carlos Luiz Alpizar treated a patient who had an inoperable, grapefruit-sized abdominal tumor with shark cartilage. The tumor stopped growing within a month, and after six months shrank to the size of a walnut.

In Panama, Dr. Ernesto Contreras, Jr. treated eight terminal cancer patients with shark cartilage over a two-month period. Seven of the eight showed a reduction in tumor size of 30 to 100 percent. A patient with an advanced liver tumor experienced complete remission after eight weeks of shark cartilage therapy.

A panel at the U.S. Office of Alternative Medicine, National Institutes of Health, recommended Dr. Simone start a formal evaluation of shark cartilage. In the meantime, the Cubans have started a new study, this time with 100 patients.

CHAPTER 36:

Would You Buy A Used Car From the FDA?

"People think the FDA is protecting them – it isn't. What the FDA is doing and what people think it's doing are as different as night and day."
— Dr. Herbert Ley, FDA Commissioner, the San Francisco Chronicle, January 2, 1970

Add the Food and Drug Administration to our list of known carcinogens. Not only does this organization betray the public trust by not investigating food products for cancer causing substances, but it gives manufacturers permission to add carcinogenic additives to our food and pesticides to our produce. How they get away with this is insidious indeed. Instead of evaluating the collective effect of all the carcinogenic additives and pesticides present in our food supply, they evaluate them individually, casually dismissing them as having a "negligible risk" of giving us cancer.

According to the FDA's national market basket survey, at least 38 percent of the food supply contains pesticide residues. This figure is probably an underestimation because routine laboratory tests can detect fewer than one-half of the pesticides applied to food (Meyerhoff, p. 51).

In 30 years, conventional pesticide use in the U.S. has doubled from 500 million to more than 1 billion pounds annually, representing one-third of the world market. Total pesticide use in 1991 (including wood preservatives and disinfectants) exceeded 2.2 billion pounds (*ibid*).

Eliminating Our Fail-Safe

The Delaney Clause of the Food, Drug and Cosmetic Act mandates that any food additive found to induce cancer cannot be deemed safe. It has been in effect since the early '70s, when one of my icons, Gloria Swanson, and I helped Congressman Delaney word the amendment. It does not, however, specify how cancerous, and this is the loophole not only the FDA but Congressional representatives are using to get out of it.

Under law, the FDA was supposed to evaluate the safety of all food, drug and cosmetic dyes by January 1963.

In 1984, the Health Research Group of Ralph Nader's Public Citizen organization sent a letter to then FDA Commissioner Frank Young saying it would take them to court if the FDA did not act to ban certain food dyes.

The Health Research Group said none of the dyes had been found safe by the FDA and that animal studies had indicated they can cause cancer. The dyes in question were Red nos. 3, 8, 9, 19, 33, 36 and 37; Yellow nos. 5 and 6; and Orange no. 17.

In 1984, a congressional report criticized the FDA and the Department of Health and Human Services (HHS) for postponing a decision on the dyes.

In 1986, according to the FDA, they approved four cosmetic dyes for which the "cancer risk was trivial." These were Orange no. 17, and Red nos. 8, 9 and 19. The agency based its approval on the legal maxim "de minimis non curat lex," meaning the law does not concern itself with trifles (Zamichow, p. 5).

In 1987 a federal appeals court ruled that the FDA violated federal law when it approved two of the dyes (Orange no. 17 and Red no. 19) after the Cosmetic, Toiletry and Fragrance Association showed they caused liver cancer in rodents.

The FDA had accepted the tests as valid, and agency scientists urged Commissioner Young to disapprove the dyes.

However, when a government review panel assessed the risks as, at worst, 1 in 19 billion for Orange no. 17, and 1 in 9 million for Red no. 19, Young overruled his scientists, ruling in 1986 that the cancer risk was trivial and implicitly exempt from Delaney.

In the 1987 appeals court ruling, Judge Stephen F. Williams said once the FDA "squeezed the scientific trigger" by recognizing a dye as a carcinogen, Delaney took effect automatically (Mintz, p. 9).

The decision came a week after the House Government Operations Committee concluded the FDA had no legal authority to declare an additive that induces cancer somehow fails to within the meaning of the Delaney clause.

In response to the court's rejection of their decision, the FDA, in a "clarification," switched its argument, saying the dyes are safe because the phrase "induce cancer in man or animal" is a "term of art."

The Justice Department agreed, repeating the phrase in the appeals brief, saying that "simply because a substance can be labeled 'carcinogenic' does not mean that its use is automatically barred by statute."

Previous FDA commissioners held that the Delaney Clause absolutely prohibits approval of dyes that cause cancer in animals, even if it can be shown that they pose a seemingly negligible risk to humans.

After all this, where does the food dye issue currently stand? You only have to look at your supermarket shelves to see for yourself.

Red No. 3, for example, has historically been the most problematic. It brightens maraschino cherries, other foods, and cosmetics; is among the most widely used, and is the color that food manufacturers and the cosmetics industry have fought the hardest for. Since 1981, the FDA has proposed to ban Red no. 3 at least 12 times, but each time the dye has been given a reprieve. According to the International Association of Color Manufacturers, Red no. 3 is widely used in industry today.

In 1986, an FDA advisory committee concluded that "Yellow no. 5, (tartrazine) may cause itching or hives." Despite this finding, they still chose not to warn the consumer. Instead, they looked for ways to justify leaving it on the market. In a December 1993 article in their publication, *FDA Consumer*, a Dr. Linda Tollefson is quoted as saying, "(These) reactions are classified as hypersensitive and are not true allergic reactions, which would be more severe." The article did not include Dr. Tollefson's credentials. I called the FDA myself to discover that she is a doctor of veterinary medicine.

The only action taken to warn the public about the possible side effects of Yellow no. 5 is a 1981 requirement that all foods products containing the dye list the ingredient on their labels. The requirement was extended to drugs as well.

Despite the years of questions regarding the safety of food and drug dyes, only recently (May 8, 1993) has there been a requirement to list all certified colors (part of the Nutrition Labeling and Education Act of 1990) on food and drug labels.

The future remains bright for food dye manufacturers, thanks to the special interest groups who wish to see agriculture continue to embrace pesticides. Representing these special interests, certain congressmen have introduced legislation that would basically nullify the Delaney Clause and allow our foods and drugs to legally contain carcinogens. Substances deemed to cause at most one additional case of cancer in one million people over a 70-year lifetime of exposure to one compound would be defined as having a "negligible risk," and thus be marketable.

According to "Red No. 3 and Other Colorful Controversies," an article from the May 1990, *FDA Consumer Magazine*, President Bush endorsed the negligible risk standard for pesticides in his October 1989 Food Safety Plan. A joint press statement issued that same day by Health and Human Services Secretary Sullivan, United States Department of Agriculture Secretary Yeutter and Environmental Protection Agency Administrator Reilly noted that while the president's plan specifically addresses pesticide residues, the principle of negligible risk is one that naturally applies to other additives to the food supply. What is happening here is the lucrative cancer market isn't satisfied with profits gained from unsuccessful and expensive treatments, it is now targeting our food supply so there will be plenty of new cancer cases to treat. And as cancer consumers we have become so used to the concept that cancer cannot be prevented, as conventional medicine would have us believe, that we accept this!

I contacted a representative of the FDA, who stated that as of November, 1993, Red nos. 8,9 and 19 are off the market, as is Orange no. 17. Red no. 37 was withdrawn by petitioners so it remains on the market. Red no. 33 is listed for drug and cosmetic use; Red no. 36 is listed for use in drugs, mouthwash and dentrifices; and Yellow no. 6 is listed for use in food, cosmetics and drugs.

In the 1992 fiscal year the FDA certified over 11.5 million pounds of color additives, most of which, no doubt, have not been tested for carcinogens. Important to keep in mind is that the FDA is not required to test for carcinogens. It depends on manufacturers, who may or may not test, to assure the agency their products are safe for consumption. There have been many, many cases of pharmaceutical manufacturers lying to the FDA about the safety of their products; discovered only after the death of their consumers. Incentive to lie is strong, as billions of profit dollars are at stake, with the only punishment being thousands of dollars in fines.

FDA's Support of Pharmaceuticals

As I've already established, pharmaceutical companies have a history of being far more interested in profits than safety. What hasn't been established is the role the FDA plays in making sure pharmaceuticals remain firmly entrenched in the conventional cancer treatment system.

Powerful and dictatorial, the Food and Drug Administration has often been referred to as a bureaucracy gone berserk. The closest thing America has had to the old Soviet commissar system, the FDA has been a thorn in the side of those seeking new and alternative cures for cancer since its birth in 1906 as the Bureau of Chemistry.

The FDA's main aim over the last 80 years has been to protect the powerful, influential pharmaceutical giants rather than the health of the American people. This credo was succinctly expressed in 1982 by Dr. Richard Crout, the director of the FDA's Bureau of Drugs: "I never have and never will approve a new drug to an individual, but only to a large pharmaceutical firm with unlimited finances."

Eleven years later the FDA, this time through a task force report, again admitted its bias when it stated, "...the task force considered many issues in its deliberations including to ensure the existence of dietary supplements on the market does not act as a disincentive for drug development..."

In 1993, David Adams, the FDA Deputy Commissioner, went even further in his support for drug conglomerates. Speaking before the Drug Information Association, he said, "...pay careful attention to what is happening (with dietary supplements) in the legislative arena...if these efforts are successful, there could be created a class of products to compete with approved drugs that are subject to less regulation than approved drugs...the establishment of a separate regulatory category for supplements would undercut exclusivity rights enjoyed by holders of approved drug applications."

One of the few FDA officials not having a love affair with the pharmaceutical companies was the FDA's first boss, Dr. Harvey Wiley. A powerful and no-nonsense administrator, Wiley was so disgusted with the Bureau of Chemistry's support of the drug cartel that he resigned in 1912. He announced that he was leaving the bureau "because the fundamental principles of the Pure Food Law have been strangled," and that he was powerless to punish manufacturers of misbranded and adulterated drugs.

In his book, *History of a Crime*, published in 1929, Wiley wrote, "If the Bureau of Chemistry had been permitted to enforce the law as it was written and as it tried to do, what would have been the condition now? No food product in this country would have any trace of benzoic acid, sulphurous acid or sulphites ... no soft drink would contain caffeine, no bleached flour would enter interstate commerce. Our food and drugs would be wholly without any form of adulteration."

FDA Persecution of Nutritional Supplements and
Alternative Therapies

If Dr. Wiley was alive today, he would see that the Bureau hasn't changed much over the past 60 years – other than its name. Descendants of the bureau's bureaucrats are still promoting the dangerous products of the drug conglomerates – while spending most of their time trying to destroy the small manufacturers of vitamins, minerals and food supplements.

In 1949 FDA Commissioner Dr. George Larrick admitted with obvious pride that "the activities of the so-called health food lecturers have increasingly engaged our attention." He also announced that his brave band of FDA agents were fighting "the good fight against dried vegetables, mineral mixtures, vitamins and similar products."

Two decades later a witness told Senator Long in a subcommittee hearing that the FDA spends a great deal of time going after little manufacturers, but that whenever a small company was purchased by a large company the harassment stopped. In 1973 FDA Commissioner Charles Edwards testified at another congressional hearing that, "It is not our policy to jeopardize the financial interests of the pharmaceutical companies."

FDA's record prompted Milton Friedman, the feisty Nobel Laureate economist, to state, "Any increase in the FDA's authority over anything is a clear and present danger to the nation's health."

The FDA Draws Its Guns

In 1963, the FDA spent millions of dollars in an unsuccessful attempt to prosecute Dr. Steven Durovic and Dr. Andrew Ivey for producing and proscribing Krebiozen, an anti-cancer substance. During the 289-day trial, government witnesses gave falsified testimony. Despite the lies, which the government later admitted, the jury found the doctors not guilty on all 240 counts.

In 1970, the cruel manner in which the FDA treats practitioners of alternative medicine affected me personally. I was watching TV when

I saw my good friend, Dr. John Richardson, handcuffed to his nurse, being dragged out of his office in Albany, California by FDA agents. In the background I could see his patients still attached to IV gurneys. John's "crime," the TV announcer stated, was that he had been using vitamins as a cancer cure. It seemed like a preposterous reason for an arrest, but within a few months this marvelous doctor was sentenced to three years in a federal prison. I was so incensed that I started a newsletter and sent it out to his patients asking for donations. We raised enough money to go back to court and fight for his freedom. Happily, we succeeded and his conviction was overturned.

In 1990, a pet food manufacturer was sentenced to 179 days in prison and fined $10,000 in a case brought by the FDA for allegedly mislabeling natural dog food. Another case had a small manufacturer in prison when the FDA accused him of making "unscientific" claims that his food supplements were beneficial to health.

On May 8, 1992, FDA officials raided the offices of my dear friend and chairman of the board of the National Health Federation, Dr. Jonathan V. Wright, a licensed physician practicing out of a Tahoma, Washington clinic. He had instigated legal proceedings against the FDA and believes this action was retaliatory.

I was in Pittsburgh doing a series of TV shows when Jonathan's wife, Holly, called me to say that the FDA had raided his office. She described how FDA agents in their flak jackets and drawn guns had broken down the door and were holding everyone in the office at gunpoint. The agents held Jonathan and his staff for 14 hours. When one woman tried to make a call, one of the agents put a gun to her head and said, "If you touch that phone I will blow your head off."

The FDA agents said they obtained a search warrant to inspect the clinic's ozone generating machine, even though it had already been inspected and approved by the Washington State Department of Industrial Hygiene. The machine was used by Jonathan to dispense his successful ozone therapy to patients with AIDS-related viruses or cancer. Many of his patients had been told by other clinics there was nothing that could be done but found themselves symptom-free thanks to Jonathan's alternative treatments.

Agents confiscated the machine and other expensive electronic equipment vital to the clinic's functioning, making it impossible for him to continue treating his patients.

I spent the next three days and nights working feverishly writing press releases and letters to National Health Federation members, rallying support for Jonathan. I think I slept six hours in those three days, but the terrible injustice spurred me on – and still does.

During the ensuing court case, FDA agents lied, claiming Jonathan was manufacturing drugs. The fact was he never manufactured anything. After two grand jury investigations, the FDA failed to indict him. But ever since they have been trying to get his employees to inform on him. And of course in its grand tradition of justice for all, the FDA is still harassing Jonathan.

The message the FDA is sending to the public is very clear: the FDA will turn a blind eye if an Upjohn, an Eli Lilly or a Johnson and Johnson manufactures drugs that kill thousands — but be warned, the FDA will get you if you try selling food supplements or promote alternative medicine.

Senator William Proxmire, writing in the National Health Federation Bulletin in 1974, noted that "The FDA is actively hostile against the manufacture, sale and distribution of vitamins and minerals as food or food supplements. They are out to get the health food industry and drive the health food stores out of business. And they are trying to do this out of active hostility and prejudice."

Powerful testimony that supported Proxmire's views was presented by Dr. Michael Janson, an orthomolecular physician and director of the Center for Preventive Medicine in Cape Code, Massachusetts, before Senator Kennedy and his Senate Labor Committee hearing in 1993. Janson told of the FDA's long history of bias against dietary supplements and alternative health care. He cited as an example the FDA's recent attempt at "removing from the market black currant oil capsules, claiming that it was an unsafe food additive. The "food" to which this "unsafe additive" was being added was the gelatin capsule in which it was packaged.

Their argument was thrown out of court by three judges who said that the FDA was using "Alice-in-Wonderland" reasoning in an effort to make an end-run around the law." Janson added that "the FDA's own scientists and toxicologists testified they were unaware of any safety problems with the oil." He also said that the FDA's goals include "steps necessary to ensure that the existence of dietary supplements on the market does not act as a disincentive for drug development." The Food and Drug Administration, formerly the Bureau of Chemistry, is, and always has been, in place solely to protect the pharmaceutical marketplace and, if necessary, force the medical consumer to "live through chemistry."

In pursuing this goal and purpose, it has taken the irrational and unsubstantiated stand that nutritional supplements, vitamins and minerals are useless. Even today, despite all the evidence to the contrary, Linus Pauling is still regarded as a charlatan for advocating vitamin C as a cold treatment.

In 1962, FDA agents arrested Dr. William Abt as he was lecturing on nutrition in Detroit. Sounding like dialogue from a Mel Brooks movie, the FDA actually said that Dr. Abt was arrested because "he sold vitamins, herbs and seasonings."

Another classic example of the FDA in action in its own personal war on vitamin and food supplements was reported by Martin Walker in *Dirty Medicine*. In it he cites the example of the Cardiac Society, a non-profit group of several hundred heart patients, formed in the 1960s. The group promoted vitamin E, and when the Society started a buyer's club for vitamin E, the FDA took action. Customers sending orders to the Society found them returned by the United States Postal Service stamped "fraudulent."

On July 29, 1993, the FDA presented a survey report to a House subcommittee hearing on dietary supplements entitled "Unsubstantiated Claims and Documented Health Hazards in the Dietary Supplement Marketplace." The report was designed to support the FDA's objections to pending legislation which would clarify the agency's regulation of dietary supplements.

An analysis of the FDA survey made by Senator Orrin G. Hatch (D-Utah) staff members reveal that "the FDA has knowingly submitted false information to Congress, and that it has willfully violated the presumption of accuracy and impartiality traditionally granted the agency. The report conclusively proves the FDA's animosity to dietary supplements," the analysis concluded.

Thirty-four of the 528 products the FDA alleged made false claims did not even exist; 25 of the 528 were listed twice; 142 of the products were attributed to distributors or manufacturers who had nothing to do with them; one of the "products" was actually a book written by a doctor; and 17 of the products had been removed from the market prior to the FDA's survey. Altogether, 42 percent of the claims made by the FDA were false.

Despite compelling scientific evidence, despite decades of usage in other countries, despite countless successes and few failures, the FDA still continues to deny the public access to nutritional therapies, and to persecute and imprison qualified physicians who choose to use them for the benefit of their patients.

The continuing antagonism of the FDA is summarized succinctly by Bernard Rimland, Ph.D., head of the Autism Research Institute in San Diego. "The FDA has a long sordid record of deceit and repression in its handling of nutritional supplements. The FDA has repeatedly shown it cannot be trusted. Congress, take note!...We don't need the FDA to protect our health. We need Congress to protect us from the FDA!"

Write Your Congressman

Strong public outcry is growing across the country to control the FDA monolith. More and more Americans are realizing that the FDA is nothing more than a tool of the pharmaceutical-medical establishment out to destroy the health food business, and, consequently, our freedom of health choice. Over 100 million Americans take food supplements. Think what could be accomplished if just half of these people called their congressional representative demanding the right to information and access to nutritional supplements.

Responding to the outcry, legislative bills are being written and sponsored attempting to guarantee the rights of the nutritional health industry and encourage alternative medical research. However, it is a long, steep, uphill battle with pharmaceutical giants buying amendments that limit, if not stop, any forward motion. For every one step forward that the health food industry makes, the pharmaceutical industry pushes it back two steps. Only a unified, resounding cry of protest by consumers of supplements and pharmaceuticals alike, loud enough to be heard by every politician in Washington, D.C., will be enough to stop the FDA's assault on our personal liberties. Much, much more needs to be done before we can enjoy true medical freedom in this country.

In view of the FDA's chilling record for approving killer drugs, its known and stated bias against nutritional supplements and its vendetta against health food stores, our legislative representatives in Washington should limit the powers of the Food and Drug Administration to monitoring drugs, giving the power to monitor supplements to the United States Department of Agriculture. One of the best organs of the federal government, the Department of Agriculture conducts meaningful research into foods and supplements at its superb facility at Tufts University. It would be an uphill battle since Tufts depends upon grants for its research and the drug cartel could quickly move in with its big money donations, but there is no doubt that the Agriculture Department has an excellent record in its food research — a record that puts the FDA's efforts to shame.

It is up to us to let Washington know the FDA is a failed agency. We must remind our representatives that the FDA abuses its power and has shown a disgraceful bias toward drugs over natural therapies and supplements.

Thomas Jefferson was once asked "what should we do when government gets out of the hands of the people?" He replied, "You educate the people. They are the sovereign power." To that end, the National Health Federation, of which I am the president, was founded. For 38 years it has been a powerful educator of the people. It has also been in the forefront for reform, choice and standing up to Big

Brother. I urge you to become a member. The NHF is the oldest and largest health freedom organization in America. Your membership dollars will guarantee not only your access to valuable information, including current legislation, bills and activities, courtesy of its publication *Health Freedom News*, but your dollars help fund political representation in Washington, D.C. for the right to nutritional and alternative medical choice in America. To win the battle against cancer, we need your help and the help of our government. Remember, politicians don't see the light; they only feel the heat. Believe me, when you write letters they will feel the heat. So I urge you to make your vote count and join me in demanding government not for the bigshot allopathic physicians and pharmaceuticals, BUT FOR THE PEOPLE.

The fee for joining the NHF is $36. The subscription rate for the *Health Freedom News* magazine is $36. Donations are accepted.

National Health Federation
P.O. Box 688
Monrovia, Ca. 91017
(626) 357-2181 phone
(626) 303-0642 fax
www.thenhf.com

REFERENCES

Ables, J.C., *Ann. Int. Med.*, 16:221, 1942.

"Air Pollution Boosts Mortality Rates," *Cancer Researcher Weekly*, December 20, 1993.

Adams, Ruth, "Versatile Vitamin E," *Better Nutrition for Today's Living*, v.53, n4, p. 14, April 1991.

Allen, G., *None Dare Call it Conspiracy*, '76 Press, Seal Beach, CA, 1975.

Associated Press: "Toxics Reportedly Added to Cigarettes," *The Sacramento Bee*, April 9, 1994.

Ballentine, R., *Diet and Nutrition, A Holistic Approach*, Himalayan International Institute: Pennsylvania, 1978.

Bayle, M. Beddow, *Cancer: The Failure of Modern Research*, London, 1936.

Beard, John, *"The Enzymes Treatment of Cancer,"* Chatoo & Windus, London, 1911.

Benet, S., Abkahasians, Holt Rinehart, New York, 1968.

Bergulas, Alexander, *Cancer Nature, Cause and Cure*, Institute Pasteur, Paris, 1935.

Beveridge, J., et al., "Dietary Factors Affecting Plasma," *Canadian Journal Biology & Phys.*, 34.441.

Bieler, H.G., *Food Is Your Best Medicine*, Vintage, New York, 1972.

Bland, J., "How Vitamin E Slows Aging," *Prevention*, March 1976.

Bland, Jeffrey, 1984-85 *Yearbook of Nutritional Medicine,* New Canaan, CT, 1985.

Block, Gladys, "Vitamin C and Cancer Prevention, the Epidemiologic Evidence," *American Journal of Clinical Nutrition,* January 1991.

Brohier, Catherine, "Diet May Shield Against Two Leading Cancer Killers," *Environmental Nutrition*, v.15, n.2, February 1992.

"Breath in Danger II," The American Lung Association, April 30, 1993.

Brooke, B.N., *Understanding Cancer,* Holt Rinehart, New York, 1973.

Buckner, N. & Swaffield, M., *Cancer Research*, 33,12, 1973.

Burk, D., *A Brief on Foods and Vitamins*, McNaughton Foundation, Marin, CA, 1975.

Burk, Dr. Dean & Yamouyanis, Dr. J., *Public Scrutiny*, June, 1979.

Burton Goldberg Group, *Alternative Medicine, The Definitive Guide,* Future Medicine Publishing, Inc., Puyallup, WA, 1993.

Burzynski Research Institute, Inc. *"The Status of Investigational New Drug Applications for Antineoplaston A10 and AS2-1,"* Stafford, TX, April 11, 1994.

Butterworth, C., Hatch, K., Gore, H., et al., "Improvement in Cervical Dysplasia Associated With Folic Acid Therapy in Users of Oral Contraceptives," *American Journal of Clinical Nutrition*, 1982.

Cameron, E. & Pauling, L., *Cancer and Vitamin C*, Linus Pauling Institute of Science and Medicine, Menlo Park, 1979.

Cameron, E. & Pauling, L., "Supplemental Ascorbate in the Supportive Treatment of Cancer," *Proceedings of the National Academy of Science,* 1978.

Campbell, James T., "Trypsin Treatment of Malignant Disease," *Journal of the American Medical Association*, January 19, 1907.

Cancer Facts and Figures 1993, American Cancer Society, Atlanta, GA.

Cancer Research, December 1979.

Carper, Jean, *The Food Pharmacy*, Bantam Books, New York, 1988.

Challem, Jack, "Vitamin Therapy Lengthens Survival of Advanced Cancer Patients," *Let's Live*, March 1994.

Charles, Dan, "A Cup of Green Tea a Day May Keep Cancer Away," *New Scientist,* v131, n1786, Sept. 14, 1991.

Cheraskin, Ringsdorf & Clark, *Diet and Disease*, Rodale Press, New York, 1968.

Cornfield, J., et al, *Journal of the National Cancer Institute*, 22:176, 1959.

Cowen, Ron, "Medicine On the Wild Side: Animals May Rely On a Natural Pharmacy," *Science News*, v.138, Nov. 3, 1990.

Crohns, Giraud R., "Disease in the Yransvaal Bantu," *South Africa Medical Journal*, 43:610-75.

Culbert M., *Freedom from Cancer*, '76 Press, Seal Beach, CA, 1974.

Cutfield, A. & Dontai, "Trypsin Treatment in Malignant Disease," *British Medical Journal*, August 31, 1907.

Davis, Adelle, *Let's Get Well*, Harcourt Brace, CA, 1965.

Davis, Adelle, *Let's Cook it Right*," New American Library, Los Angeles, 1970.

Dawson, E., Nosovitch, J. and Hannigan, E., "Serum Vitamin and Selenium Changes in Cervical Dysplasia," *Fed. Proc.*, 1984.

Delver, E., & Pence, B.C., "Effects of Dietary Selenium Level on UV-Induced Skin Cancer and Epidermal Antioxidant Status," Texas Technical University Health Sciences Center, Lubbock, Texas, *Cancer Researcher Weekly*, July 12, 1993.

"Disease Prevention: Flax Seed Endorsed by the FDA," *Total Health*, October 1993.

Duprey, H., "Trypsin in Epithelioma of Larynx," *New Orleans Medical and Surgical Journal*, v.68.

Eastwood, M., *Lancet*, Dec. 6, 1969.

Ells, G.W., et al, "Effect of Temperature and Oxygen Tension on Gamma-Linolenate Toxicity Towards Human Breast Cancer Cells," *Cancer Researcher Weekly*, August 30, 1993.

The Encyclopedia of Common Diseases, Rodale Press, Inc. Emmaus, PA, 1976.

End Results of Cancer, U.S. Government, H.E.W., Report No.4, 1972.

Faelton, Sharon, *The Complete Book of Minerals for Health*, Rodale Books, Emmaus, PA, 1981.

"FDA, Others Offer New Tamoxifen Warnings," *Science News*, v.145, April 16, 1994.

Fein, G. G., et al., "Prenatal Exposure to Polychlorinated Biphenyls: Effects on Birth Size and Gestational Age," *Journal of Pediatrics,* August 1984.

Feinblatt, H.M. & Gant, J.C. "Palliative Treatment of Benign Prostatic Hypertrophy: Value of Glycine, Alanine, Glutamic Acid Combination," *Journal of the Maine Medical Association,* 1958.

Fenzau, C. J. and Walters, Charles, *An Acres USA Primer,* Kansas City, MO, 1992.

Franklin, Byjay, Tirelee, Ritnin: *"Correct Approach to Cancer Therapy."* Lotta Workana Research, March 8, 1908, p. 381.

Fredericks, C. & Bailey, *Food Facts and Fallacies,* Arc. Giant, New York, 1969.

Geoth, Richard A., "Pancreatic Treatment of Cancer With Report of A Cure," *Journal of the American Medical Association,* March 23, 1907.

Gerson, M., *A Cancer Therapy,* Totality Books, New York, 1977.

Gerstenberg, F. Krebsf. u. Kr. Beh., Bd. V, 1964.

Golley, F.B., "Two Cases of Cancer Treated by the Injection of Pancreatic Extract," *Medical Record,* New York, December 8, 1906.

Golley, F.B., "Two Cases of Cancer Treated With Trypsin," supplementary report to the foregoing in *Medical Record,* May 8, 1909.

Greeley, Alexandra, "Dodging the Rays," *FDA Consumer,* v.27, n.6, July-August 1993.

"Green Tea Shown to Have Anti-Cancer Effect in Rodents," *Food Chemical News,* v.36, n.11, CRC Press, Inc., May 9, 1994.

Greenstein, J.P. *"Biochemistry of Cancer,"* Academic Press, 1954.

Griffen, E., *"World Without Cancer,"* American Media, CA, 1976.

Griffiths, Keith, Dr., "Talc and Carcinoma of the Ovary and Cervix," *Journal of Obstetrics and Gynecology,* March 1971.

Gurchot, C., "The Trophoblast Theory of Cancer," *Oncology,* v.31, n.5 & 6, 1975.

Halstead, B.W., *Amygdalin Therapy,* Committee for Freedom of Choice, CA, 1977.

"Harnessing Fatty Acids to Fight Cancer," *Science News,* v133, n21, May 21, 1988

Harder, Joan, "Defense Against Breast Cancer," *Bestways,* September 1986.

Hart, James P. & Cooper, William L., "Vitamin E in the Treatment of Prostate Hypertrophy," Lee Foundation for Nutritional Research, Milwaukee, WI, *Report No. 1,* November 1941.

Hegsted, D.M., *Nutrition,* v.1, Beaton, New York, 1971.

Hematology/Oncology Clinics of North America, 1991.

Herber, V., *American Journal of Clinical Nutrition,* 21 7 746, 1968.

Herbert, Victor, Genell J. Subak-Sharpe, *The Mt. Sinai School of Medicine Complete Book of Nutrition,* St. Martin's Press, New York, 1990.

Herbert, Victor, M.D., et al, *The Mount Sinai School of Medicine Complete Book of Nutrition,* St. Martin's Press, New York, 1990.

Herbert, Victor, The Health Robbers.

Herbst, A.L., "DES Clear Cell Cancer-1992," *Cancer Weekly,* April 19, 1993.

Hoffman, F., *The Mortality From Cancer Throughout the World,* 1915.

Hunter, B.T., *Food Additives,* Keats, Ohio, 1972.

Hur, R., *Food Reform, Our Desperate Need,* Heidelberg Pub., Texas, 1975.

Irving, D., *Ann. Internal Medicine,* 16:221, 1942.

Jaffe, Richard, Esq., "Burzynski Wins Latest Round of Medical Licensing Case," Editorial, *Townsend Letter for Doctors,* June 1994.

Jaret, Peter, "Bet on Broccoli," *In Health,* v.5, n.5, Sept-Oct, 1991.

Kintish, Lisa, "Sun Protection: Vitamin A Derivatives, Antioxidants Endorsed At Skin Cancer Foundation Conference," *Soap-Cosmetics-Chemical Specialties,* v.65, n.5, May 1989.

Kittler, G.D., *Control for Cancer,* Warner, New York, 1963.

Kittler, G., *Laetrile Control for Cancer,* Pa. B. Lib, New York, 1963.

Kono S., Ikeda, M., Tokudome S., et al, "A Case-Control Study of Gastric Cancer and Diet in Northern Kyushu, Japan," *Japan Journal of Cancer Research,* 1988.

Krakowski, Wien, Klin. W., 1965/15.

Krebs, Ernst T., Jr., & Bouziane, N.R., *Laetriles in the Prevention of Cancer,* McNaughton Foundation, Sausalito, CA, 1967.

Krebs, E.T., Speech to National Health Federation, Los Angeles, 1979.

Krebs, E.T., Jr., *Unitarian or Trophoblastic Thesis of Cancer.*

Kugler, Hans, et al, *Life Extenders and Memory Boosters*, Health Quest Publications, Reno, Nevada, 1993.

Kunin, Richard, *Mega Nutrients*, McGraw-Hill, New York, 1981.

Langer, Stephen, *Solved: The Riddle of Illness,* Keats Publishing, Inc., New Canaan, CT, 1984.

Langer, Stephen "Selenium Is Instrumental in Cancer Prevention," *Better Nutrition,* v.51, n.11, November 1989.

Lappe, T., *Diet for a Small Planet*, Ballantine, New York, 1971.

Lavik, P. & Bauman, C., *Cancer Research*, 3 11 749, 1943.

Leuchtenberger, R., Science, 101:46, 1945.

Lieberman, Shari, "Good Nutrition Can Prevent Colon Cancer," *Better Nutrition*, v.51, n.7, July 1989.

Life Extenders and Memory Boosters, Health Quest Publications, Reno, Nevada, 1993.

Loma Linda U., Dept. of Nutrition, 1977.

MacDonald, E.S., *Cancer Bulletin*, 25 2 4, 1973.

Manner, H., *The Death of Cancer,* Advanced Publishing Co., Illinois, 1978.

Marsden, Aspinall, "Carcinoma of Cervix Uteri Successfully Treated With the Pancreatic Ferment," *General Practitioner,* January 11, 1908.

McCance & Widdowson, E.M., *The Composition of Foods*, HEW Mag. Sta. Off., 1960.

McGuire, Rick, "Cancer Prevention Under the Sun," *Total Health,* v.13, n.2, April 1991.

Medical Hotline, v.5, n.1, January 1984.

Meggitt, Henry, "The Pancreatic Treatment of Cancer," *General Practitioner*, March 21, 1908.

Meyerhoff, Al, "We Must Get Rid of Pesticides in the Food Supply: Exposure to These Deadly Chemicals Can Cause Cancer, Birth

Defects, and Neurological Damage," *USA Today,* v122, n2582, November 1993.

Miller, Clinton, "EPA Ordered to Reinstate Fluoride Whistle-Blower," *Townsend Letter for Doctors,* June 1994.

Mintz, Morton, "Court Bans Cancer-Causing Dyes FDA Passed," *The Washington Post,* October 24, 1987.

Mitchell, et al., Cooper, *Nutrition in Health and Disease,* n.15, Lippincott, New York, 1968.

Moertel, *NCI Report on Non-Toxicity of Amygdalin.*

Mora, John M., "Foods That Contain Cancer-Preventive Compounds," *East West Natural Health,* v.22, n.2, March-April, 1992.

Morgan, Brian, *Nutrition Prescription,* Crown Publishers, New York, 1987.

Murray, Frank, "Zinc: Healing Mineral," *Better Nutrition for Today's Living,* v.54, n.9, September 1992.

Nagy, M., *Journal of the American Medical Association,* 226-8, Nov. 19, 1973.

Namalas, J. *Cancer Answer,* Wioulp, CA, 1981.

Oden, C., *Thank God I Have Cancer!,* Arlington House, NY, 1976.

Null, Gary, *The Complete Guide to Health and Nutrition,* Dell Publishing Co., New York, 1984.

"Nutrition and Cancer Study," Melbourne, Australia, University of Melbourne, Department of Medicine, 1989.

Oguni, I., Chen S. J., Lin, P.Z., et al, "Protection Against Cancer Risk by Japanese Green Tea," *Preventive Medicine,* 1992.

Ondeviecer, *Help on Diet,* Bood Farm Manor, Illinois, 1980.

Orr, J., Wilson, K., Bodiford, C. et al., "Nutritional Status of Patients With Untreated Cervical Cancer, II Vitamin Assessment," *American Journal of Obstetrics and Gynecology,* 1985.

Pack, G.T., *Tumors of the Gastrointestinal Tract,* Peters, New York, 1962.

Paul, John A., "Urban Air Quality: The Problem," *EPA Journal,* January, February 1991.

Pauling, Linus, *How to Live Longer and Feel Better,* W.H. Freeman & Co., New York, NY, 1986.

Pauly, Michelle M & Talbert, Lee, *Colon Cleansing,* American Institute of Health and Nutrition, 1992

Pfeiffer, C.C., *Mental and Elemental Nutrients,* Keats Publishing Co., Connecticut, 1975.

Physician's Handbook of Vitamin B17 Therapy, McNaughton Foundation, Science Press International, CA, 1973.

Pinoci, E. Sid. Sc. Bul., June 1980.

Poydock, M.E., et al., "Inhibiting Effect of Vitamins C and B12 on Mitotic Activity of Ascites Tumors," *Experimental Cell Biology,* v.47, n.3, 1979.

Pozniak, P.C., The Carcinogenicity of Caffeine and Coffee: A Review," *Journal of the American Dietetic Association,* 1985.

Pritikin, N., *Pritikin Program for Diet and Exercise,* Grosset and Dunlap, New York, 1979.

Quillin, Patrick, *Healing Nutrients,* Contemporary Books, Chicago, IL, 1987.

Rennam & Asi & Duarf, *"In Cancer Research,"* V.C.I., CA, 1980.

Rennam & Tonsir & Ohtua, *"Crisis Protocol For Cancer,"* V.C.I., CA, 1980.

Rice, Clarence C.: "Treatment of Cancer of the Larynx By Subcutaneous Injections of Pancreatic Extract," *Medical Record,* New York, November 24, 1906.

Robertson, W., & Kahler, National Cancer Institute, 2 595, 1942.

Schlegel, J.U., et al, "The Role of Ascorbic Acid in the Prevention of Bladder Tumor Formation," *Journal of Urology,* 1980.

Schmidt, Karen F., "Extending the Healthy Lifespan," *U.S. News & World Report* v114, March 8, 1993.

Schweitzer, A., *How White Man's Diet Affects Natives of Africa,* 1954.

Selbert, Pamela, "A Modern Investment In Age-Old Cures," *Americas,* v.43, July-August, 1991.

Shute, Wilfred E. & Tab, Harold J., *Vitamin E for Ailing and Healthy Hearts,* Pyramid House, New York, 1969.

Silverstone, H. & Tannenbaum, A., *Cancer Research,* 11:443, 1951.

"Skin Savers: Shade Your Hide From the Inside?", *Prevention,* v.46, n.2, February 1994.

Spencer, J.G.C., "The Influence of the Thyroid In Malignant Disease," *British Journal of Cancer,* 1954.

Stahelin, H.B.,; et al, "Cancer, Vitamins and Plasma Lipids: Prospective Basel Study," *Journal of the National Cancer Institute,* 1984.

Stefansson, Vilhjalmur, *Cancer: Disease of Civilization,* Hill and Wang, New York, 1969.

Steiner, P.E., *Cancer Research,* 2:425, 1942.

Steiner, P.E., *Cancer Research,* 3:385, 1943.

Steinman, D., *Diet for A Poisoned Planet,* Ballantine Books, New York, 1990.

Stix, Gary, "Back to Roots: Drug Companies Forage for New Treatments," *Scientific Americar* .268, January 1993.

Sugiura, Kanematsu, *A Summary of the Effect of Amygdalin Upon Spontaneous Tumors in Mice.* Extracted from confidential Sloan-Kettering report suppressed but leaked by staff members.

Sunday Express, London, England, December 27, 1931.

Sunzel, H., et al, "The Lipid Content of Human Liver," *Metabolis,* 13:1469-74.

Tannenbaum, A., *The Physiopathology of Cancer,* Hoeber, New York, 1959.

Tannenbaum, A., *Annals of the New York Academy of Science,* 49:9 & 49:10, 1947.

Taylor, Renee, "Hunza Health Secrets," *Award,* 1974.

Teresi, Dick, "Wanted: 40 More Years," *Health,* v21, n10, October 1989.

The Practical Encyclopedia of Natural Healing, Rodale Press, Inc., Emmaus, PA, 1983.

Townsend Letter for Doctors, June 1994.

Treating Prostate Problems, an informational booklet, Krames Communications, 1991.

Trowell, H., *American Journal of Clinical Nutrition,* 25:926, 1972.

U.S. Government Printing Office Document #89471.

U.S. Public Health Service U.S.D.A., Handbook #8, 1963.

U.S. Public Health Service Bulletin 1103, 1964.

Warburg, A., *The Prime Cause of Cancer,* English edition by Dean Burk, N.C.I., Bethesda, MD.

Warburg, Otto, *"Concerning the Ultimate Cause and Contributing Causes of Cancer,"* Lindau Germany, July 1966.

Wassertheil-Smoller, S., Ronmey, S., Whylie-Rosett, J., et al., "Dietary Vitamin C and Uterine Cervical Dysplasia," *American Journal of Epidemiology*, 1981.

Wiggin, Frederick H., "Case of Multiple Fibro-sarcoma of the Tongue," *Journal of the American Medical Association,* December 15, 1906.

Williams, W.R., *The Natural History of Cancer,* 1927.

Williams, R.S., *Nutrition in a Nutshell,* Doubleday, New York, 1962.

Williams, R.S., *Nutrition Against Disease*, Bantam Books, New York, 1971.

Willis, G.C. & Fishman, S., *Canadian Medical Association Journal,* 72:500, 1955.

Wlodyga, R.R., *Health Secrets from the Bible,* Triumph Publishing Co., CA, 1979.

"Women Doing Poor Job of Breast Self-Examination," News Feature, University of Southern California News Source, November 1988.

Wright, Jonathan, M.D., *Dr. Wright's Book of Nutritional Therapy*, Rodale Press, Emmaus, PA, 1979.

Wynder, E. L., et al., "Nutrition and Metabolic Epidemiology of Cancers of the Oral Cavity, Esophagus, Colon, Breast, Prostate and Stomach," *Nutrition and Cancer: Etiology and Treatment,* Raven, New York, 1981.

Zamichow, Nora, "FDA Expected to Postpone Decision, For 30th Time, on Banning Food Dyes," *Washington Post,* June 4, 1986.

Index

This book was written to the glory of God and for Jesus Christ, who saved my unregenerate soul.